PRACTICAL ATLAS OF NUTRITION

AND FEEDING IN CATS AND DOGS

VOLUME 1

Roberto Elices Mínguez

Doctorate in Veterinary Medicine from the Universidad Complutense de Madrid (UCM), Spain.

Professor of Animal Nutrition and Companion Animals.

Veterinarian in the Small Animal Medicine Department (Endocrinology and Obesity) of the Veterinary Clinical Hospital of the School of Veterinary Medicine of Madrid (UCM), Spain.

Clinical Veterinarian –medicine and surgery– of companion animals in private centers.

For this English edition:

Practical atlas of nutrition and feeding in cats and dogs. Volume I

Plaza Antonio Beltrán Martínez nº 1, planta 8 - letra I
(Centro empresarial El Trovador)
50002 Zaragoza - Spain

First printing: December 2016

This book has been published originally in Spanish under the title:
Atlas de nutrición y alimentación práctica en perros y gatos. Volumen I.
© 2010 Grupo Asís Biomedia, S.L.
ISBN Spanish edition: 978-84-92569-40-3

Translation:
Anna Frandsen

Illustrator:
Jacob Gragera Artal

ISBN: 978-84-16818-41-9
D.L.: Z 1615-2016

Design, layout and printing:
Servet editorial - Grupo Asís Biomedia, S.L.
www.grupoasis.com
info@grupoasis.com

Warning:

Veterinary science is constantly evolving, as are pharmacology and the other sciences. Inevitably, it is therefore the responsibility of the veterinary surgeon to determine and verify the dosage, the method of administration, the duration of treatment and any possible contraindications to the treatments given to each individual patient, based on his or her professional experience. Neither the publisher nor the author can be held liable for any damage or harm caused to people, animals or properties resulting from the correct or incorrect application of the information contained in this book.

To my parents, family, and pets

Acknowledgments

To Arancha for her support, understanding, patience and love.

To my right hand, Mercedes Morán Cuesta, for sharing her time. Thank to you, Mer, without your help and efforts, this would not have been possible.

To my colleague at the HCV, Dr. Lola Pérez Alenza, for her advice.

To my dear friends, Cristina Ortiz Díez de Tortosa and Mar Sanz Luengo, from the Library of the School of Veterinary Medicine of Madrid (UCM). Without your work and affection, collecting the bibliography would have been impossible.

To the editing and design teams at the Servet publishing house, especially to Tatiana Blasco, for all of the hours shared sending emails back and forth, and to Javier Nuviala. I send my congratulations to the graphic designers for their magnificent work.

To all of my friends, but especially to Pablo Mantilla and Silvia Miguélez.

Prologue

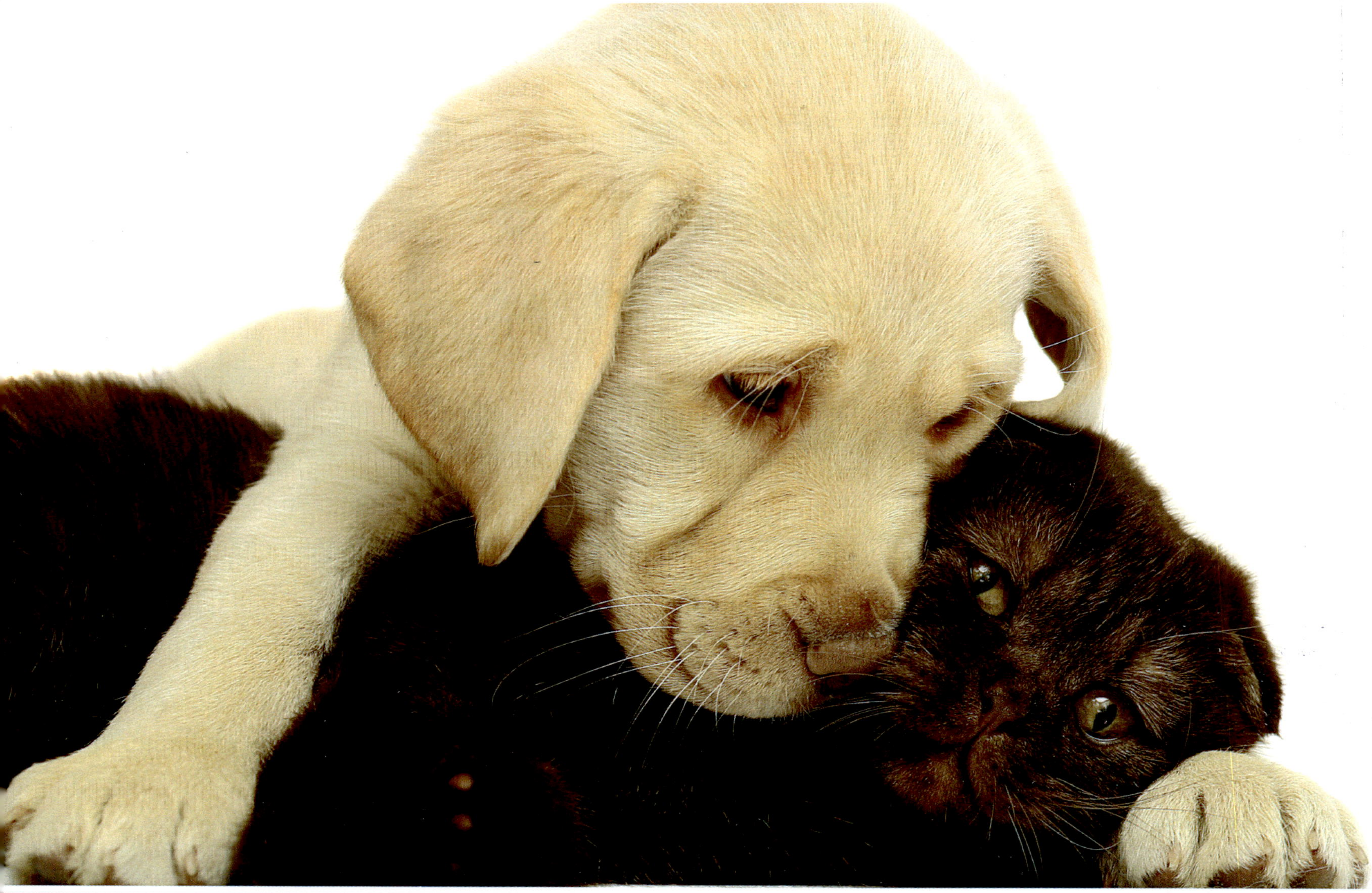

When we came up with the idea of creating a nutrition atlas, it seemed just as interesting as it did complicated. We found the idea interesting because providing images, drawings, diagrams and other graphic elements with the text could facilitate reading and comprehension about nutrition in pets, a discipline of great clinical relevance that can sometimes be arduous and complex. However we knew it would be complicated due to the difficulty of synthesizing and visually expressing certain content, such as all references to the energy of foods and their metabolism, as the intention was to make it easier to understand and more enjoyable to read. We hope that the reader feels that we have met these objectives.

Aside from his experience and knowledge, we would also like to acknowledge the commitment and enthusiasm that the author brought to this project from the very beginning. Together with other members of the creative department, he was key in the final result which you currently have in your hands.

Without further ado, our only wish now is that you read this book and enjoy it.

Editorial Servet
[Servet publishing house]

Preface

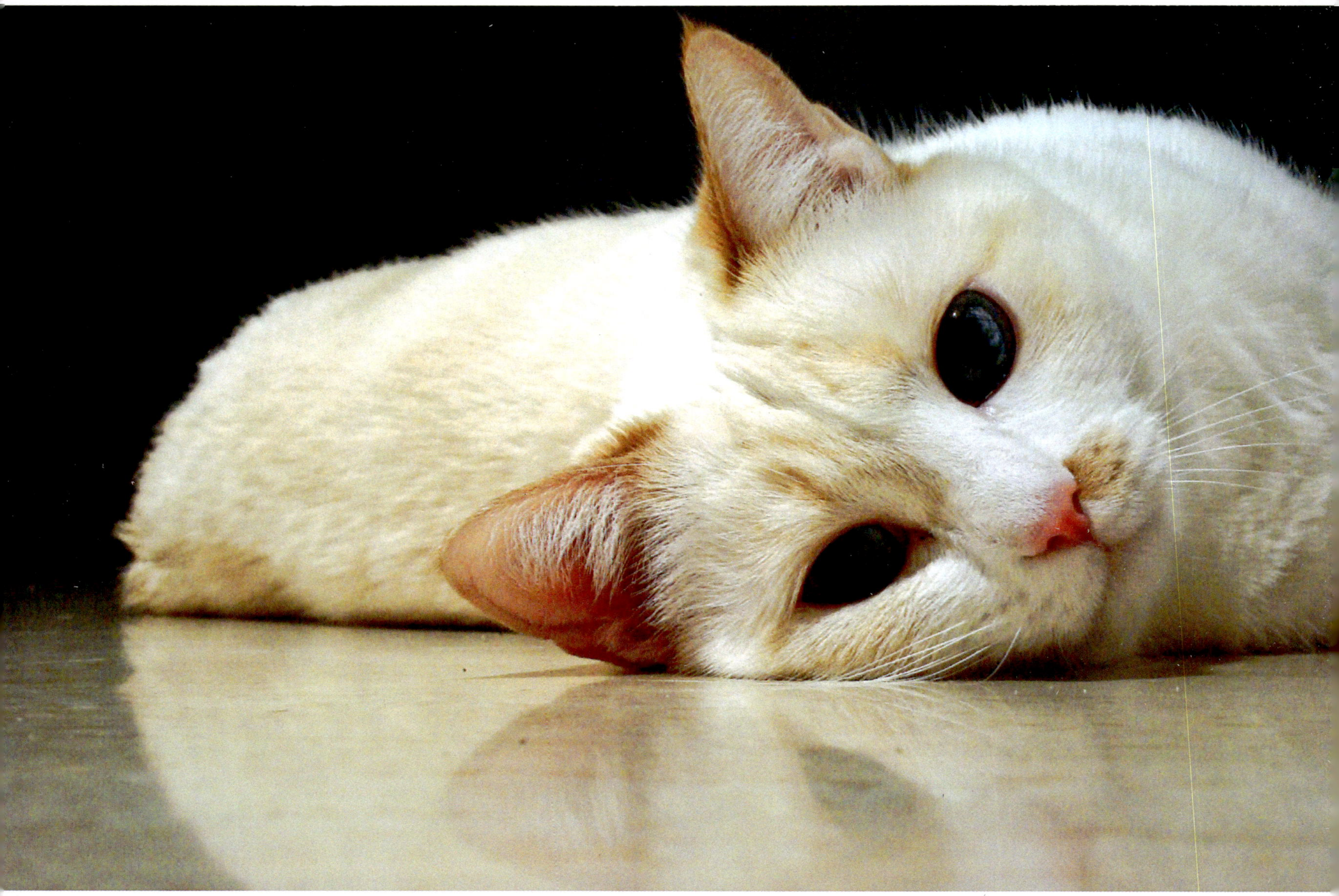

Dogs and cats represent the exception among the animal kingdom. They are our number one house pets, and have become so important in developed countries that they are considered core members of the family. They live with us in exchange for affection. The benefits from this symbiosis to pet owners' health have been described in literature. Therefore, the longevity of the pets' lives directly benefits the lives of their "guardians".

In the middle of the 19th century, the first commercial foods for pets were developed. Currently, estimates show that there are more than one thousand two hundred manufacturers of pet food around the world. Feeding these two species (cats and dogs) is unique within animal nutrition. Their nutrition needs have not been established according to any productive criteria, however, they have been based on the prevention and improvement of the quality of their lives, from the very first stages. In fact, specific foods are available for the treatment of certain pathologies. The nutrition of these two species integrates science and clinical practice. These circumstances have led to greater well-being and increased life expectancy of our small animal friends. This way, we close the circle.

In veterinary medicine, we are not used to understanding the importance of nutrition in the health of the patient. But, unlike humans, our patients accept our recommendations, more or less enthusiastically, and the results are usually satisfactory. However, most veterinarians that work with dogs and cats are not especially interested in nutrition.

There is abundant literature on nutrition and feeding, biochemistry, physiology, and veterinary anatomy regarding pets. We have tried, with the most recent information available, to create a book that is easy to use and that can serve as a tool for daily clinical practice. For this reason, all recommendations should be taken into account at this moment as the science of nutrition continues to advance.

I have been lucky enough to share my life with a small four-legged, whisker-bearing family and learn from them. I believe I owe them a lot. This is my small contribution to the endless hours of gratuitous love that they have given me.

We hope and desire that this book will help to stimulate veterinarians' interest in this area of knowledge.

Roberto Elices Mínguez

Index

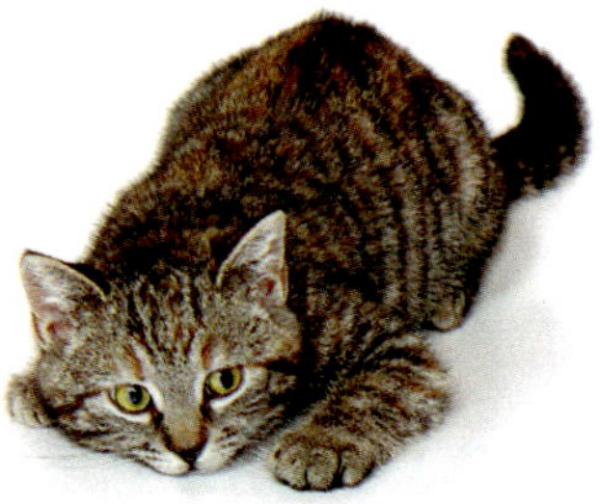

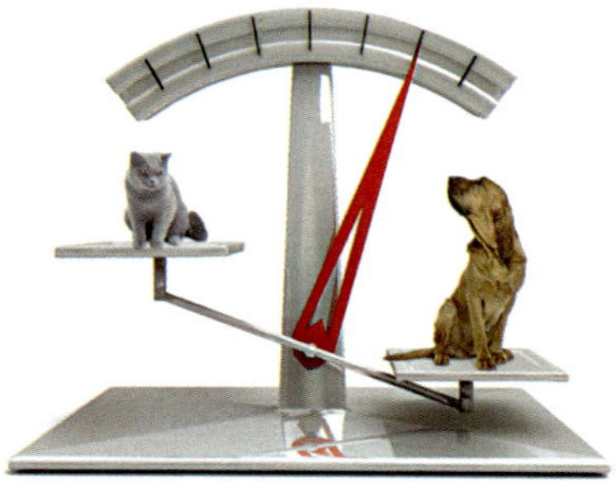

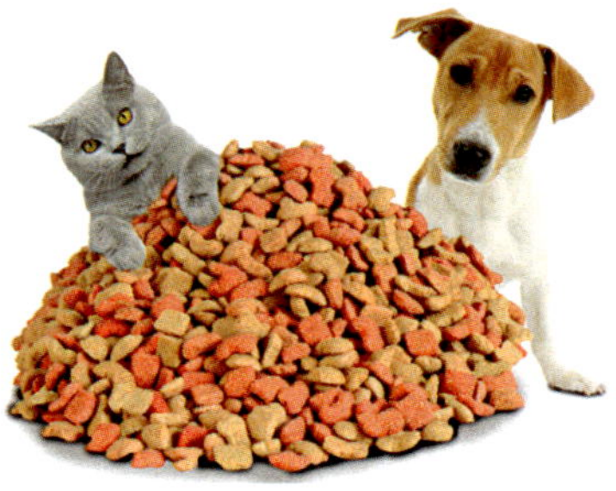

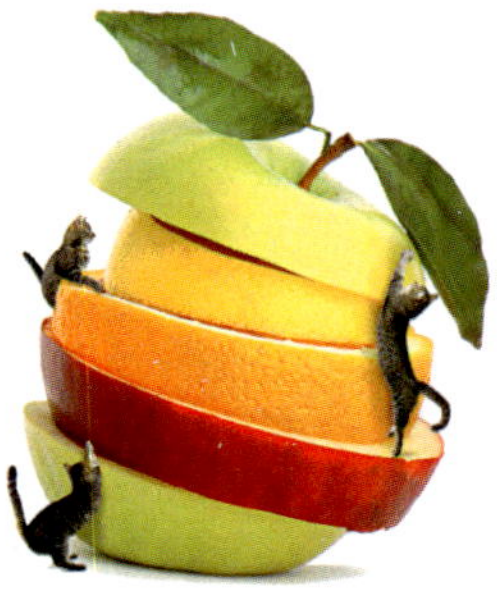

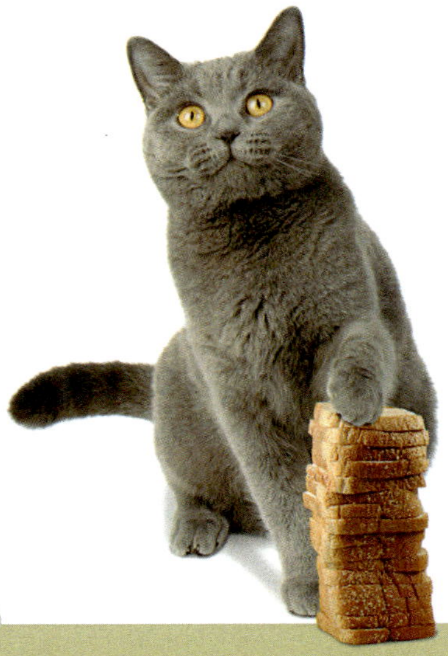

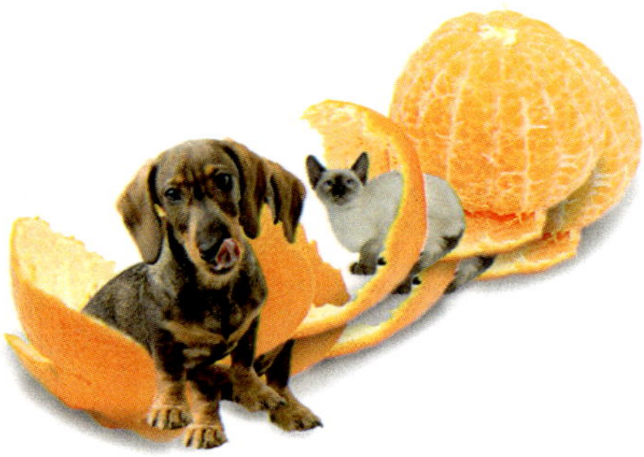

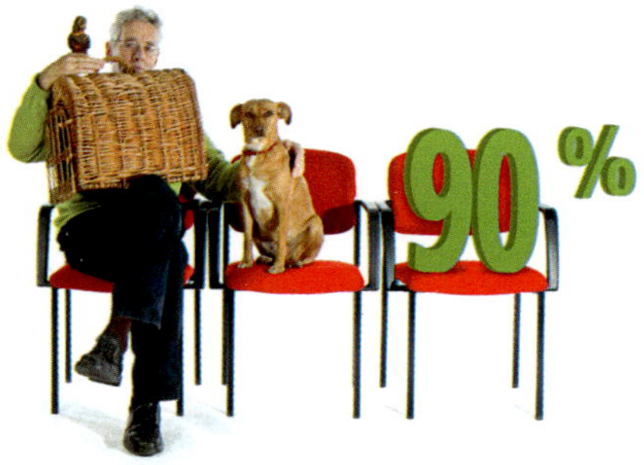
90 %

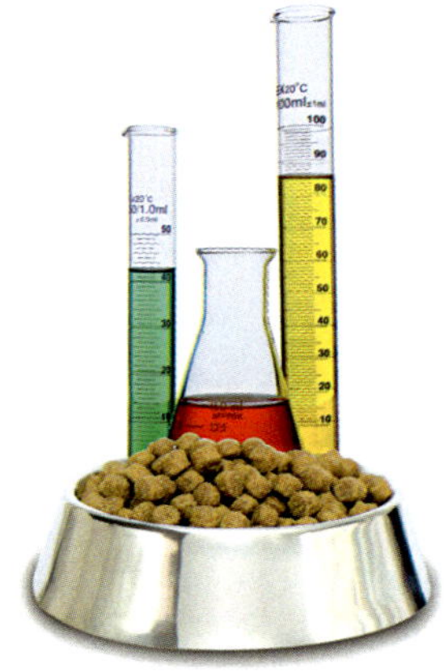

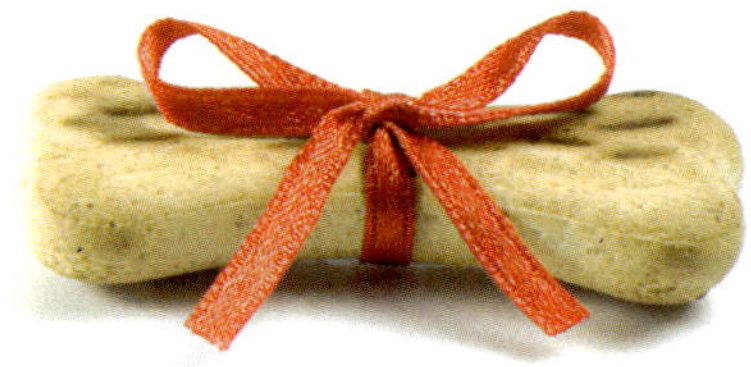

Carnivores

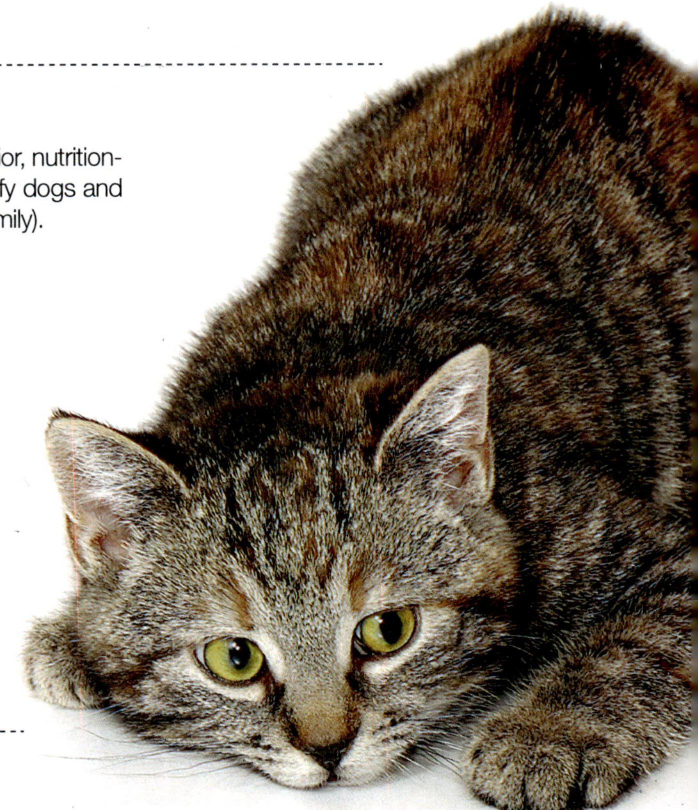

1 Cats are carnivores and dogs eat everything

Different studies have shown us that from natural ingestive behavior, nutritional needs, and metabolism and digestive anatomy, we can classify dogs and cats as strict carnivores (Felidae family) or omnivores (Canidae family).

Kingdom Animalia → **Phylum** Chordata (vertebrata) → **Class** Mammalia → **Order** Carnivore →
- **Family** Canidae → **Genus/species** *Canis lupus familiaris*
- **Family** Felidae → **Genus/species** *Felis silvestris catus*

2 The digestive system in dogs is longer

Dogs and cats have a similar digestive system although the relative length is around 30 % greater in dogs. The length is directly correlated with the duration of digestion and the efficiency of the use of the different types of foods.

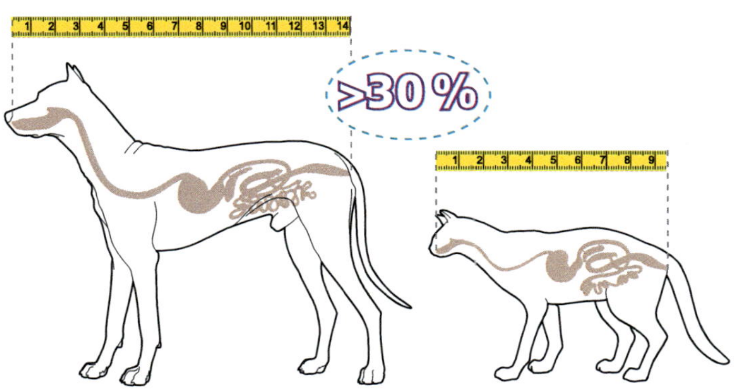

Average food transit time

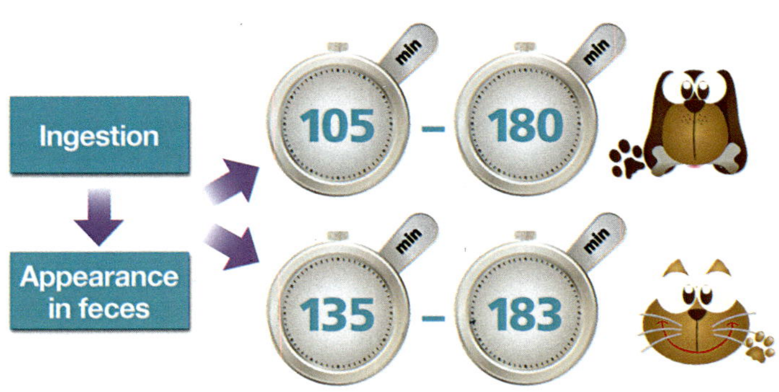

3 The digestibility is affected by the age and breed (weight) of the dog

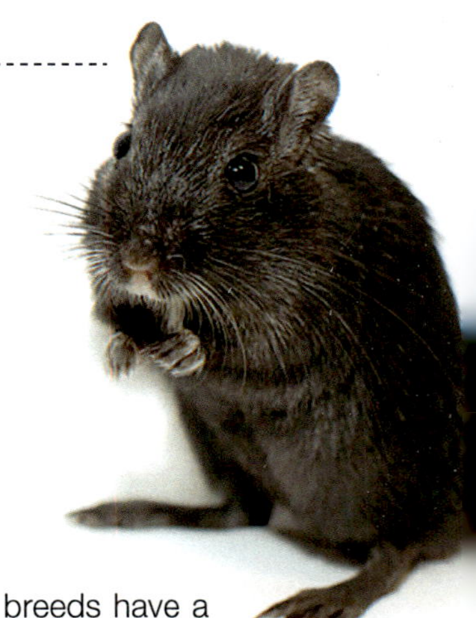

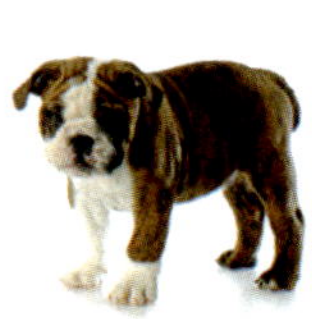

Young animals (< 12 months)

Digestion of nutrients

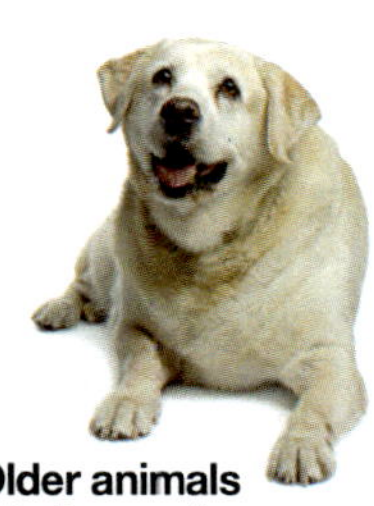

Older animals (> 9 years)

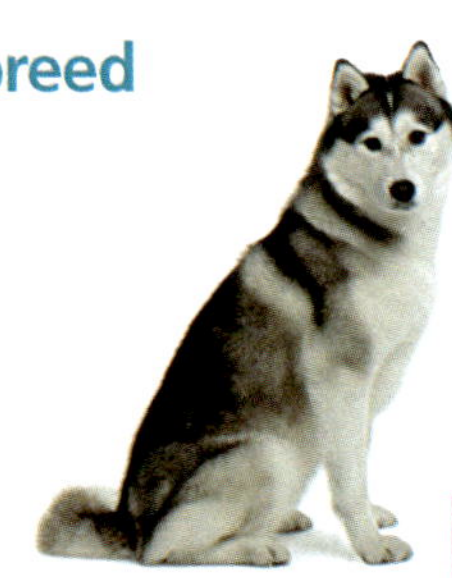

Adults (2-4 years)

Digestion of nutrients

✔ Fat is the only nutrient of which the digestibility increases with age up to 24 months. Changes over time regarding enzymes and their activity conditions feeding. For example, amylase activity is greatly reduced in dogs under 12 months, while lactase is at a maximum in the two first months of life.

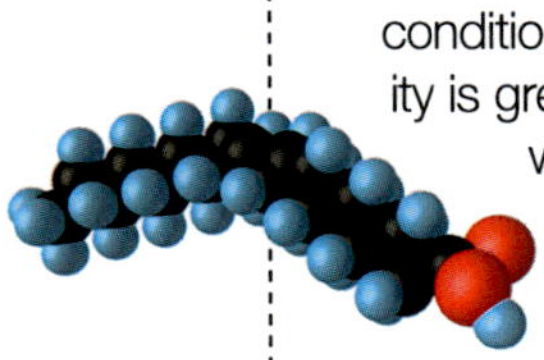

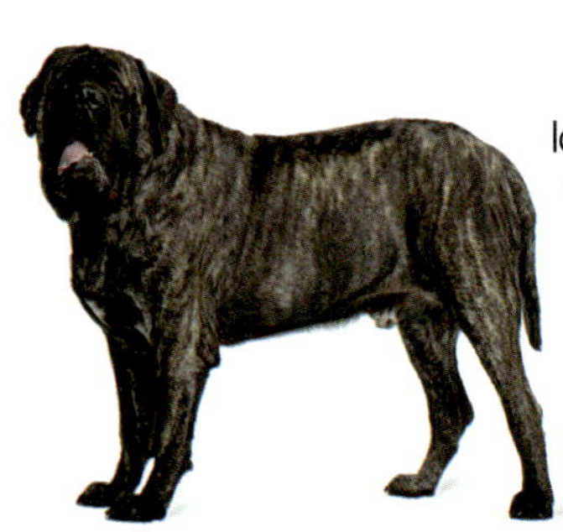

✔ Large and giant breeds have a lower relative proportion of digestive system (approximately half), but the digestibility of nutrients, regardless of age (between 3 months and 5 years), is greater.

and omnivores by nature

Ingestion behavior

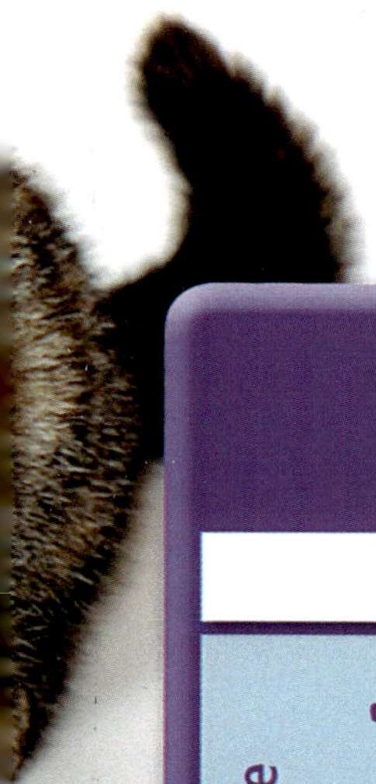

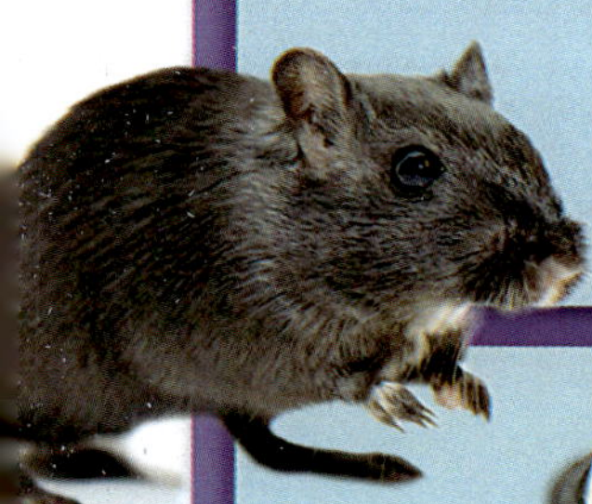

	Dog	Cat
Attitude	✔ Group hunters with a wide range of raw materials in their diets (opportunist consumers), which include other middle to large sized animal species, fruits, berries, manure from herbivores, and cadavers.	✔ Solitary hunters. Their prey include animals from small grasshoppers to young rabbits. ✔ They are natural hunters. They can stop eating at a given moment if the opportunity arises to hunt another animal. This behavior may seem confusing, as it is not related to hunger. Feeding reduces the time they dedicate to hunting but it does not eliminate this characteristic.
Food	✔ In line with their hunting techniques, this species ingests large volumes of food in short periods of time, until their daily requirements are satisfied. They consume both the muscle mass as well as the viscera of their catches.	✔ They eat small meals 10 to 20 times per day. **10-20 times** ✔ They eat the muscular portions of their catches and avoid eating the hollow organs. They do not like the flavor of plant matter ✔ and they prefer their food at body temperature (38.5 °C).
Water	Ingestion / kg body weight **>** ✔ This species drinks in a compulsive manner: they can ingest a volume that corresponds with the loss from dehydration in one hour.	Ingestion / kg body weight ✔ Greater capacity to concentrate urine. ✔ They can rehydrate themselves from sea water. ✔ They drink slowly, taking breaks. ✔ Unlike dogs, their re-hydration can take place over a span of 24 hours.
Biological rhythm	✔ Their daily biological rhythm is regulated by a daily cycle of activity and rest.	✔ It follows an irregular pattern with periods of activity and rest both during the day and during the night. These characteristics have been observed in natural settings (depending on the prey to be hunted) and in house cats, which are stimulated to eat food by the presence of their owners and/or artificial light.

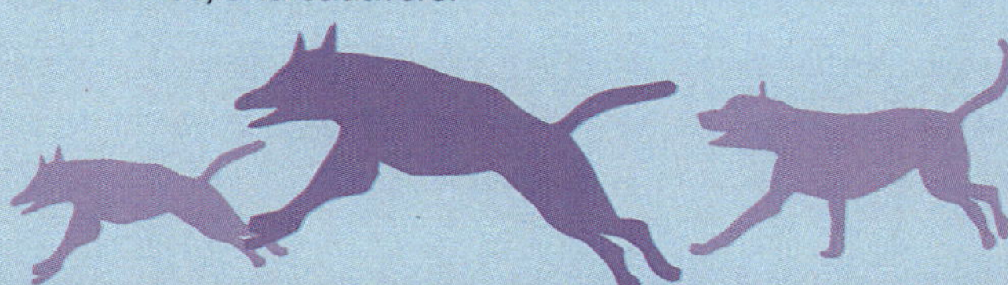

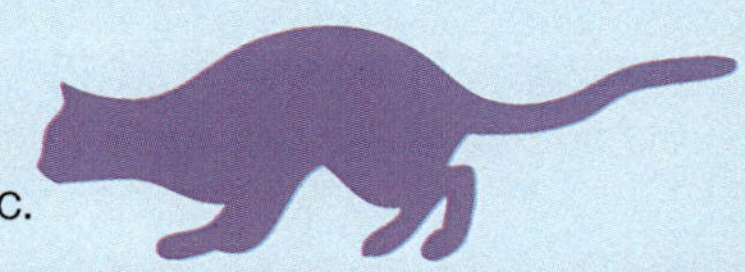

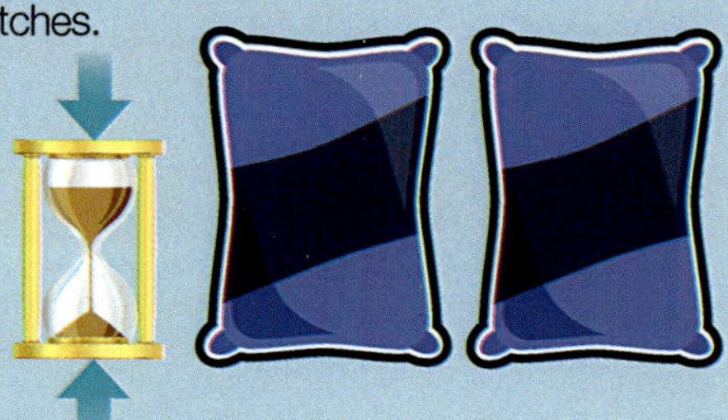

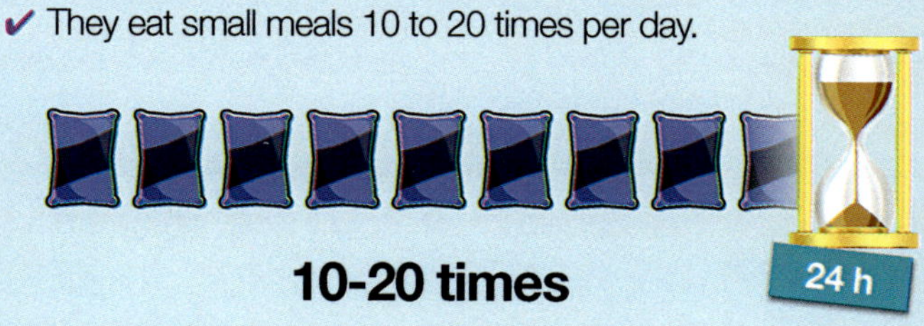

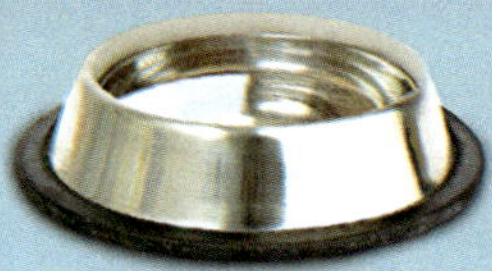

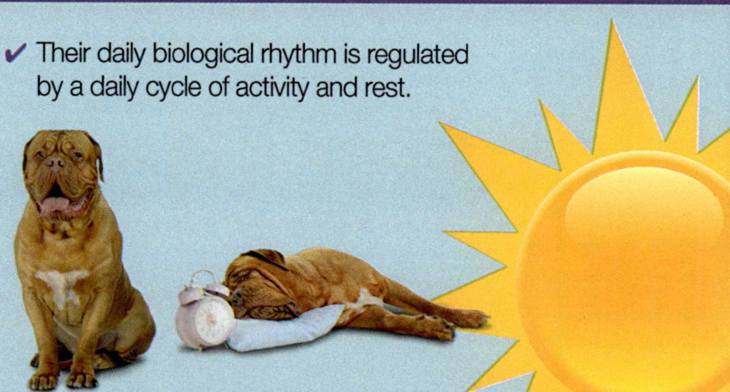

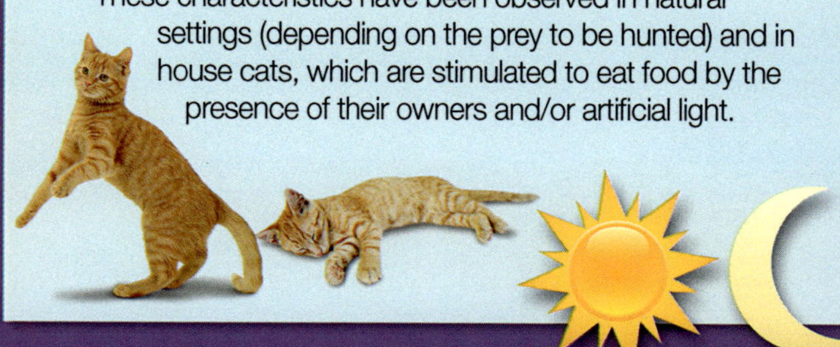

The digestive process (I):

The oral cavity

The oral cavity provides information about the feeding behaviour of the dog or cat, while dental development helps to determine their age: this is very important to establish their needs and determine what type of diet can be used to feed them. Young cats and dogs are immature at all levels; this includes their digestive system. The figure below shows the different changes that take place according to the animal's age.

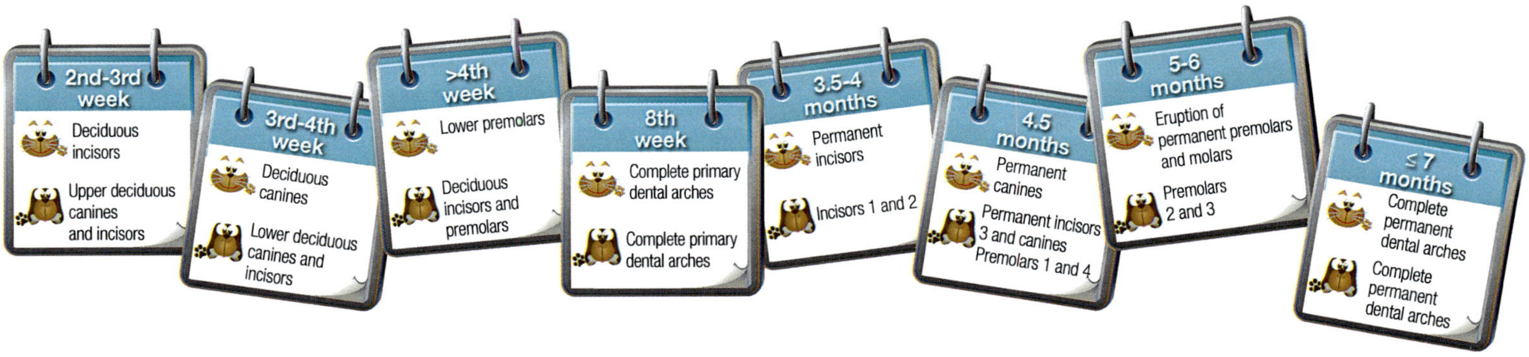

1 Dental arches in an adult animal

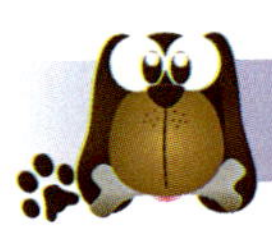

42 PERMANENT TEETH

Dental arches with mixed characteristics of an omnivore and carnivore:

Premolars
With a correct biting surface.

Canines
Long to hold onto prey.

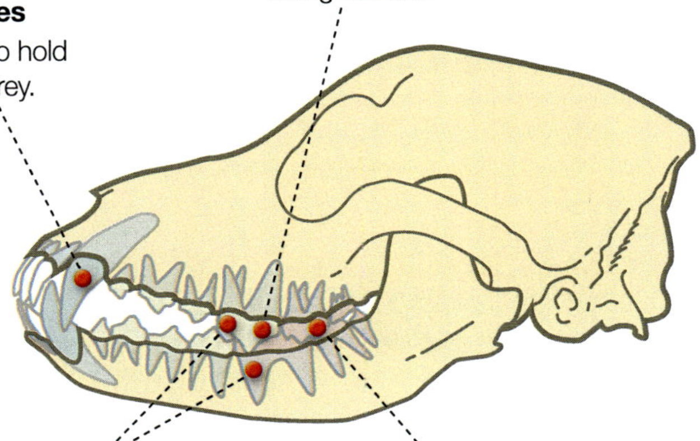

Carnassial teeth
4th upper PM and 1st lower M.

Molars
With large crested occlusal surfaces adapted to mastication.

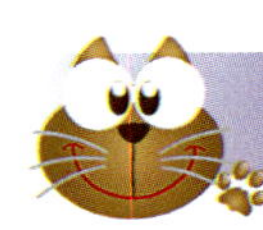

30 PERMANENT TEETH
(lower number or premolars and molars)

The lateral and craniocaudal movements of the mandible are very limited. Their teeth are those of a carnivore:

Canines
Long, slightly curved and sharp.

Premolars
Conical, adapted to cutting.

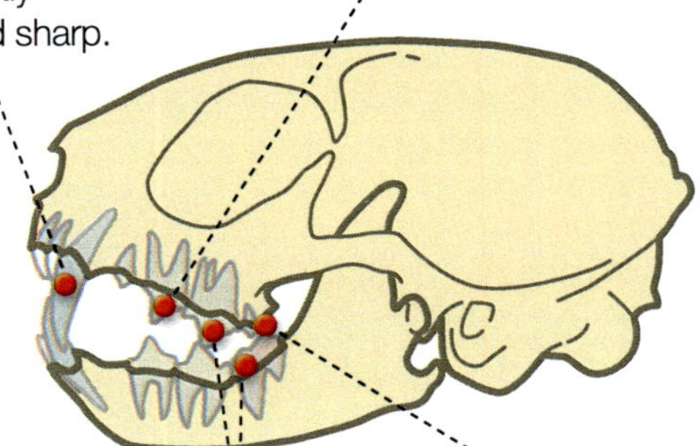

Carnassial teeth
Large.

Molars
Conical, adapted to cutting.

2 Chewing and salivation

The only digestive process that takes place in the oral cavity is mastication and mixing with saliva. The composition of saliva includes water and inorganic ions such as sodium, chloride, potassium and bicarbonate. Its pH is slightly alkaline (pH=7.5). Both species lack the enzyme α-amylase (which degrades starch).

The functions of saliva are lubricating the food and cooling the organism down by evaporation, which is very important.

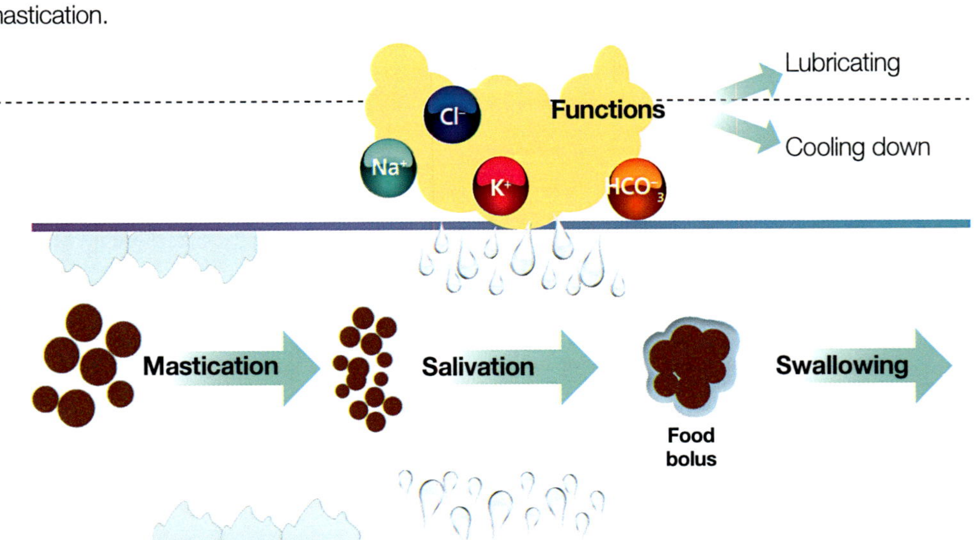

mouth and stomach

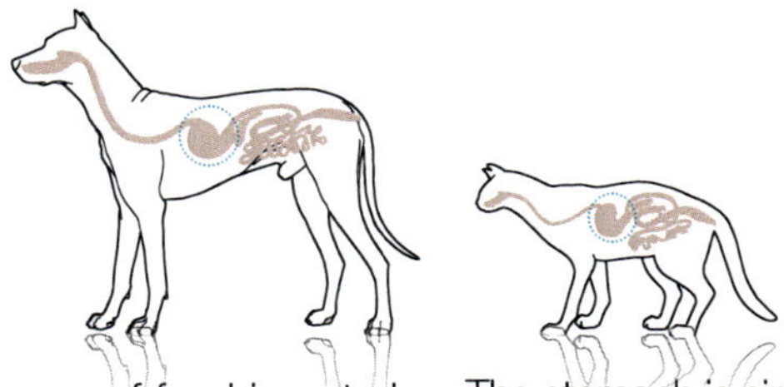

The stomach

The stomach of dogs is adapted to hold large volumes of food ingested without prior appropriate mastication. This capacity conditions the ingestion of food and its passage through the small intestine.

The stomach is simpler in cats (smaller size and uniform surface).

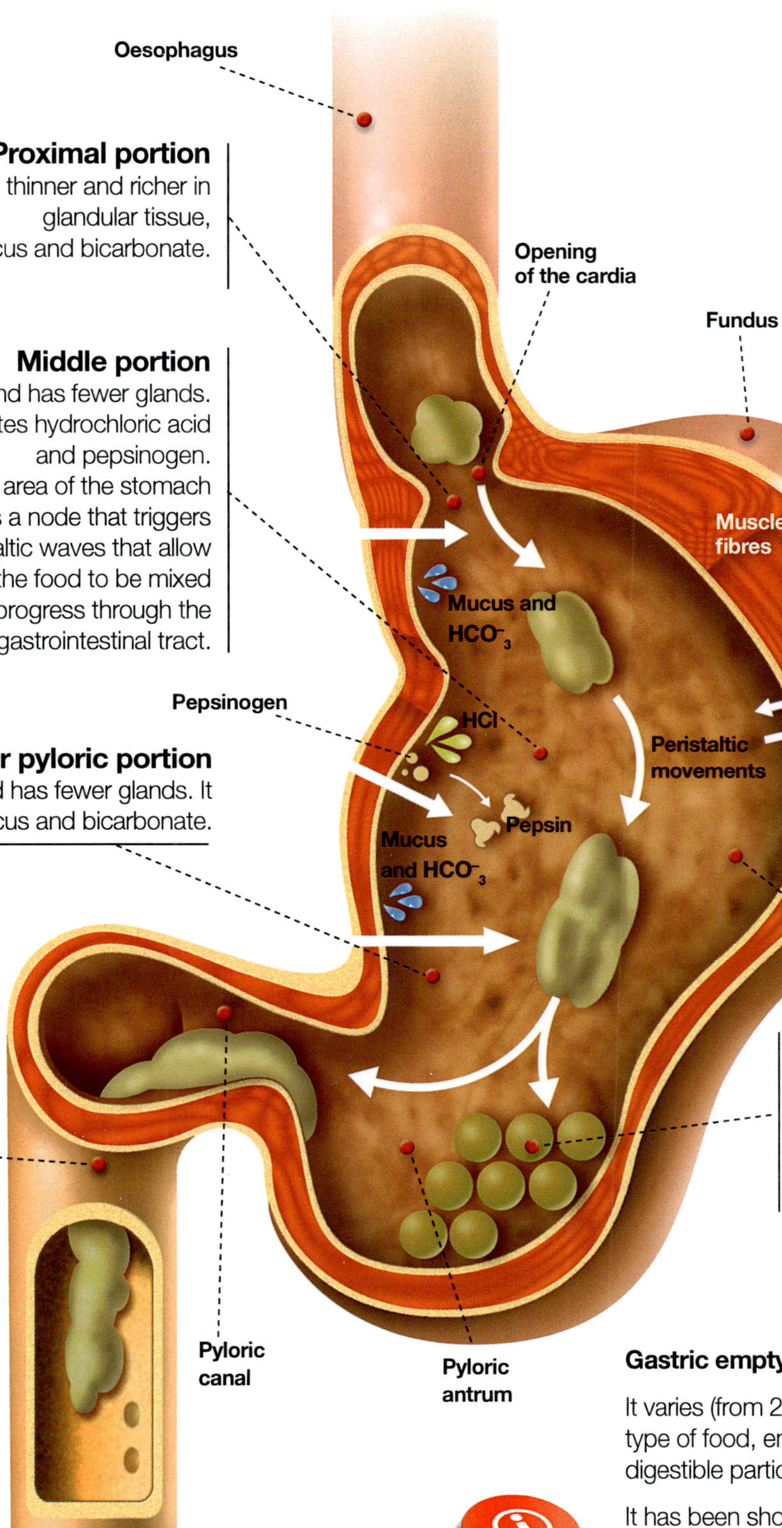

Digestion

Hydrochloric acid, pepsin and, to a lower extent, lipase participate in the process. These secretions depend on:

- ✓ The volume of the ration.
- ✓ The cephalic, gastric and intestinal phases of digestion.
- ✓ The protein content (the activity of pepsin is greater against collagen-rich tissue).

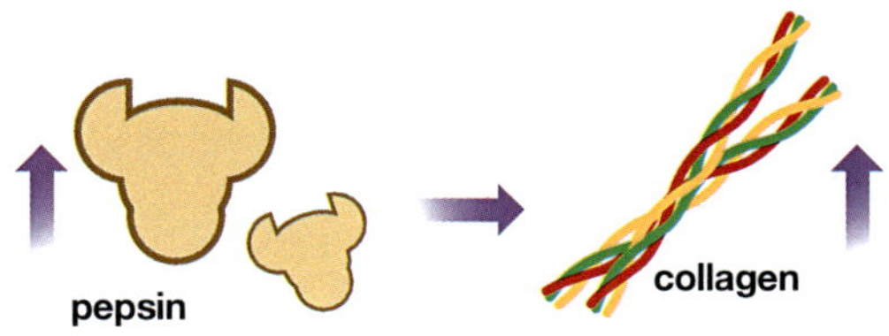

- ✓ The activity of some hormones (e.g. ACTH increases and secretin decreases hydrochloric acid secretion).

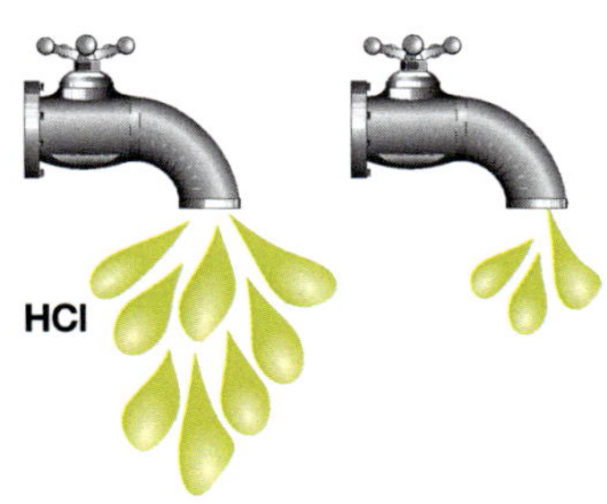

Indigestible particles or those that are too large are retained in the stomach until the other nutrients are completely digested. They are eliminated with the first contractions that occur during fasting. This effect is interesting for the control of satiety and of some nutrients (e.g. glycaemia).

Gastric emptying time.

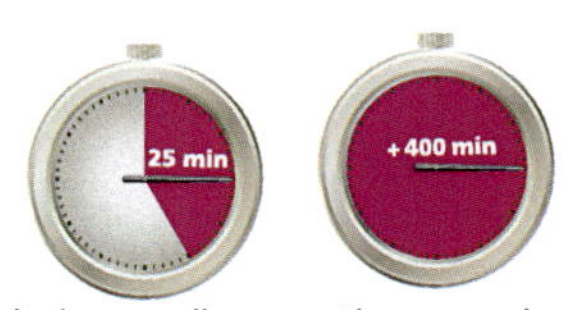

It varies (from 25 to more than 400 minutes) depending on the species, type of food, energy density, viscosity, particle size, presence of non-digestible particles and fasting time.

It has been shown that the osmotic effect of monosaccharides and fatty acid esters at the duodenum actively participates in this process: the greater the concentration, the longer gastric emptying will take.

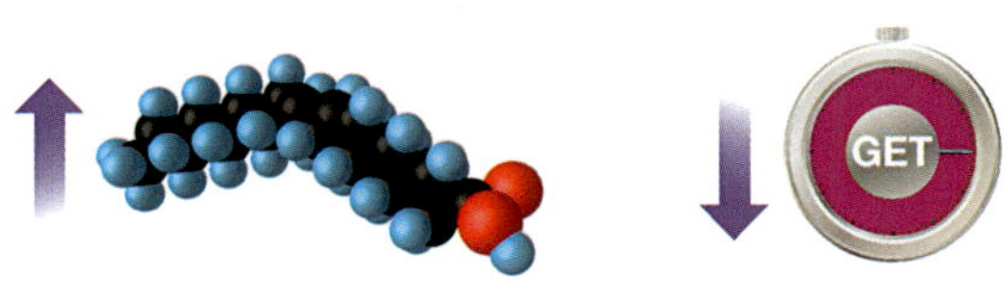

Aspects to take into account

The concentration of saliva varies with the speed of secretion: it is slightly hypertonic when it is secreted abundantly. This fact should be taken into consideration in animals under conditions of exercise, when temperatures are high and in those canine breeds that secrete a lot of saliva.

The digestive process (II):

Small intestine

1 Digestion in the small intestine

The small intestine consists of the duodenum, jejunum and ileum. Once the food (chyme) enters the small intestine, bicarbonate is released from the pancreas to neutralise the acid pH.

Enzymatic digestion starts by the action of pancreatic enzymes (amylases, lipases and proteases), under the hormonal control of cholecystokinin (CCK) and secretin; by the enzymes from the brush border of the villi; and by the presence of bile.

The presence of partially digested food, especially fat and some peptides rich in phenylalanine, stimulates CCK secretion.

The secretion of bile stored in the gallbladder starts 30 minutes after the ingestion of food and lasts for the following two hours. Its release is stimulated by the presence of fat from the diet.

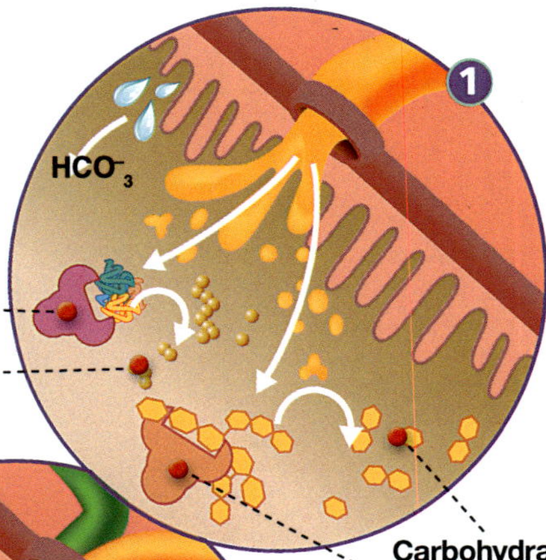

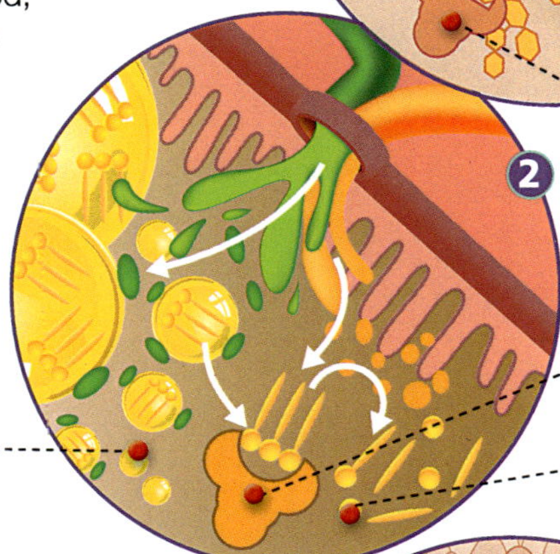

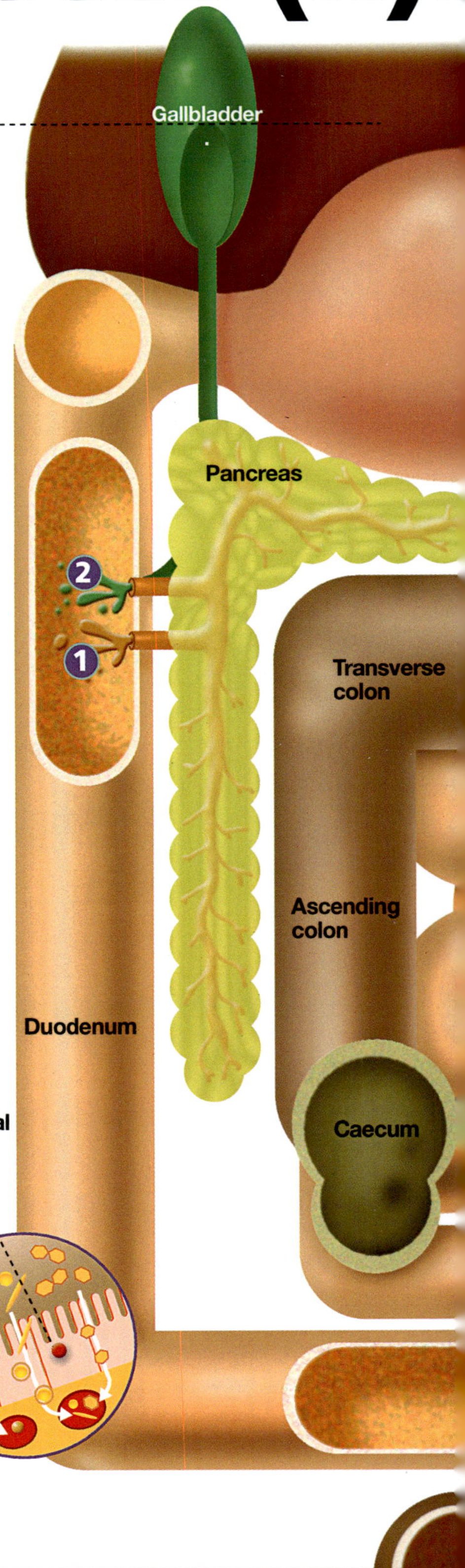

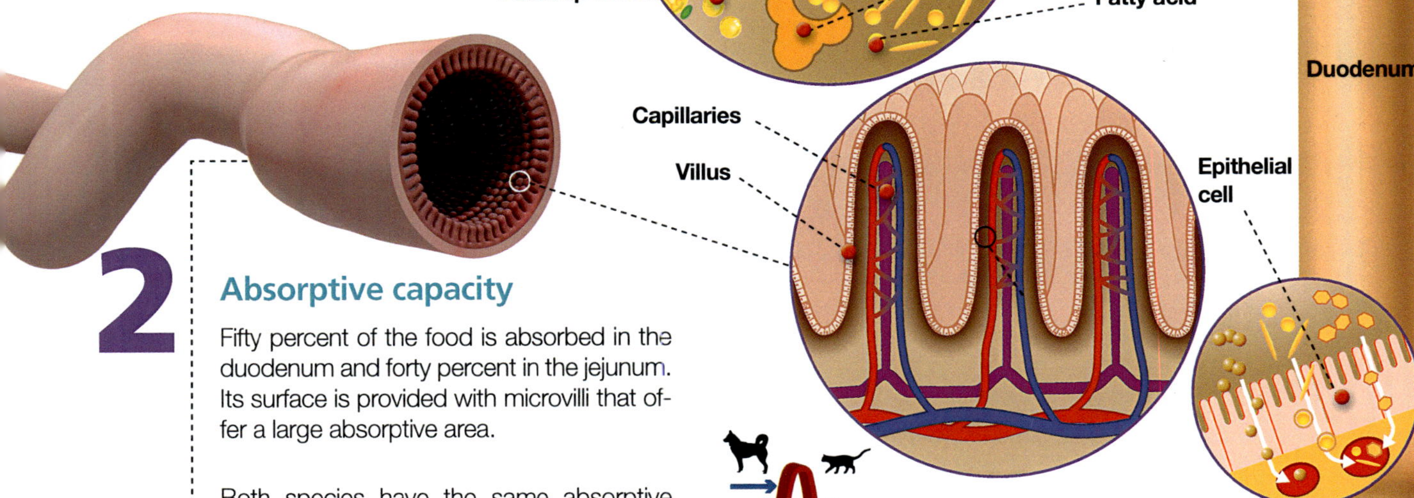

2 Absorptive capacity

Fifty percent of the food is absorbed in the duodenum and forty percent in the jejunum. Its surface is provided with microvilli that offer a large absorptive area.

Both species have the same absorptive surface per cm²; however, cats' absorptive capacity is 10 % lower.

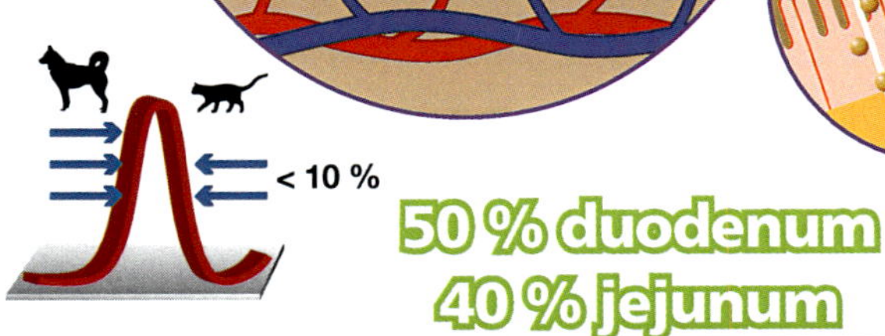

Digestive microflora

The type and quantity of digestive microflora varies depending on the area:

	Stomach	Small intestine	Large intestine
Population	Very low	Medium	High
Yeasts	Yes	No	Yes
Facultative anaerobes: *Lactobacillus, Streptococcus* and Enterobacteriaceae	Yes	Same	One thousand times lower
Strict anaerobes: *Bacteroides* spp., *Bifidobacterium* spp., *Clostridium, Atopobium* spp., *Fusobacterium* spp. and *Peptococcus* spp.	No	Same	Dominant

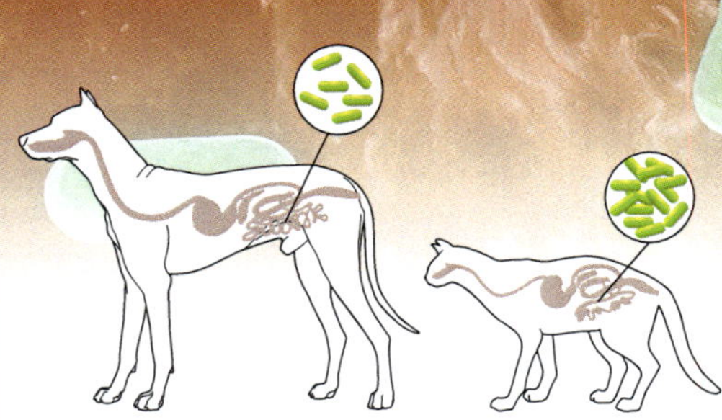

There are differences between species. Cats have a greater flora population in the small intestine in comparison with dogs. Both are the species with the lowest concentration of bifidobacteria.

The factors that play a role on their adherence to the mucosa and colonisation are:

- ✓ Bactericidal effect of the pancreatic juice.
- ✓ Acid pH.
- ✓ Biliary secretions.
- ✓ Intestinal motility.
- ✓ Availability of nutrients.

The main function of this microflora is to act as a defence barrier against pathogenic microorganisms through the production of antibacterial substances, by modifying oxygen concentrations and by competing for nutrients.

small and large intestine

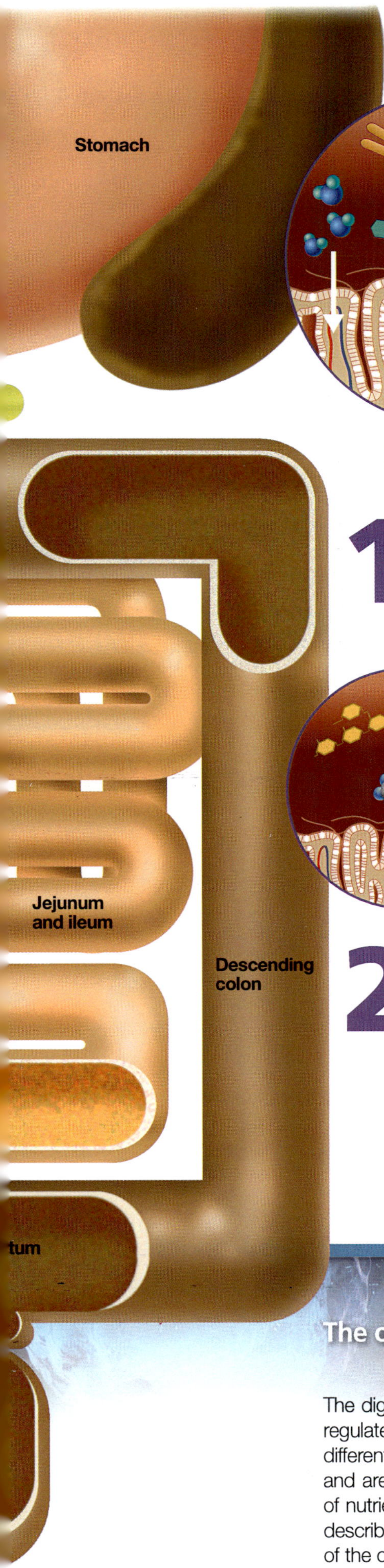

Large intestine

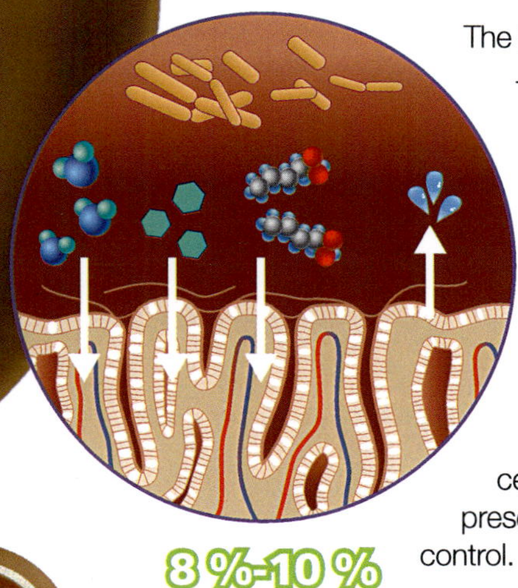

The large intestine is composed of the caecum (vestigial in cats), colon and rectum.

The mucosa of this part of the digestive tract lacks villi, it is rich in mucus-secreting cells and it is relatively short when compared with the portion that precedes it: it represents approximately 15 % of the total. Most of the diet's water and minerals, as well as the fatty acids released by microbial fermentation, are absorbed in the large intestine. Only 8-10 % of the food is absorbed at this point.

The food remains in this portion for 12 hours before defecation, although the location varies depending on the species. In cats, it takes place in the transverse colon, while in dogs it does so in the caecum and ascending colon. Large intestinal motility depends on the presence and type of fibre, as well as on neurohormonal control.

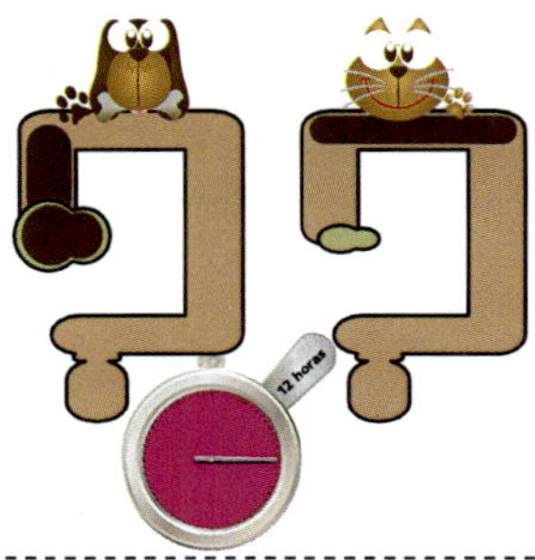

1

Nutrient fermentation

The microflora living in the large intestine is responsible for the fermentation of nutrients (products of the food and endogenous secretions), thereby giving rise to different compounds. The proportions of short-chain, or volatile, fatty acids (SCFA) depends on the substrate and microflora.

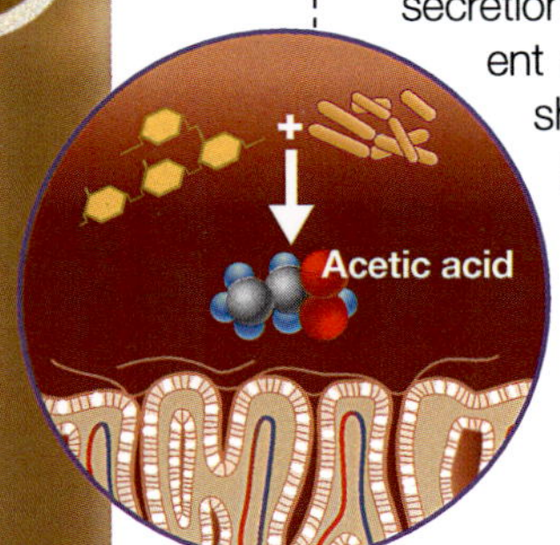

Products of fermentation	Generated compounds
✓ Non-digested protein	✓ SCFA: acetic acid, propionic acid and butyric acid
✓ Resistant starch	✓ Lactate
✓ Disaccharides	✓ Carbon dioxide
✓ Fermentable fibre	✓ Hydrogen
✓ Non-starch polysaccharides	
✓ Enzymes and mucus	

Carbohydrates are fermented in the initial portions (e.g. bifidobacteria and lactobacilli, with production of acetic acid).

Proteins are fermented in the final portions (e.g. clostridia and eubacteria, with production of butyric acid).

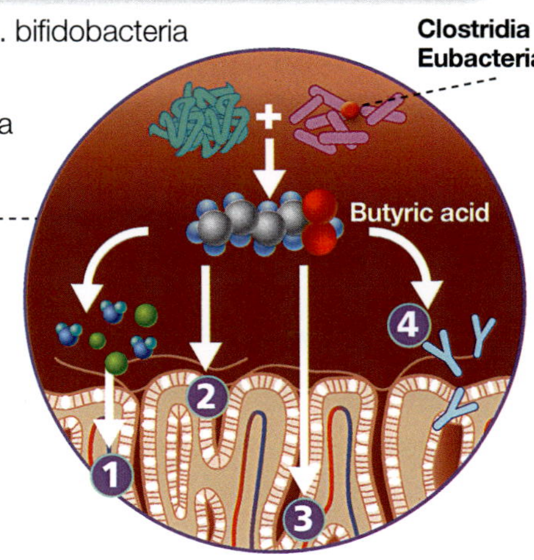

2

Butyric acid

Of all SCFA, butyric acid participates most actively in the structure and function of the mucosa. Its importance lies in the following aspects:

1. It stimulates the absorption of water and electrolytes (Na^+).
2. It is the energy substrate of colonocytes.
3. It stimulates the proliferation of intestinal cells through GLP-2.
4. This cell proliferation constitutes a physical barrier against bacterial overgrowth.

The organism's largest endocrine organ

The digestive process and metabolism are regulated by several hormones that have different origins, functions and activities and are stimulated depending on the type of nutrient. The digestive system has been described as the largest endocrine organ of the organism due to its multitude of cells of different types with an hormonal activity. Some of these hormones are:

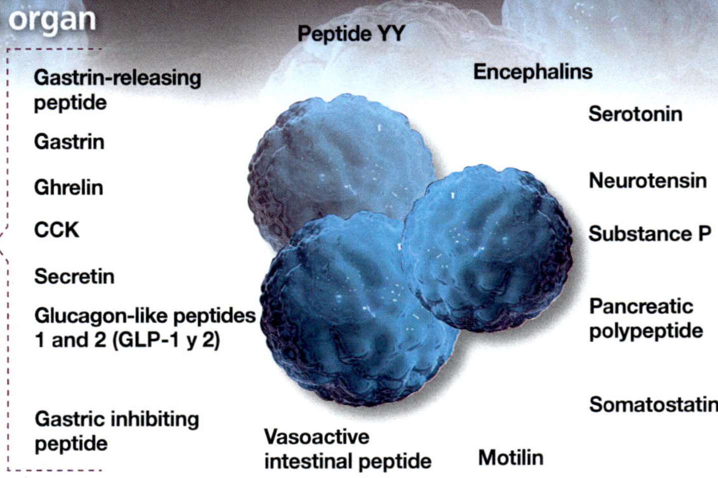

Evaluation of

1 Dogs and cats at their ideal weight present a lean:fat tissue ratio of 80:20

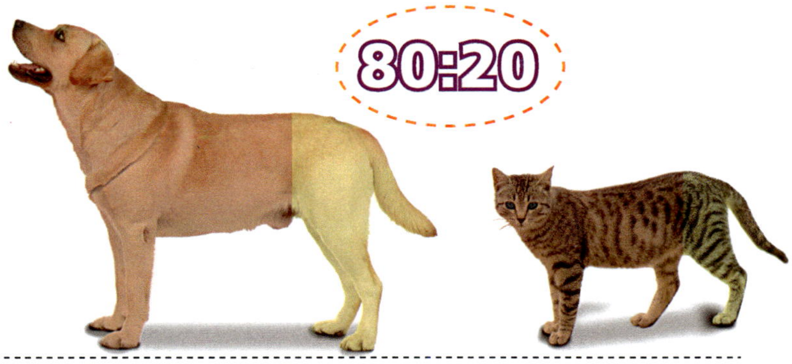

Knowing if a dog or a cat's weight and body condition are adequate is essential to understand and establish their nutritional requirements.

In overweight animals, there is no point in estimating their needs based on their current weight given that fat is an inert tissue from a metabolic point of view. Likewise, knowing these proportions is of great interest to avoid the use of muscle tissue as an energy source.

2 30 % of pets are overweight

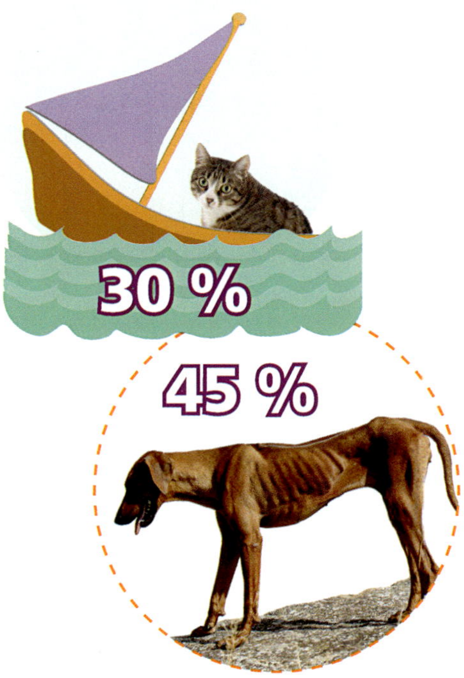

Records can be kept of the weight modifications of patients from when they are puppies or kitten to when they are adults. However, this information is not always known. Sometimes animals present a weight or body condition that does not coincide with their age and physical state: it is estimated that 30 % of pets are overweight and nearly 45 % of geriatric pets suffer some kind of disease that derives in episodes of cachexia. This highlights the importance of performing a physical examination of the animal.

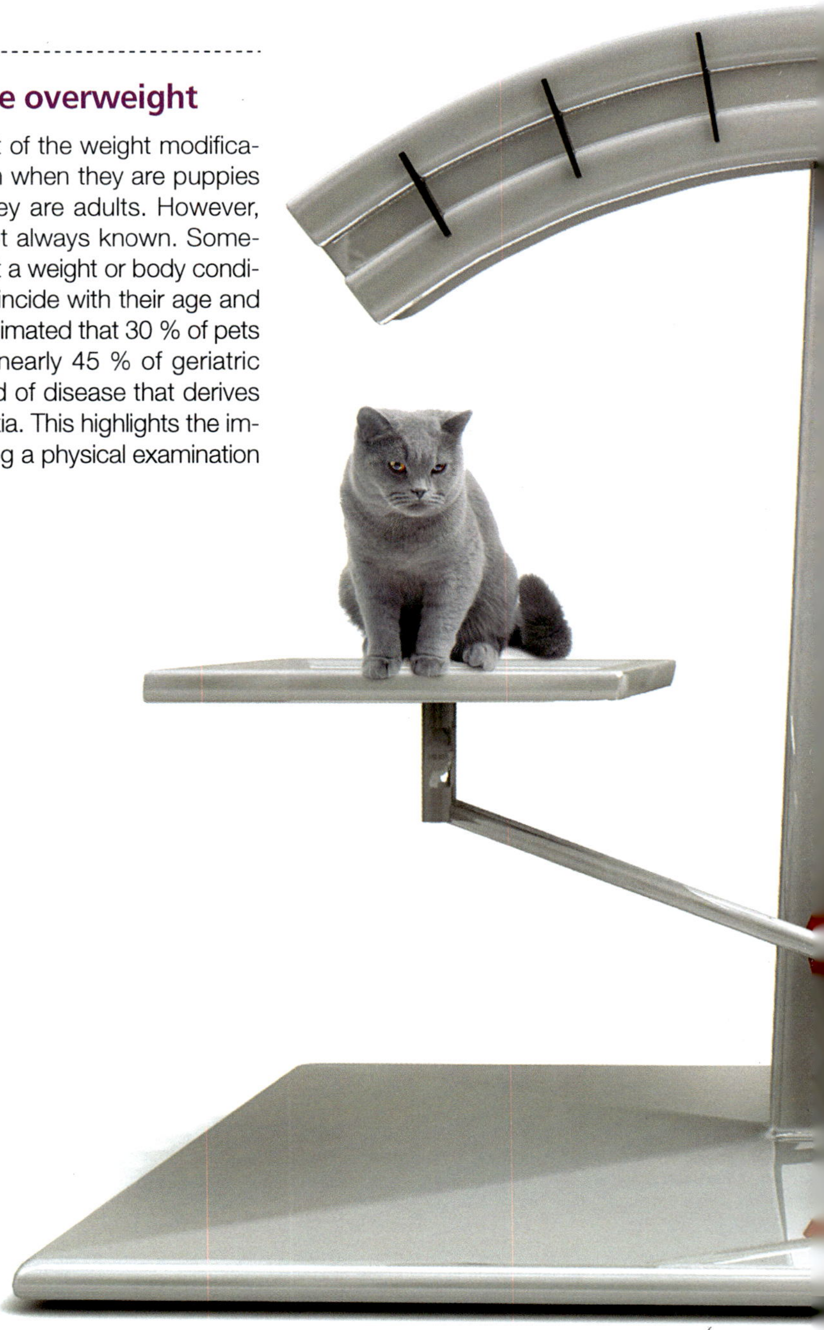

3 There should be no weight variations greater than 3.5 % in a period of 3 months

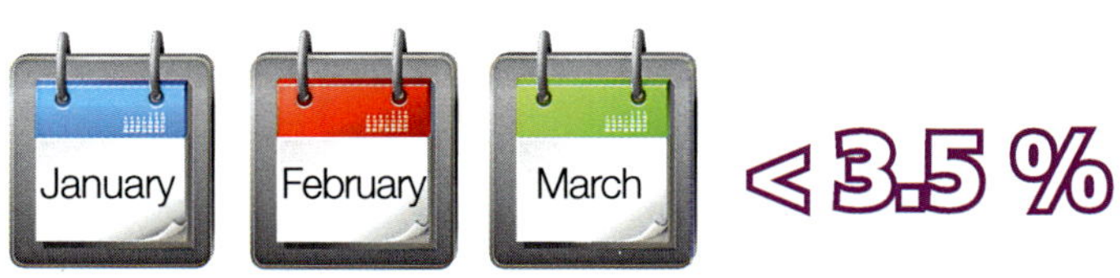

Knowing the optimal weight of an animal allows us to predict whether or not there are signs of disease, given that weight is one of the first variables to change. As a general rule, there should be no weight variations greater than 3.5 % in a period of 3 months. When the factor of this variation is not due to changes to the animal's maintenance needs (for example, exercise or rest) with poor adjustment of the daily portions, a pathology should be suspected.

BODY EVALUATION	VARIATION OF WEIGHT	TIME
Healthy animal	2 %	1 month
Healthy animal	3.5 %	3 months
Suspicions of cachexia/overweight	5 %	6 months
Cachexia/overweight	>10 %	<6 months

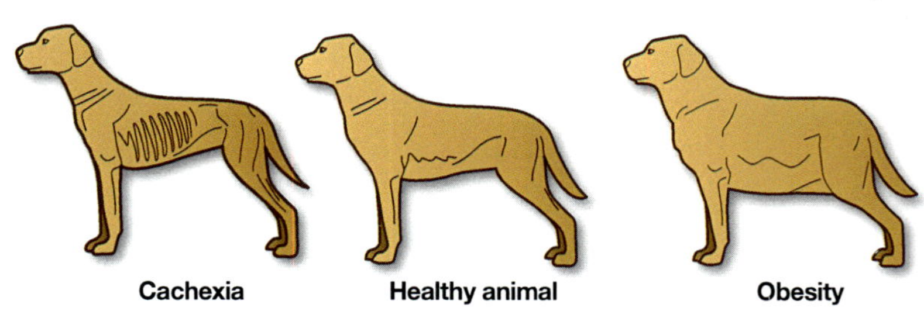

body condition

4

With the proportion of lean:fatty tissue, the dosage of medication can be better adjusted

Another advantage is more precise calculation of the dose of certain medications, as they are used with an ideal lean:fatty ratio in mind. For example, in a 25 kg dog, without taking into account their body score of 8/9, 150 mg of propofol would be used for induction, when 115 mg could achieve the same effect.

In the case of weight loss, it must be kept in mind that it is the primary prognostic factor for survival and evaluation of treatment.

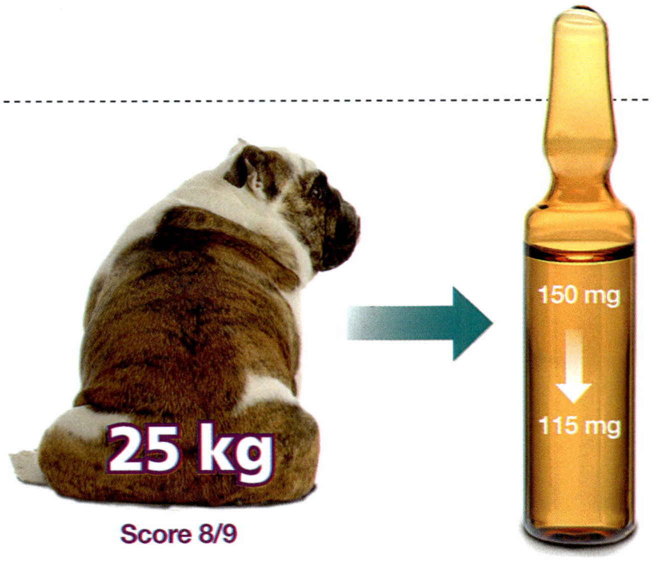

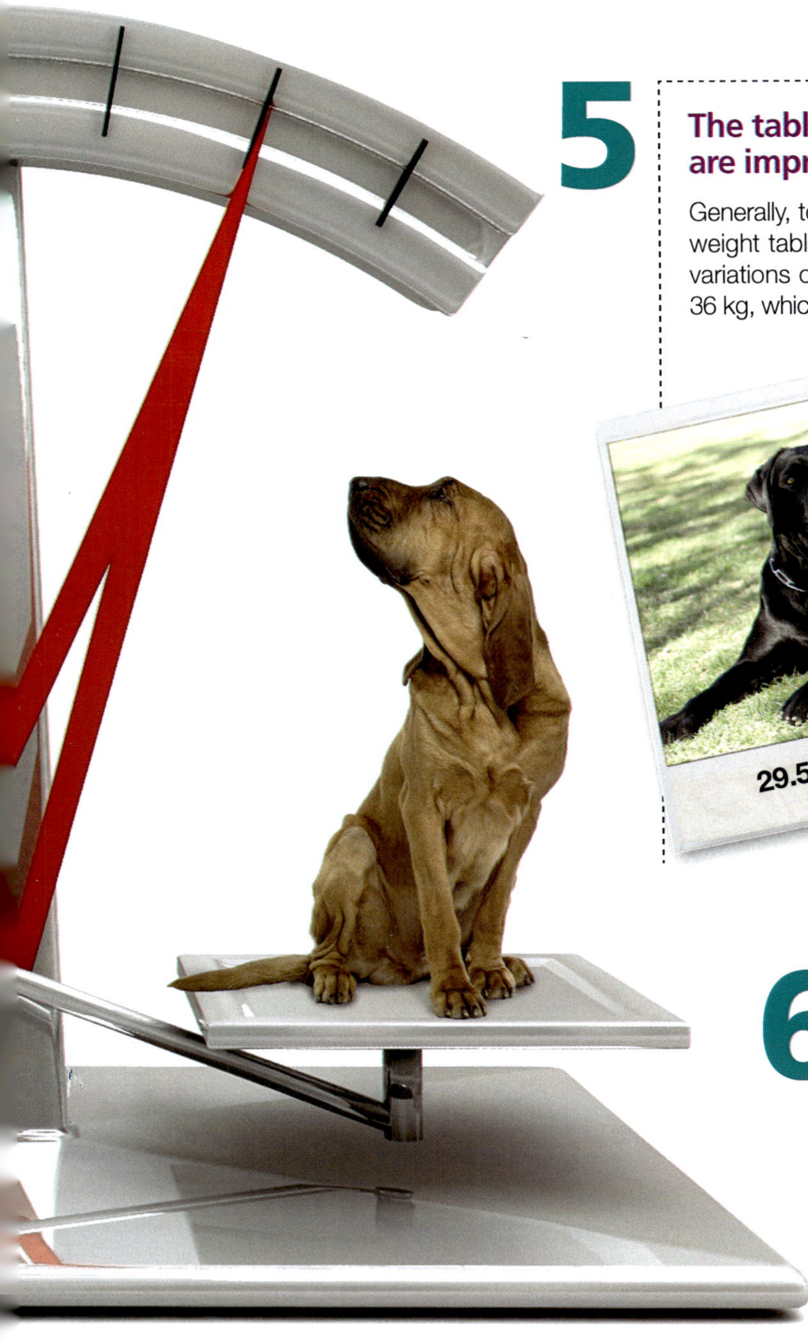

5

The tables of the standard body weight for different breeds are imprecise

Generally, to determine whether an animal is at its correct weight, we use the standard body weight tables for different breeds. However, upon a closer look, we can see that there are variations of up to 15-20 %, for example: A male Labrador that weighs between 29.5 and 36 kg, which leads us to estimate erroneously.

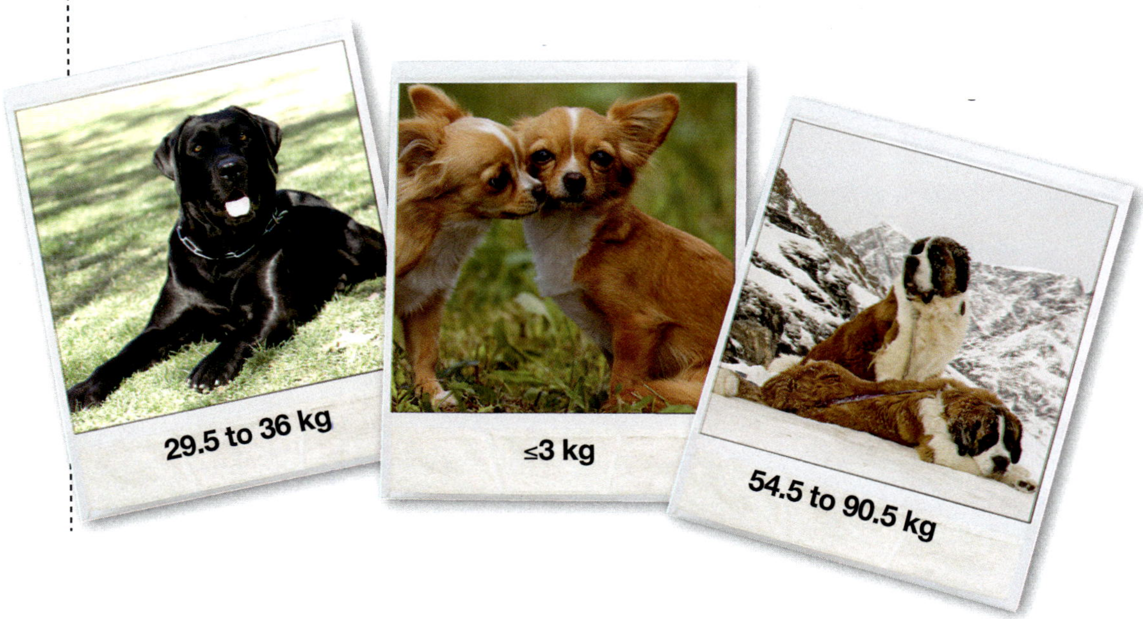

6

A practical method for daily practice must be established

The determination of the body composition can be done using other more precise diagnostic methods:

- ✓ Ultrasound of lumbar fat.
- ✓ Bioelectric impedance.
- ✓ Radioactive isotopes.
- ✓ Biochemical markers.
- ✓ Densitometry (DEXA, *dual energy X-ray absorptiometry*).

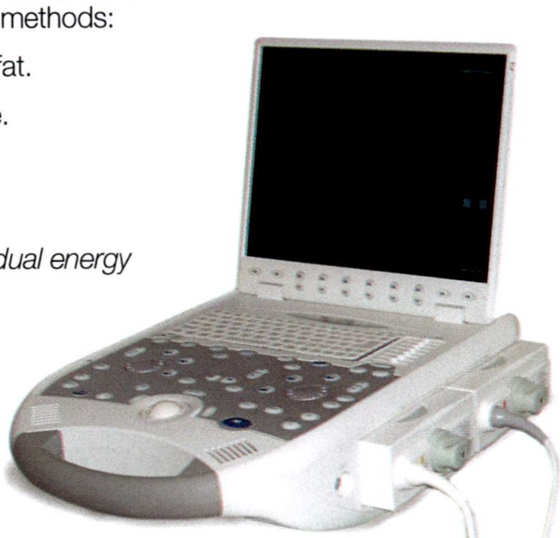

Their use has yet to be established in daily clinical practice. However, there are certain simple methods for daily use in clinical practice that allow us to estimate the body weight and optimal body condition of a pet (see next page).

Body score system

1 Body score scale

D. Laflamme (1997) developed a subjective and simple system to estimate the body condition of a pet, for dogs or cats, called the body score scale, which makes it possible to predict their ideal weight. Laflamme compared the results obtained with diagnostic imaging equipment –DEXA, dual energy X-ray absorptiometry– that evaluated the density of the different tissues, with the observation and palpation of certain bony prominences (see image) and their fat covering.

It is a system with a 90 % reliability rate, in spite of having a standard deviation of ±5 %. The scale establishes grades of 5 or 9, where 3/5 or 5/9 is the ideal weight for the animal. Each value in the scale represents a modification of 10 % or of 5 % of the total body fat (BF), depending on the scale. These modifications translate into variations of the weight of the animal.

SCALE OF9	1	2	3	4	5	6	7	8	9
Body fat (%)	<5	10		15	20	25	30	35	≥40

SCALE OF5	1	2	3	4	5
Body fat (%)	<5	10	20	30	≥40

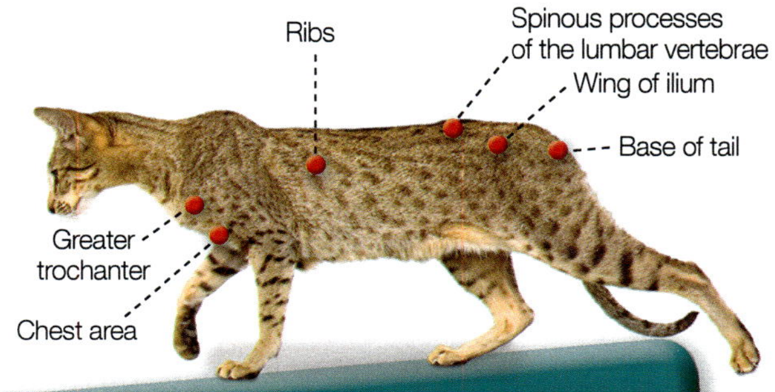

Body condition diagram

Weight lower than normal

1 The ribs, lumbar vertebrae, pelvis, and other bony prominences are clearly visible. There is no fat and the loss of muscle tissue is obvious.

2 The ribs, lumbar vertebrae, pelvic bones and other bony prominences are easily visible. There is no fat and the loss of muscle tissue is obvious.

3 The ribs are palpated and easily visible. There is no palpable fat. The spinous processes of the lumbar vertebrae are visible and the pelvic bones are prominent. The abdomen is contracted and the waist is obvious.

Ideal weight

4 The ribs are easily palpated and have minimal fat covering. The waist is easily noted, viewed from above. The abdomen is contracted and firm.

5 The ribs are palpated without excess fat. The waist is observed behind the ribs when viewed from above. Laterally, the abdomen is visibly contracted.

Overweight

6 The ribs are palpable with slight layer of fat. The waist is discernible only when viewed from above, but is not prominent. There is a certain degree of abdominal tuck.

7 The ribs are palpable with difficulty and there is a thick layer of body fat that is more noticeable in the lumbar area and base of tail. There is no waist or it is barely visible. The abdomen is only slightly tucked.

8 The ribs are only palpable under a thick fat layer when using significant pressure. Large fat deposits are observed in the lumbar area and the base of the tail. There is no waist. The abdomen is flaccid and presents a certain degree of distension.

9 Massive fat deposits are observed on the thorax, spine and base of tail and there is also fat on the neck and limbs. There is no waist and the abdomen hangs loose.

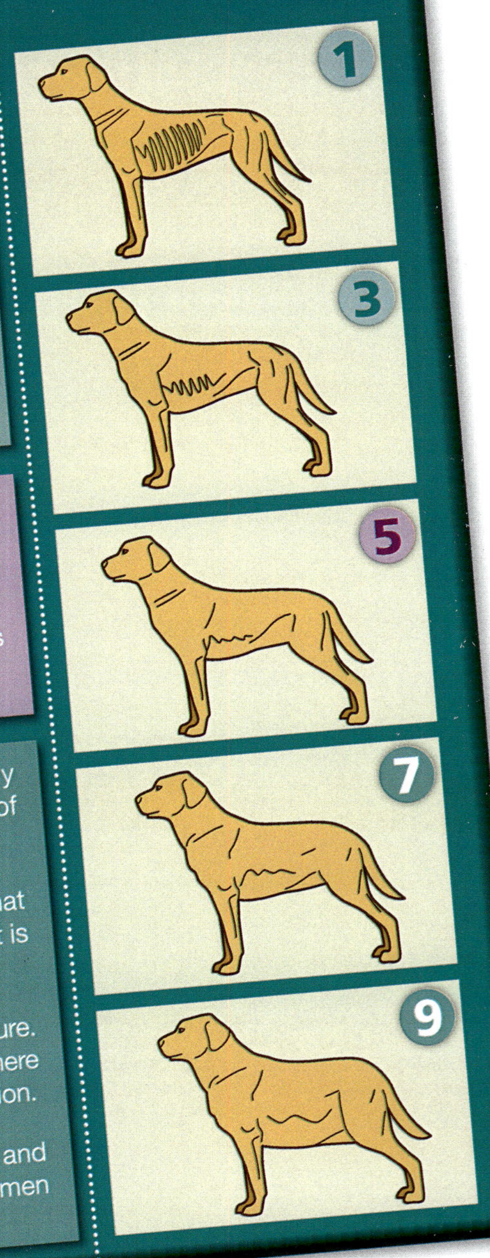

2 Cats have more body fat

Dogs have 15-20 % body fat of their total weight, although certain breeds, like Labradors, have more, and others, like Boxers, have less. Cats present a slightly higher average value, with 25 to 30 % body fat. On average, it is estimated that our pets have 80 % lean body mass and 20 % fat.

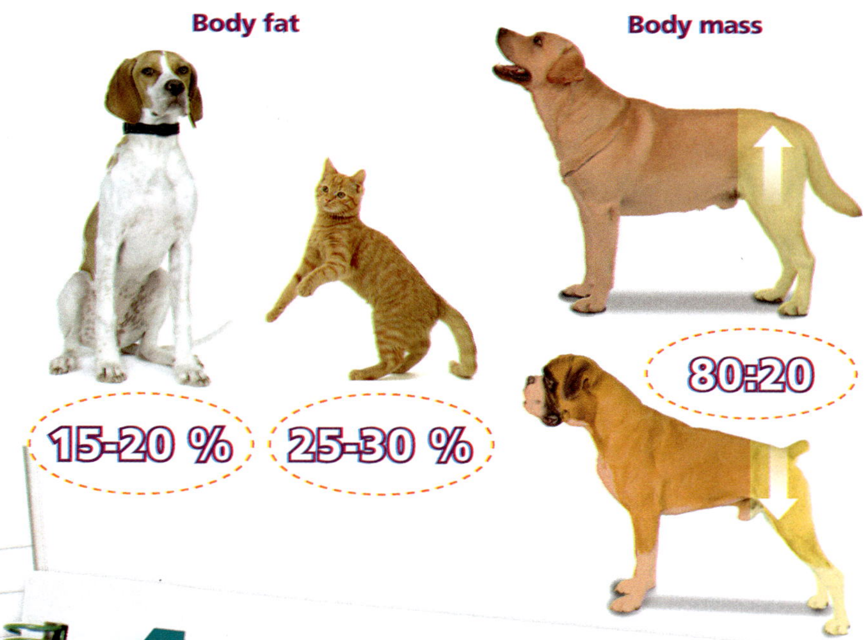

3 Calculating optimal weight

Calculating the optimal weight is done using the following equation:

$$\text{Optimal weight (OW)} = \frac{\text{current weight (CW)} \times (100 - \%\ \text{body fat})}{0{,}80}$$

Examples:

For a dog that weighs 12.5 kg with a body score of 7/9 (30 % BF), what would its optimal weight be?

✓ OW = CW x (100 - % BF) / 0.80

✓ OW = 12.5 x (100 - 30) / 0.80

✓ OW = 10.9 kg

For a cat that weighs 3.8 kg with a body score of 2/9 (10 % BF), what would its optimal weight be?

✓ OW = 3.8 x (100 - 10) / 0.8

✓ OW = 4.3 kg

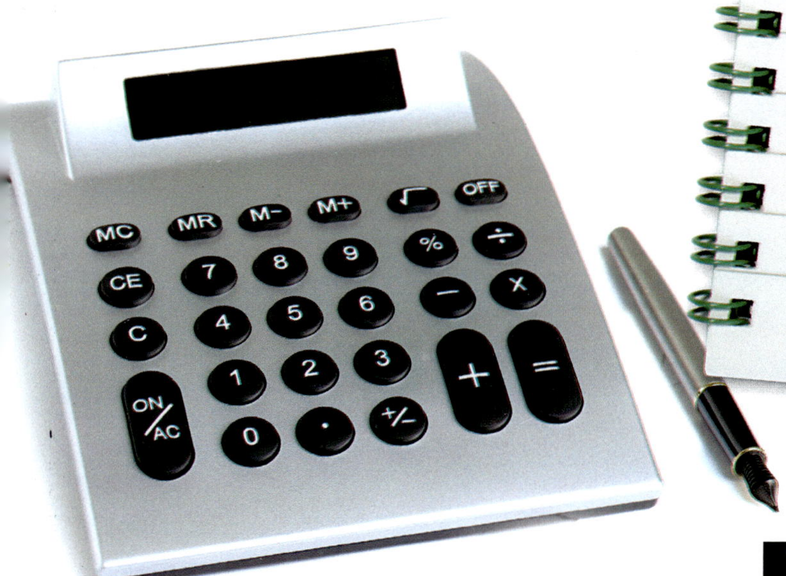

4 Calculation by means of the variations over the optimal weight

From a practical point of view, it is easier to use variations (increases or decreases) that take place over the ideal/optimal weight:

SCALE OF9	1	2	3	4	5	6	7	8	9
Variations of the ideal weight (%)	-18.7	-13.6		-6.3	Optimal	+6	+14	+23	+33
Traditional system	-20	-15		-5	0	+10	+20	+30	+40

The advantage of using the traditional values is found in how easy they are to remember. The slight variation that is produced regarding the estimations of the ideal weight or the prediction equation is small (± 4.2 %), and does not affect the energy requirements of pets in a significant manner.

Examples:

If we use the same examples above as a reference:

A dog that weighs 12.5 kg and has a body score of 7/9 (30 % BF):

✓ CW = OW + 14 % OW

✓ 12.5 = 1.14 OW

✓ OW = 12.5/1.14

✓ OW = 10.9 kg

Also, and much more practical, the traditional system can be used:

✓ 12.5 = 1.20 OW

✓ OW = 10.4 kg

A cat that weighs 3.8 kg and has a body score of 2/9 (10 % BF):

✓ CW = OW + 13.6 % OW

✓ 3.8 = 0.86 OW

✓ OW = 4.4 kg

And also:

✓ 3.8 = OW – 15 % OW

✓ 3.8 = 0.85 OW

✓ OW = 4.4 kg

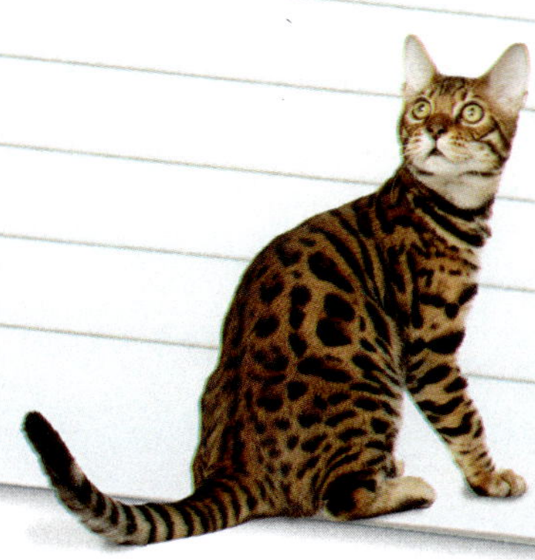

To be taken into account

There are other equations created by different researchers to predict these weight modifications, but it makes no sense to reflect them here in this atlas.

Morphometric measurements

1 Correlation of fatty content with weight and/or with specific body measurements

This is another system to evaluate the percentage of body fat. It is similar to the body mass index, or Quetelet index, used for humans. It attempts to correlate the fatty content with the weight and/or with specific body measurements.

In veterinary medicine, there are certain limitations due to the species, breed and the particular factors of the person measuring. In spite of these limitations, they serve as a good working instrument and are very affordable (only requiring a metric measuring tape and a scale).

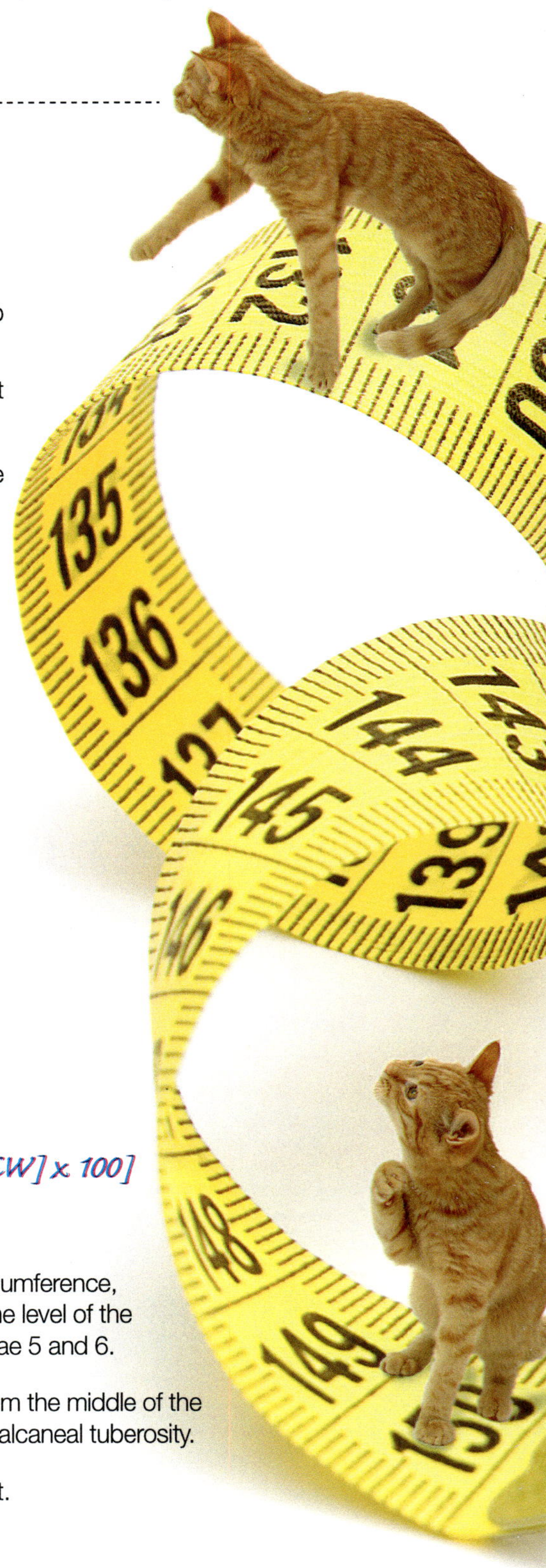

2 Equations to calculate the percentage of body fat

As adipose tissue deposits vary between species, the measurements also vary.

Cats

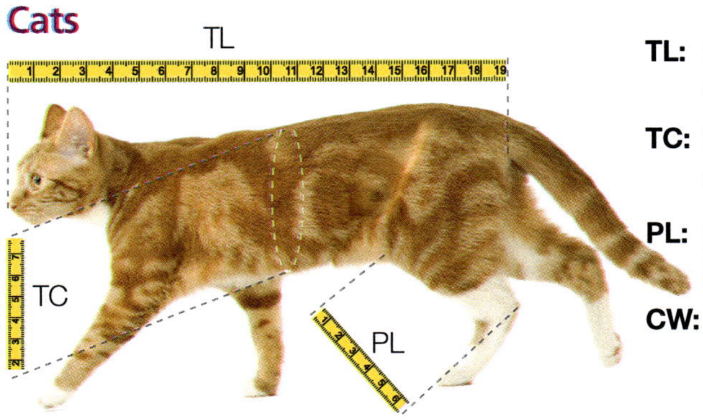

TL: total length, measured from the tip of the nose to the base of the tail.

TC: thorax circumference, measured at the level of the 9th rib.

PL: paw length, from the middle of the patella to the calcaneal tuberosity.

CW: current weight.

Some of the equations used are as follows:

- ✓ $\% \text{ body fat (BF)} = [[(TC / 0.7067) - PL] / 0.9156] - PL$
- ✓ $\% \text{ BF} = 66.715 - 0.061 \times [(TL^2) / CW]$

Dogs

The equations used are as follows:

- ✓ $\% \text{ BF} = [-12.937 + (0.696 \times AC)]$
- ✓ $\% \text{ BF male} = [(-1.4 \times PL) + (0.77 \times AC) + 4]$
- ✓ $\% \text{ BF female} = [(-1.7 \times PL) + (0.93 \times AC) + 5]$
- ✓ $\% \text{ BF} = [[(-0.0034 \times PL^2) + 0.0027 \times AC^2) - 1.9) / CW] \times 100]$

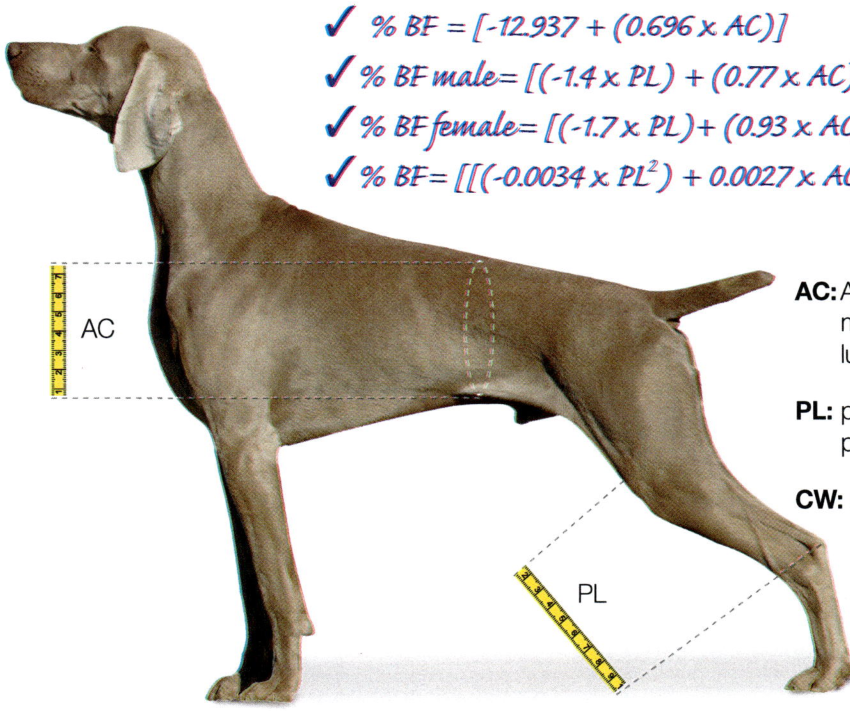

AC: Abdominal circumference, measured at the level of the lumbar vertebrae 5 and 6.

PL: paw length, from the middle of the patella to the calcaneal tuberosity.

CW: current weight.

We can determine an animal's ideal weight from the percentage of body fat using the previously described methods or correcting for a lean:fat body composition of 80:20.

Examples

1. A dog weighs 18.4 kg and presents an AC measurement of 54.5 cm and a PL of 12.5 cm. What would its percentage of fat and ideal body weight be?

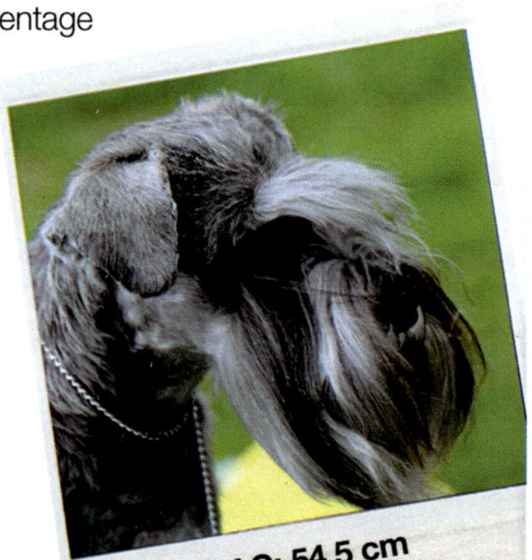

AC: 54.5 cm
PL: 12.5 cm

✓ $\% BF = [-12.937 + (0.696 \times AC)]$

$\% BF = [-12.937 + (0.696 \times 54.5)] = 25\ \%$

✓ $\% BF_{male} = [(-1.4 \times PL) + (0.77 \times AC) + 4]$

$\% BF_{male} = [(-1.4 \times 12.5) + (0.77 \times 54.5) + 4] = 28.47\ \%$

✓ $\% BF = [[(-0.0034 \times PL^2) + 0.0027 \times AC^2) - 1.9) / CW] \times 100]$

$\% BF = [[(-0.0034 \times 12.5^2) + 0.0027 \times 54.5^2) - 1.9) / 18.4] \times 100] = 30.37\ \%$

Using the previously described equations to estimate the ideal weight, the average optimal weight for this animal would be 16.48 kg. That is, we have a pet classified as 7/9 with an average body fat content of 28 %.

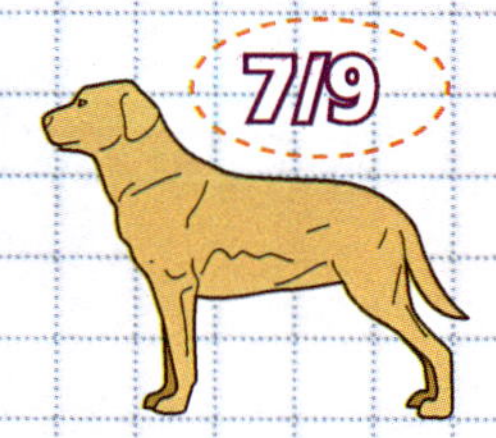

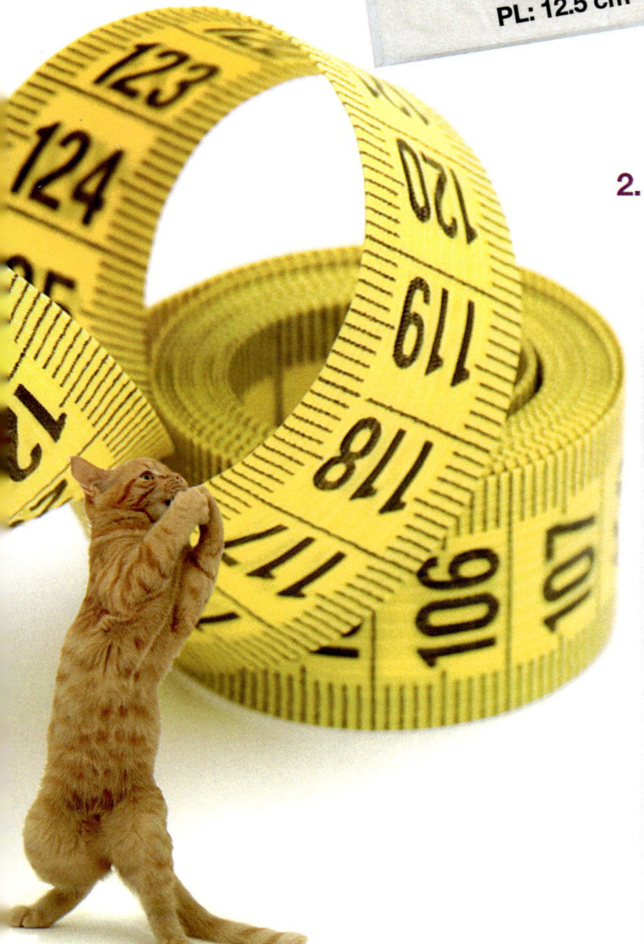

2. A cat currently weighs 8.6 kg and its measurements are as follows: TC of 53 cm, PL of 15 cm and TL of 51.5 cm. What would its ideal weight be?

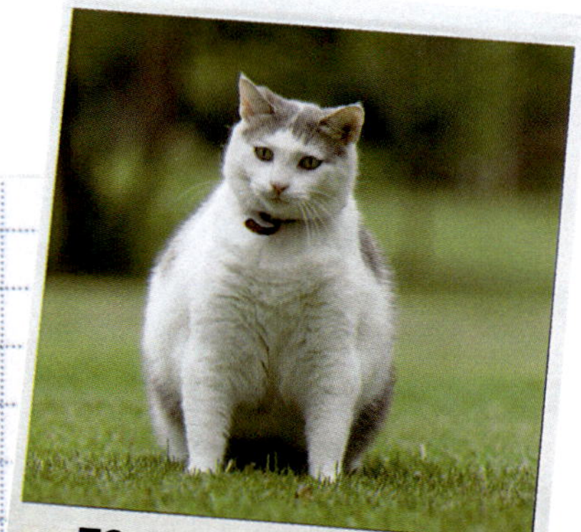

TC: 53 cm; PL: 15 cm;
TL: 51.5 cm

✓ $\% BF = [[(TC / 0.7067) - PL] / 0.9156] - PL$

✓ $\% BF = [[(53 / 0.7067) - 15] / 0.9156] - 15 = 50.53\ \%$

✓ $\% BF = 66.715 - 0.061 \times [(TL^2) / CW]$

$\% BF = 66.715 - 0.061 \times [(51.5^2) / 8.6] = 47.90\ \%$

If we apply the previous equations again, the average optimal weight would be 6.4 kg. We would classify this cat as a 9/9 with an average content of body fat of 49 %. In the case of cats, these values must be considered as inferior given that their average body fat content is higher (around 10 points higher), just as we previously noted, this pet would be an 8/9.

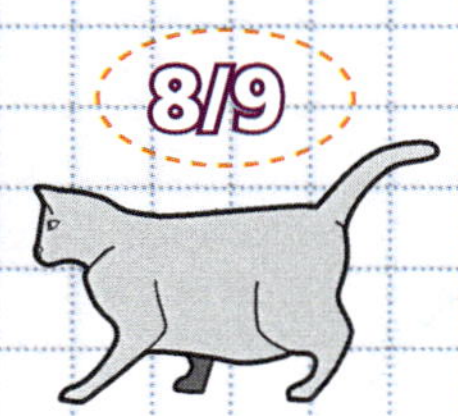

3 Other indexes to evaluate an animal's nutritional status

There are two interesting indicators of our pet's health.

✓ **Fatty mass index** (Baez, 2007).

✓ **Muscle mass index** (Mitchel, 2004).

It is a subjective system. Both indexes classify the pets on a scale of 0 to 3, where 0 is absence and 3 is an obvious or normal increase of tissue.

Both are predictive, especially in pathologies that lead to episodes of cachexia. This allows for us to modify the maintenance needs of the animals.

DEGREE	FATTY MASS INDEX	MUSCLE MASS INDEX
0	Absence on ribs and back	Severe loss: lack of musculature
1	Decrease on ribs	Moderate loss: hard-to-distinguish muscle
2	Normal	Mild loss: lacking some muscle
3	Increase	Normal

The body areas that are evaluated are:

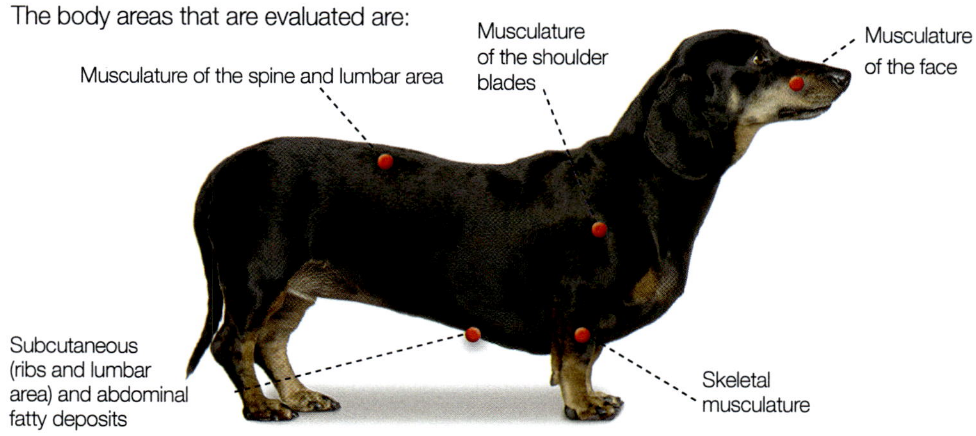

Water

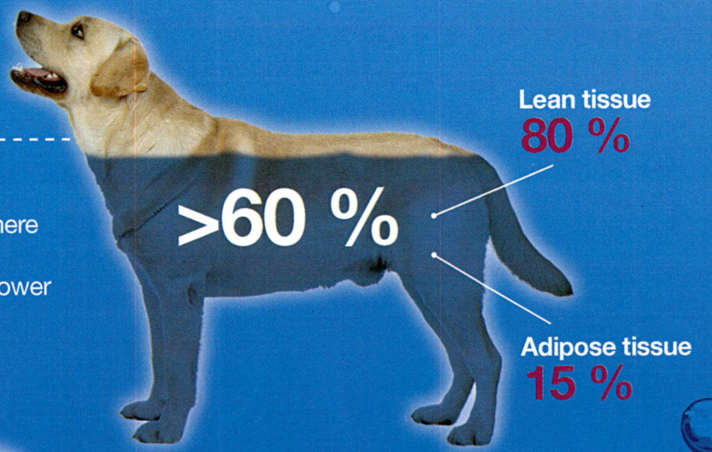

1 An essential nutrient for life

Its proportion in the organism is very high and constant although there are variations depending on the species and age.
Most of it is concentrated in lean tissue, while the proportions are lower in adipose tissue.

2 It participates in several organic functions

Some of these functions are as follows:

- Universal solvent
- Reactions of hydrolysis
- Regulates body temperature
- Responsible for the texture of the different tissues
- Controls gastric emptying

3 Quality conditions for consumption

The quality is determined by the following:

- **Salinity** (concentration of sodium chloride)
- **Mineral content** (primarily calcium and magnesium)
- **Nitrates/nitrites**
- **Presence of chemical agents**
- **Microbial contamination**

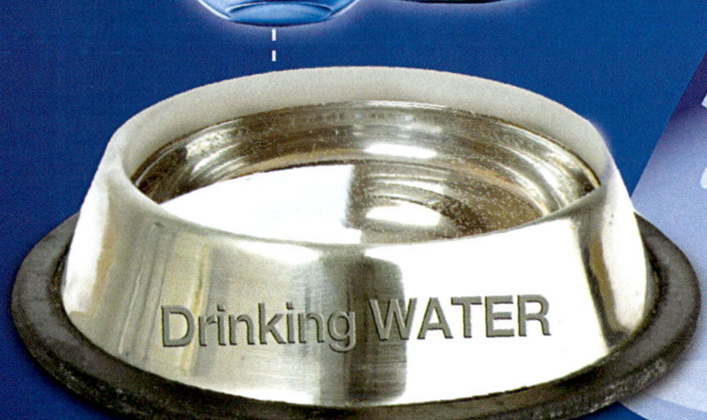

- ✓ Salinity < 250 ppm.
- ✓ Nitrogen content (nitrates + nitrites) <10 ppm.
- ✓ Absence of total coliform bacteria.
- ✓ Free of toxic and chemical contaminants (for example, pesticides).

4 Situations that require calculation of water requirements

Although the water requirements of pets can be estimated, in a practical manner they are not taken into account as the general rule is to provide them with free access to good quality, fresh, and clean drinking water. However, understanding said needs and how to calculate them is important in some situations:

- ✓ Transportation of pets.
- ✓ Environmental conditions.
- ✓ Boarding.
- ✓ Exercise and work.
- ✓ Certain pathologies.

If having water available continuously is not possible (for example, while traveling), pets must have access to water for one hour twice daily.

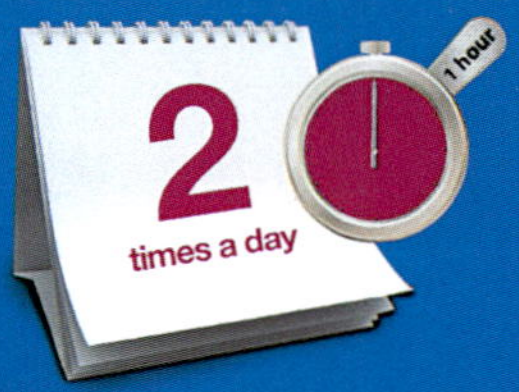

5 Losses of water

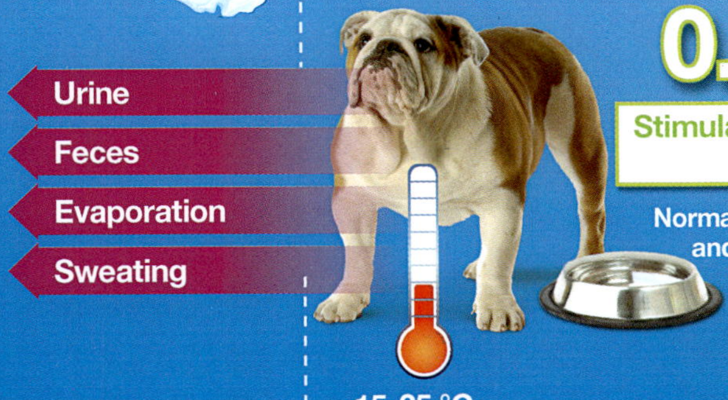

0.5-1 %

Stimulates the consumption of water

Normal loss due to evaporation and one hour in a neutral temperature zone

Losses are continuous and the feeling of thirst depends on the degree of dehydration; dehydration, at the same time, depends on the modifications of the body water: the plasma osmolarity ratio. The antidiuretic hormone, or vasopressin, participates in this process. Other factors that regulate ingestion are the oropharyngeal receptors and the physical receptors of the digestive apparatus.

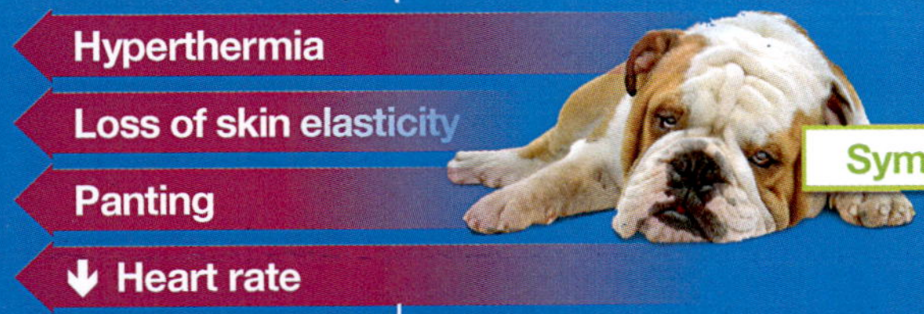

5 %

Symptoms of dehydration

The symptoms of dehydration are compensatory and attempt to preserve the organism's water content and temperature. The lethal rectal temperature for dogs is **41.7 °C,** and for cats, **43.4 °C**. In this sense, the evaporation of water in dogs and cats depends on the atmospheric temperature and of the degree of hydration/dehydration.

>15 %

Multi-organ failure

When dehydration is over 15 %, the capacity to eliminate heat by evaporation is lost, and the body temperature in these conditions increases by 7 °C per hour, leading to death by multi-organ failure.

6 Species particularities

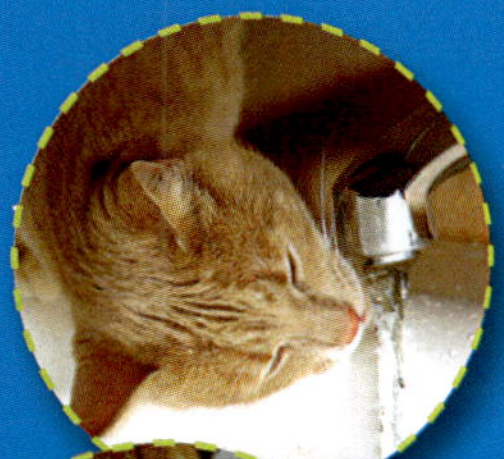

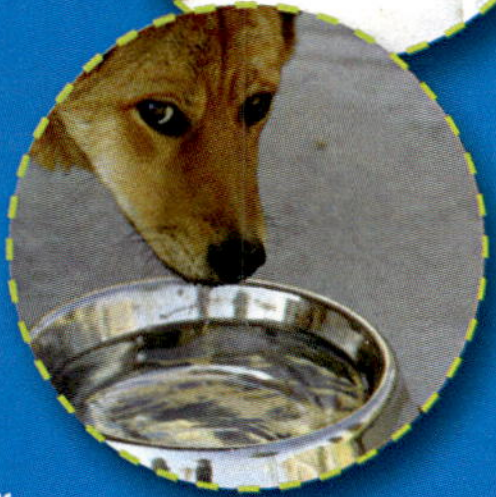

The use of running water has been observed to stimulate drinking water in cats.

Dogs ingest small volumes of water throughout the day, but when faced with a situation of thirst, they can ingest very large amounts of liquid.

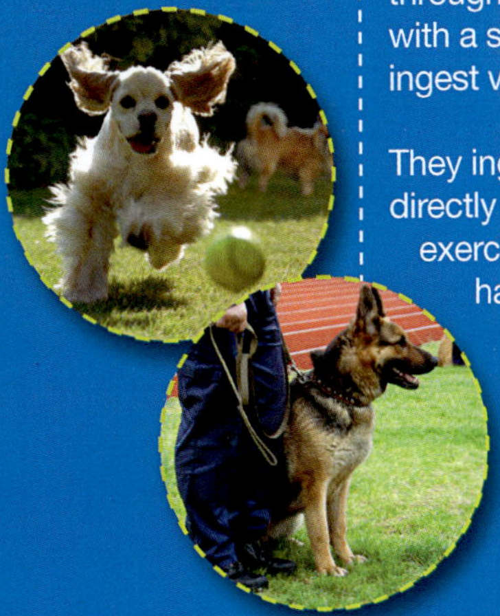

They ingest water in a compulsive manner directly after exercising. Five minutes after exercising, dogs ingest water only if they have lost between 0.5-1 % of their weight.

Working dogs drink before starting to exercise.

To be taken into account:

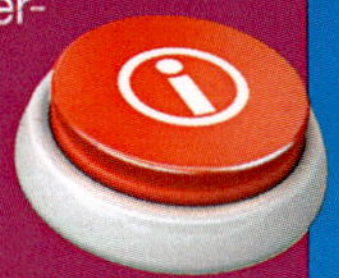

As we have seen, there are certain situations where an animal's drinking habits must be controlled. In these cases, the self-regulation of the ingestion of water does not impede rapid re-hydration. Ingesting large amounts of liquid in the organism causes hydropic degeneration and rupture of nervous system cells and red blood cells.

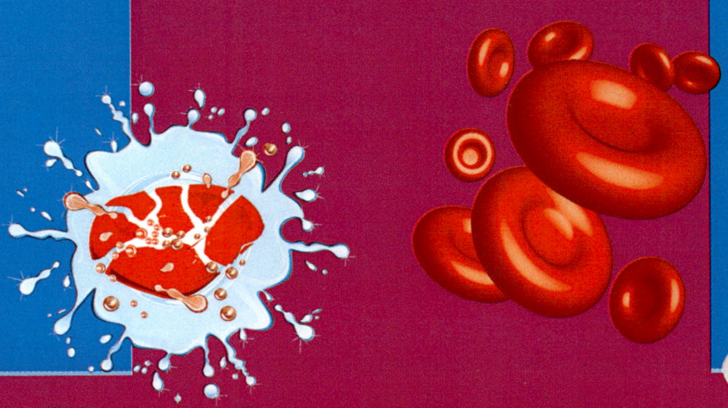

Water requirements

1 Water intake

The water found in pets' bodies comes from three sources:

Metabolic water
Represents only 5-10 % of the total requirements of water.

Water found in foods

Drinking water

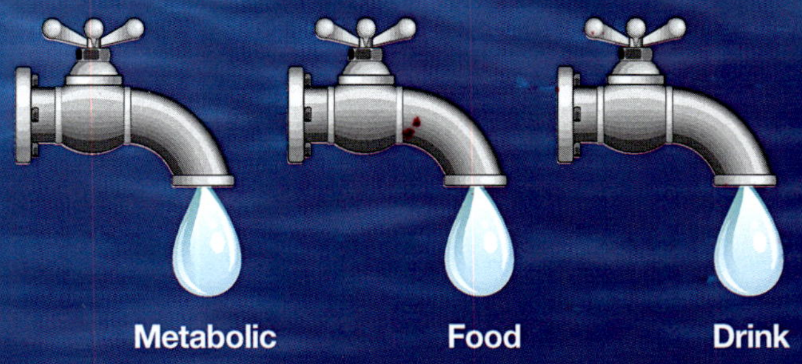

The ingestion of water is correlated with breath humidity. Animals who are fed primarily dry food ingest more water than those who are fed wet food. This process ensures the maintenance of the water balance of the organism. However, when food is restricted, their water ingestion decreases by 30-50 % from normal levels. On the contrary, animals that receive a wet diet will increase their water intake. In either case, in fasting situations, the elimination of urine is reduced, but its values are close to those of the ingestion of liquids. This effect allows us to differentiate between episodes of polydypsia/polyuria in our patients.

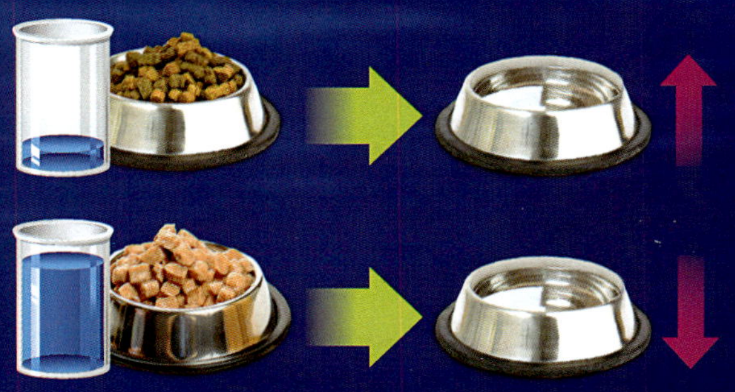

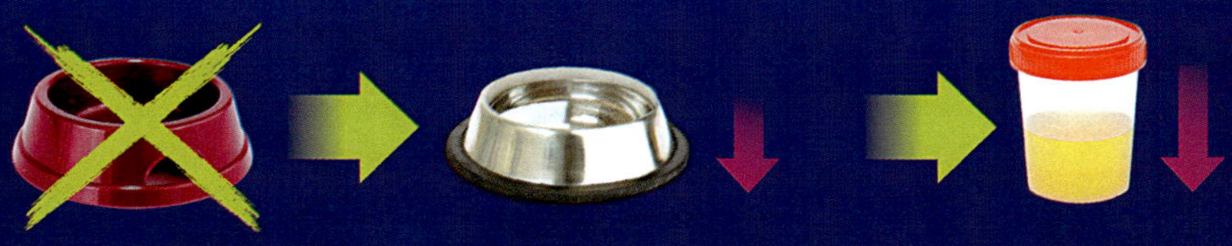

2 Factors that determine the daily requirements

The daily requirements for water are affected by other factors that are not dependent on the animal's food (see drawing).
Depending on the composition of the food, those rich in protein, carbohydrates, and salt will increase water intake as they present a greater concentration of solutes. That said, with foods rich in fat, the ingestion of water is less due to various factors:

- ✔ The quantity of DM (dry material) ingested is lower, and therefore so is the ingestion of the other nutrients.
- ✔ Water loss through the feces is lower.
- ✔ Greater contribution of metabolic water.

The water requirements for the comfort zone are 0.5-1 % of the animal's body weight per hour. In adult dogs and cats, the neutral temperature zone is found between 15-20 °C (maximum 30 °C) and in cold-weather dog breeds, between 10-15 °C. The upper and lower limits of the neutral zone are called critical temperatures.
The corresponding corrections will need to be made for values above or below the aforementioned temperatures given that modifications are produced in the MER (metabolizable energy requirements) and water requirements. Above 30-35 °C, the daily requirements must be increased. These values, when the temperatures reach 45 °C, are doubled in dogs and multiplied by three or seven in cats: as an average, it is estimated that the water requirements should be 2 % of the animal's body weight per hour, or, 20 ml/kg of body weight per hour.
It is very important to keep this data in mind for working dogs that work outdoors (hunting dogs), or in countries with warm climates.

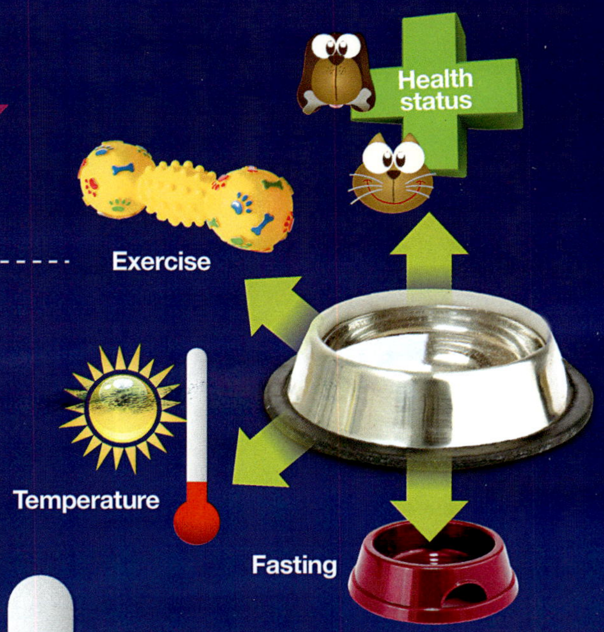

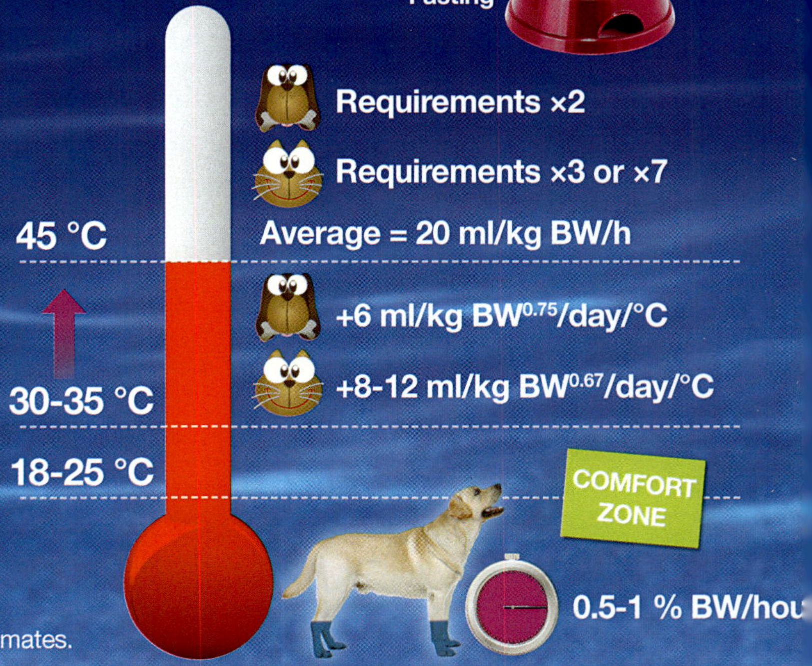

3 How to determine a pet's water requirements

There are several ways to determine a pet's water requirements:

- ✔ The daily water recommendations (ml/day) are equal to the maintenance energetic requirements (kcal ME/day). There is a ratio of ml water:kcal ME whose value is 1.
Cats, due to their desert origins, are adapted to water restrictions: they have a high capacity to concentrate their urine and they better endure dehydration. In this sense, their water:energy ratio is between 0.6-0.7. Generally speaking, we can use a 1:1 rule taking into account that we are overestimating the true requirements for cats.

ml water : kcal ME = 1

(cat) → : = 0.6-0.7

- ✔ Water requirements, expressed in liters per day, are close to 7 % and 5.5 % of body weight in dogs and cats, respectively.

(dog) 7 % BW (cat) 5.5 % BW

- ✔ They can also be determined using the 50-60 ml (and up to 72.3 ml) equation of water per kilogram of body weight.

50-60 ml × kg BW

- ✔ On the other hand, due to the fact that there is a relationship between the dry material and water ingested, it is estimated that the daily amount of water ingested represents 2.5 to 3 times the dry material ingested as food (with a mean energetic concentration of 3,500 kcal/kg DM). This method of determining the drinking water can lead to errors due to the variability in the energetic concentration of the foods ingested. The increase in the energetic density for the same levels of dry material produces an underestimate of the true water requirements of our pet: the estimated amount of water is reduced in approximately the same proportion as the increase of the density.

Water DM → 3,500 kcal/kg DM

↑ Energy density = ↓ (water)

Examples:

Weight: 15 kg
Temperature zone: neutral

Weight: 5 kg
Temperature zone: neutral

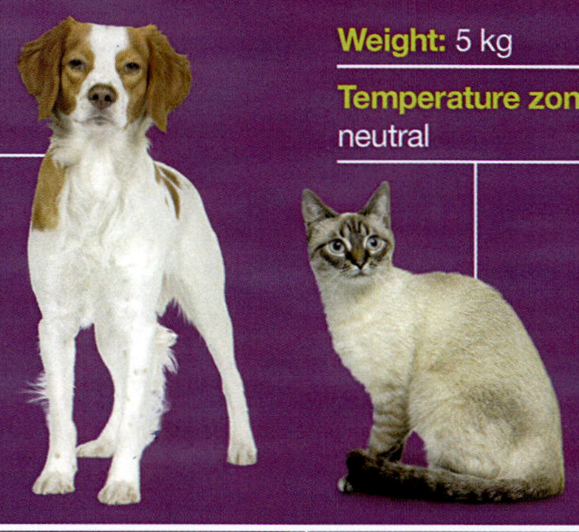

	Dog	Cat
kcal ME/d	1,006 kcal ME/d	294 kcal ME/d
ml/d	1,006 ml/d	290 ml/d
% BW	15 (kg) × 7 % → 1 l/d	5 (kg) × 5 % → 0.25 l/d
50-60 ml × kg BW	15 × 50-60 ml → 750-900 ml/d	5 × 50-60 ml → 250-300 ml/d

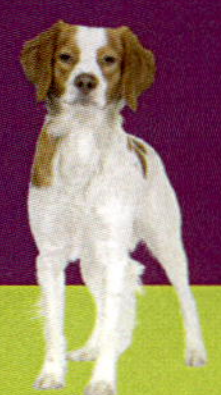

Food	A	B
Humidity	8	8
kcal ME/kg DM	3,500	4,300
kcal ME/kg	3,220	3,864
Requirements (kcal ME/day)	1,006.1	1,006.1
Food ingested (g/day) (requirements/food energy)	312.45	254.32
DM ingested (g) (ingested × % DM)	287.45	233.98
Water requirements (l) (DM ingested × 2.5-3)	0.72-0.86	0.58-0.7

Once we know our pet's water requirements, we can estimate their drinking water requirements taking into account the composition in humidity of their food. We will not take the metabolic water into account given that its contribution is very low. Following with our example of a cat that weighs 5 kg:

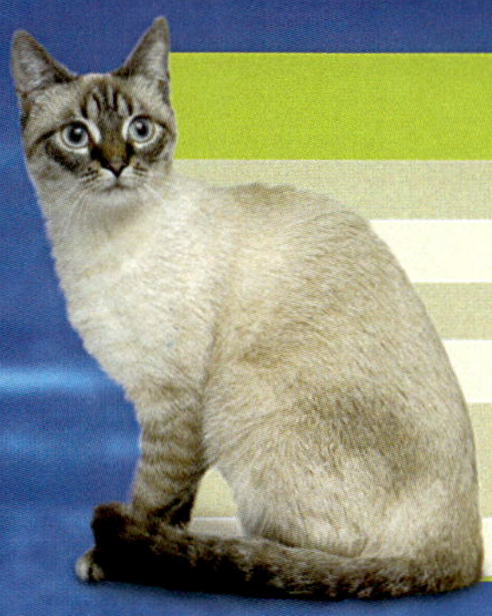

Food	A	B
Humidity	8	75
kcal ME/kg DM	3,500	3,500
kcal ME/kg	3,220	875
Requirements (kcal ME/day)	294	294
Food ingested (g/day) (requirements/food energy)	60.97	224.36
DM ingested (g) (ingested × % DM)	56.09	

Food	A	B
Water requirements (ml)		
(ml:kcal ME); ratio 0.6:1*	294 (176-205)*	
(% body weight)	275	
(50-60 ml/body weight)	250-300	
(DM ingested × 2.5-3)	140-168	
Water from food (ml)	4.8	170
Drinking water (ml) (average)	245	81

*The value 294 represents the ingestion in a ratio of 1:1, but in cats, to avoid overestimating, a ratio of 0.6-0.7 ml/kcal ME is used (values in parenthesis).

Energy requirements

Energy as an organic fuel

All animals need the energy contained in foods as fuel for the processes that take place in the organism during maintenance, growth, reproduction, lactation and exercise: primarily in the sodium/potassium pump, molecular synthesis and in the activation of contractile proteins. However, the energy found in these foods is not completely used by the organism.

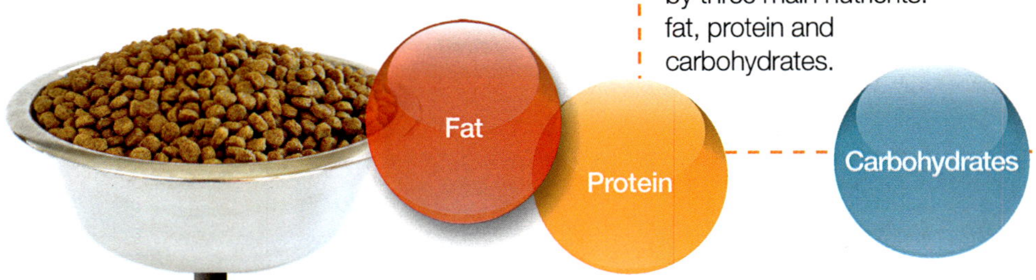

Energy is not a nutrient itself, however, it is represented by three main nutrients: fat, protein and carbohydrates.

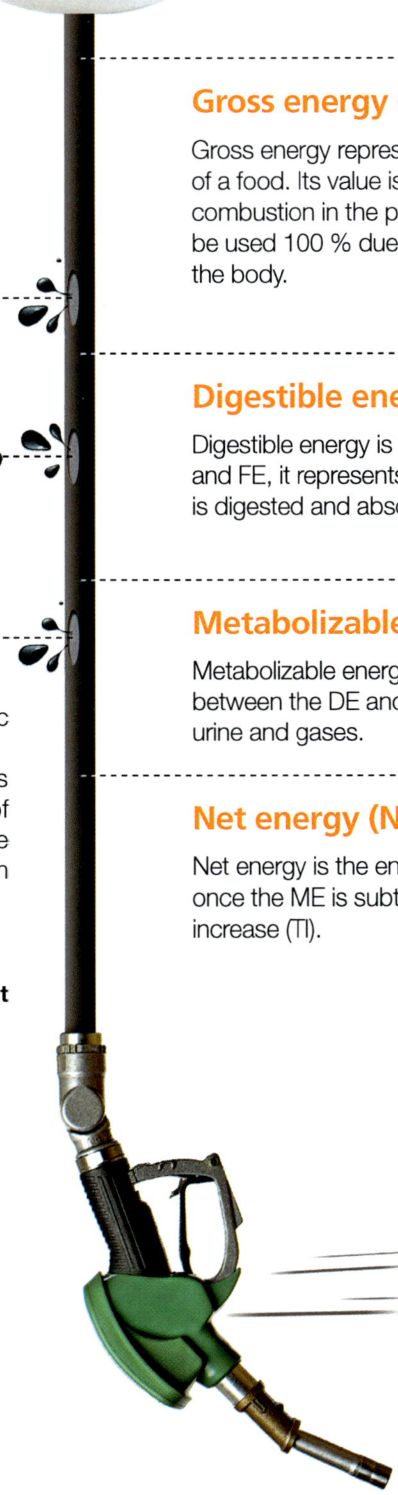

Gross energy (GE)

Gross energy represents the potential energy of a food. Its value is obtained by the complete combustion in the presence of oxygen. It cannot be used 100 % due to losses that take place in the body.

Energy lost through feces (FE)

Digestible energy (DE)

Digestible energy is the difference between GE and FE, it represents the fraction of the GE that is digested and absorbed to be used.

Energy lost through urine and gases

Metabolizable energy (ME)

Metabolizable energy (ME) is the difference between the DE and the energy lost through urine and gases.

Temperature increase (TI)

TI are the losses due to digestive and metabolic processes.

The TI takes places every time an animal eats and its value increases with the number of meals. Also, the TI varies depending on the nutrient. The efficiency of use of energy from different nutrients is as follows:

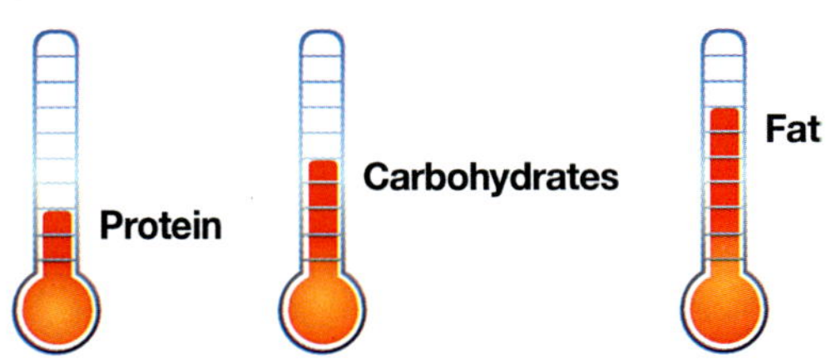

Protein has the lowest efficiency. For this reason, when the food portions have high levels of protein, the TI value is higher. It is also affected by the animal's level of anxiety, exercise and cold temperatures.

Positive effects of the TI:

- Regulates body weight when presented with large meals, decreases the energy available for the synthesis of fatty tissue.
- Maintains body heat in cold weather conditions.

Net energy (NE)

Net energy is the energy used directly by the cell once the ME is subtracted from the temperature increase (TI).

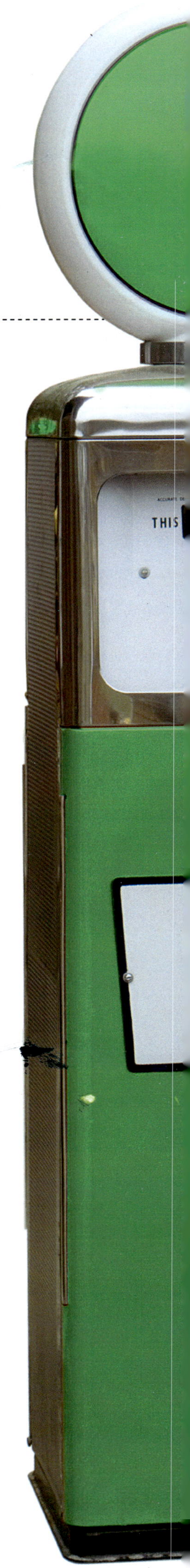

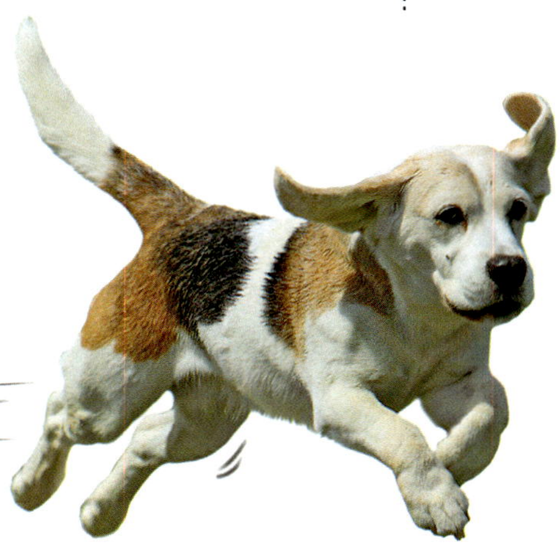

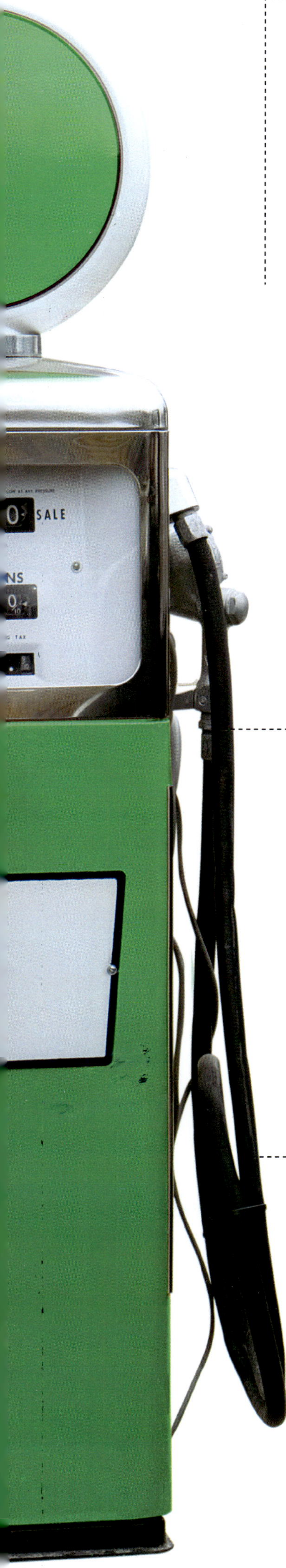

Energetic balance/imbalance

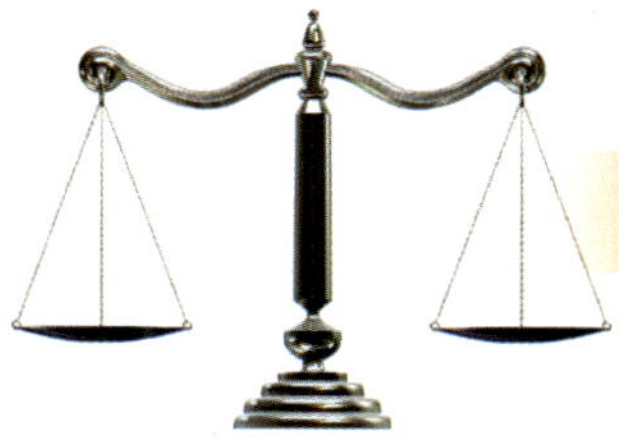

Zero balance

Energy consumed = Energy used

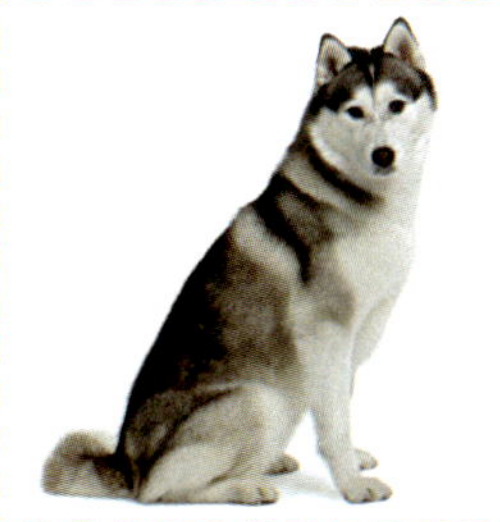

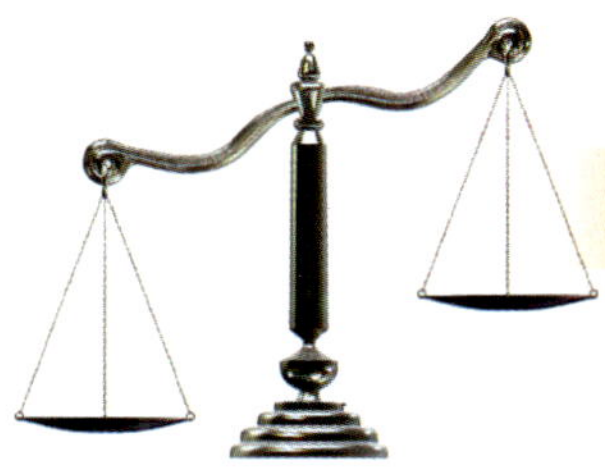

Positive balance

Energy consumed > Energy used

- Overfeeding.
- Changes to ingestion.
- Rest after an orthopedic surgical procedure.

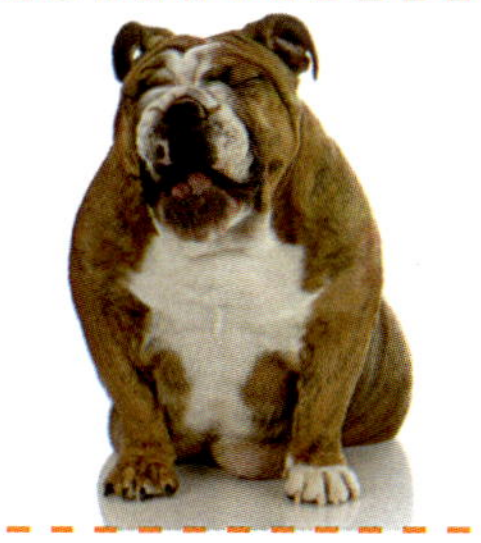

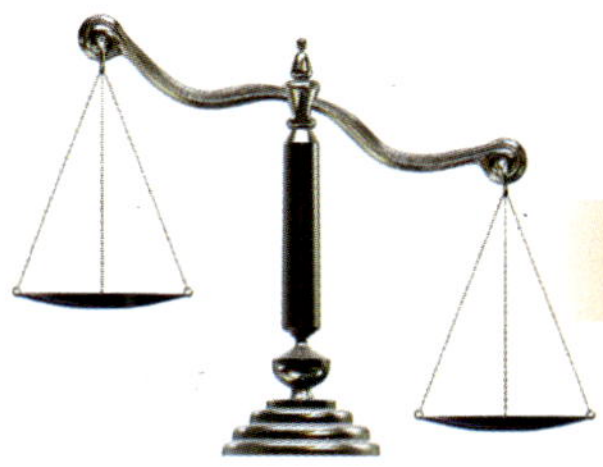

Negative balance

Energy consumed < Energy used

- Underfeeding.
- Animals used for sports.
- Chronic diseases.

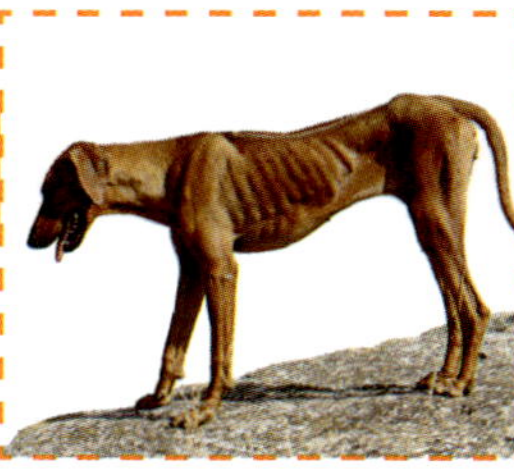

Baseline energy requirements

Basal metabolic rate (BMR)

The basal metabolic rate is the minimum amount of energy each day in an animal at rest, without activity or ingestion of food.

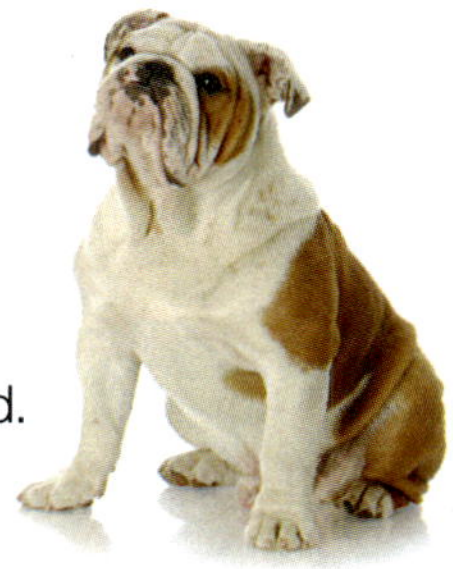

Resting basal metabolism rate (RBMR)

The basal metabolic rate at rest is the temperature increase that takes place when an animal ingests food. This increase in heat has two fractions: TI and one derived from the autonomic nervous system.

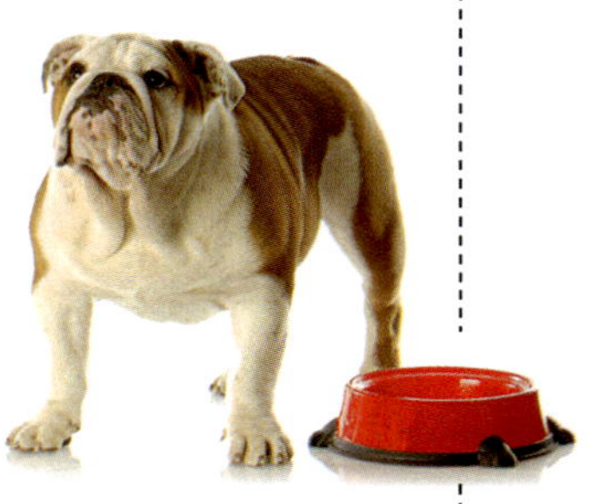

Metabolizable energy requirements for maintenance (MER)

The metabolizable energy requirements for maintenance represent the energy needed to place the organism at a zero energy balance, including the RBMR, normal activity and thermoregulation.

Daily energy requirements

The daily energy requirements are those that include exercise, productions (growth, gestation and lactation) and special situations (pain, disease, surgery...).

The ME is the energy unit in pets

The requirements and composition tables reference said unit.
It is expressed in kilocalories (kcal) or in kilojoules (kJ).
The entire scientific community, except for the Anglo-Saxons, uses the kcal as a unit.

1 kcal → 4.184 kJ

1 kJ → 0.239 kcal

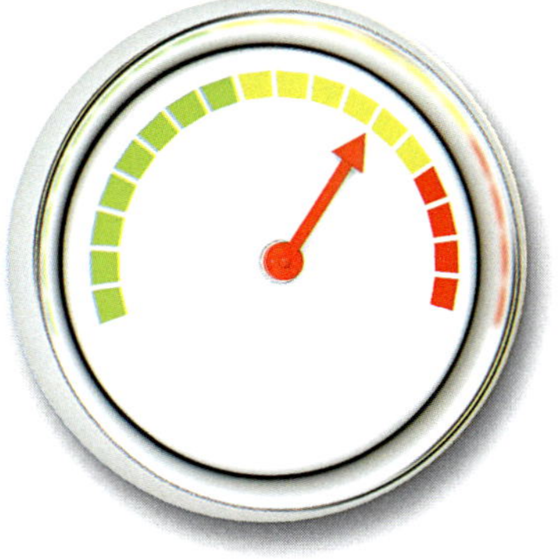

How are energy requirements

1

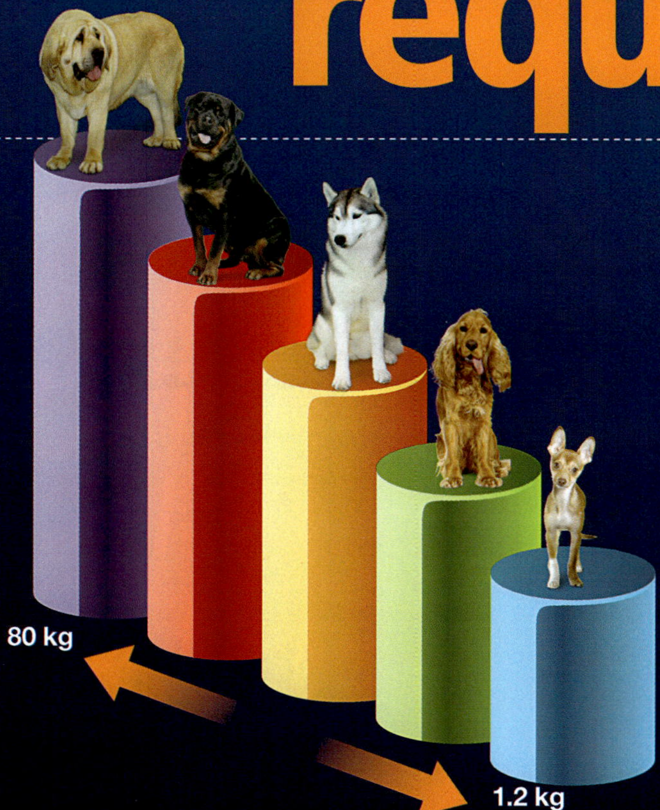

The allometry of the species must be taken into account

We can determine the energetic requirements of animals of different sizes and geometric forms by taking into account the allometry of the species.
For dogs, this fact is obvious: there are breeds that weigh as little as 1.2 kg and others that surpass 80 kg with different withers and hip widths or abdominal organ and brain weights.

2

The requirements vary with the different body weights

We can achieve more precise estimates of an animal's requirements if we take into account their metabolic weight.
The **metabolic weight (MW)** is obtained by raising the body weight to the 0.75 power: this defines the relationship that exists between the mass and energy in dogs. This factor is known as the **inter-specific allometric coefficient**.
Therefore, the determination of the basal metabolism rate (BMR) in dogs is 70 × $BW^{0.75}$. Later, we will describe what happens in the case of cats.

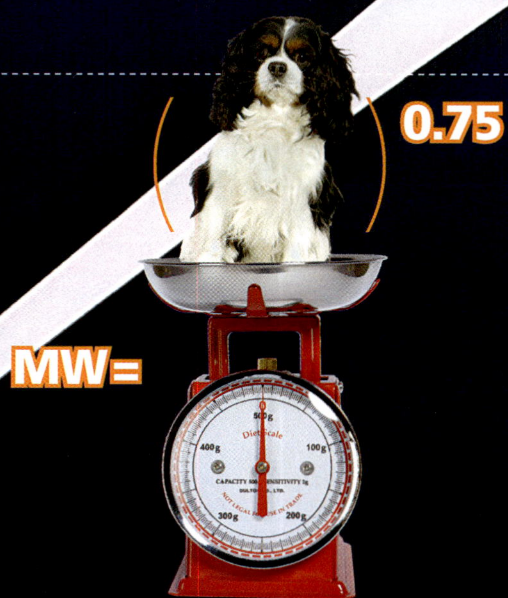

3

The values obtained for the basal metabolism are lower than the true values

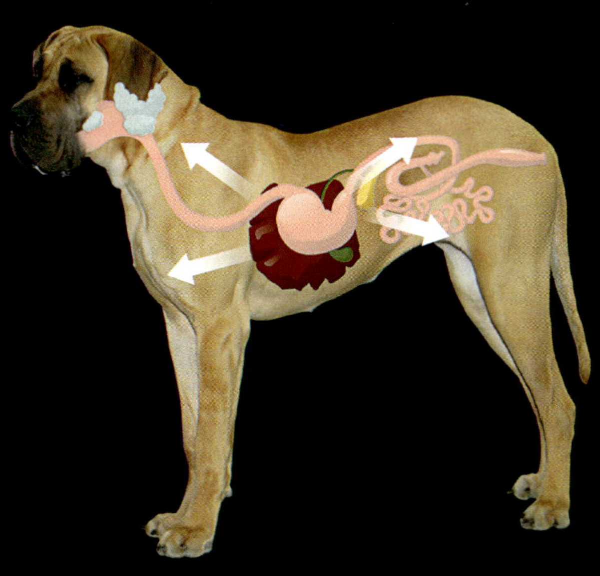

This happens due to different digestive and food assimilation processes. Using the resting basal metabolism rate (RBMR, 10-15 % higher than the BMR) or the metabolizable energy requirements for maintenance (MER) is therefore more useful, which include an animal's normal processes (they are 75 % greater, on average, compared to the RBMR).

It is important to take into account the fact that the requirements are determined for lean tissue given that fat is a tissue that has little metabolic activity. Therefore, no energy changes per unit of lean tissue are produced if we take into account the body condition.

determined?

4 Studies to calculate the energetic requirements for maintenance

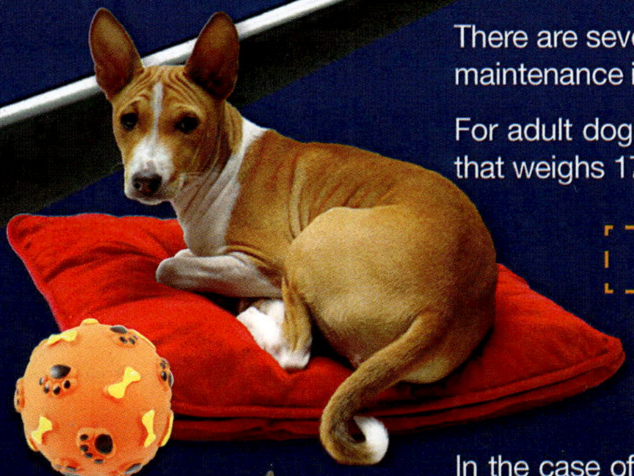

There are several studies that establish different equations to calculate the energetic requirements for maintenance in pets.

For adult dogs living in homes, stimulated to play and exercise frequently, using, for example, a dog that weighs 17 kg, is taken as an average value:

$$\text{MER (kcal ME/day)}_{dog} = 132 \text{ (kcal)} \times \text{body weight (kg)}^{0.75}$$

$$\text{MER (kcal ME/day)} = 132 \text{ (kcal)} \times 17 \text{ (kg)}^{0.75} = 1{,}105.1 \text{ kcal/day}$$

In the case of cats, due to the fact that they are animals with similar geometry and there are no great weight differences between the breeds, the mass:body surface ratio or intra-specific allometric coefficient is 0.67.

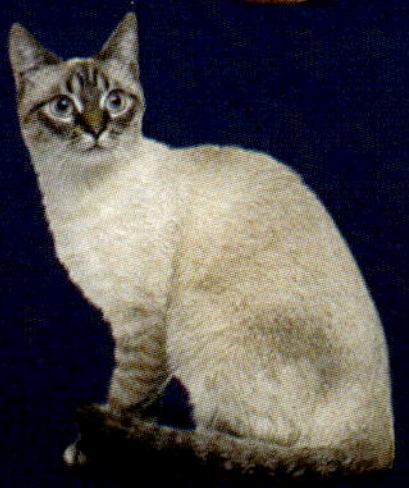

A

A. Adult cats with good body condition 3/5 or 5/9:

$$\text{MER (kcal ME/day)}_{cat} = 100 \text{ (kcal)} \times \text{body weight (kg)}^{0.67}$$

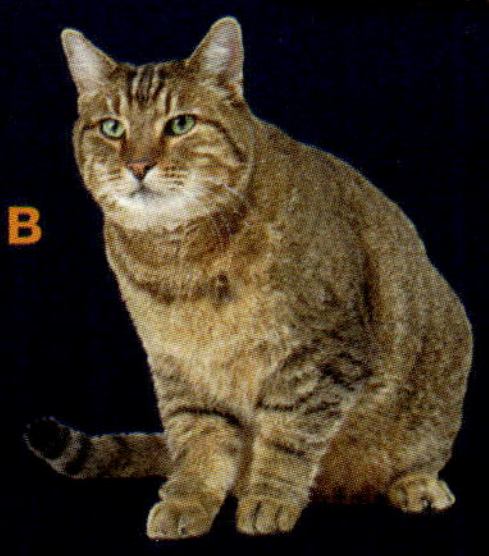

B

B. In this species, the use of a specific equation is recommended for cases where the animal is overweight (score >5/9):

$$\text{Requirements (kcal ME/day)} = 130 \text{ (kcal)} \times \text{body weight (kg)}^{0.4}$$

Its use in clinical practice makes little sense. It is easier to estimate the optimal weight and apply the previous equation. The differences between the two determinations are 0.4-3 % when the score is >8/9, while for values of 5 or 6/9, the specific equation is 9-10 % more restrictive.

5 Factors that modify the daily energy requirements (DER)

There are certain factors such as breed, activity, age and temperature that require us to correct these equations to estimate the daily energy requirements (DER) in a more precise manner; some examples in pets are as follows:

DOGS (17 kg of live weight)	CORRECTION FACTOR	EXAMPLES	
		CORRECTION FACTOR	DER (kcal ME/day)
Normal	–	MER (kcal ME/day) = 132 (kcal) × 17 (kg)$^{0.75}$	1,105.1 kcal/day
Not very active	0.72	0.72 × MER	795.7 kcal/day
Active	1.06	1.06 × MER	1,171.4 kcal/day
Very active	1.36	1.36 × MER	1,502.9 kcal/day
Anxiety	1.20	1.20 × MER	1,326.1 kcal/day
Geriatric	0.8	0.8 × MER	884.08 kcal/day
Great Danes that weigh 80 kg	1.5	1.5 × MER	5,296.35 kcal/day
Exterior temperature: >35 °C	1.1-3	3 × MER	3,315.4 kcal/day
Exterior temperature: 7.6 °C	1.6-1.9	1.6 × MER	1,768.16 kcal/day
Exterior temperature: -17 °C	1.7	1.7 × MER	1,878.67 kcal/day
CATS (5 kg of live weight)			
Normal (5/9)	–	MER (kcal ME/day) = 100 (kcal) × 5 (kg)$^{0.67}$	294 kcal/day
Overweight (7/9)	–	MER (kcal ME/day) = 100 (kcal) × 5/1.20 (kg)$^{0.67}$	260-269 kcal/day
Overweight (7/9)	–	MER (kcal ME/day) = 130 (kcal) × 5 (kg)$^{0.40}$	247 kcal/day

Other factors that modify the daily needs include different physiological states (growth, gestation and lactation), exercise and pathologies.
A few examples of these modifications, due to increases or decreases of MER, are listed below:

- ✓ Sterilization: 0.75-0.8.
- ✓ Obesity: 0.45 to 0.6.
- ✓ Chronic diseases: 1.2 to 1.8.
- ✓ Fractures: 1.1 to 1.5.
- ✓ Pain or severe injuries: 1.2 to 2.
- ✓ Simple surgery: 1.25.
- ✓ Burns: 1.2 to 2.
- ✓ Sepsis: 1.2 to 1.5.
- ✓ Treatment with corticosteroids: 1.1-1.2.

Proteins and

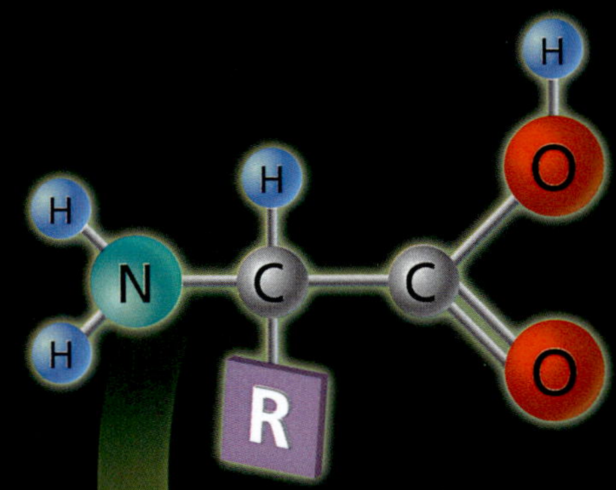

1 Composition of amino acids

The structure of amino acids includes carbon, hydrogen, a carboxyl group and an α-amino group as well as a side-chain (R), which gives them their different properties.

The average nitrogen content is 16 %.

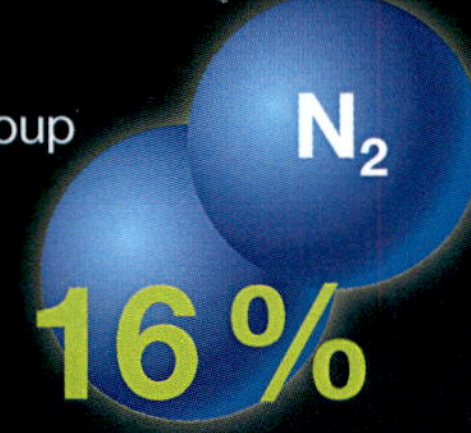

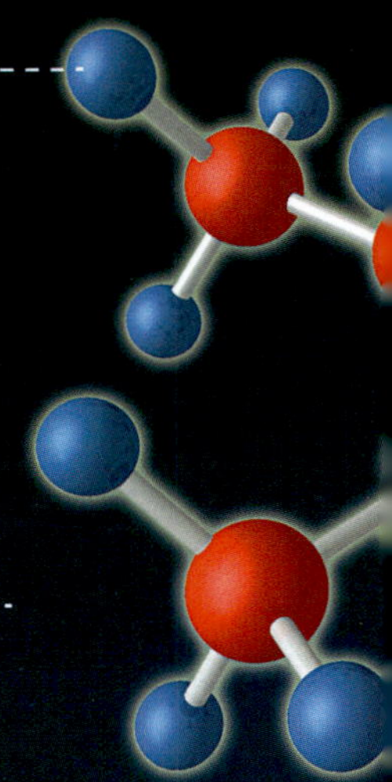

2 Structure of proteins

Proteins are linear macromolecules consisting of amino acids joined together by a peptide bond.

They have four well-defined structures:

✔ Primary ✔ Secondary ✔ Tertiary ✔ Quaternary

They have been known to be essential to life since 1816.

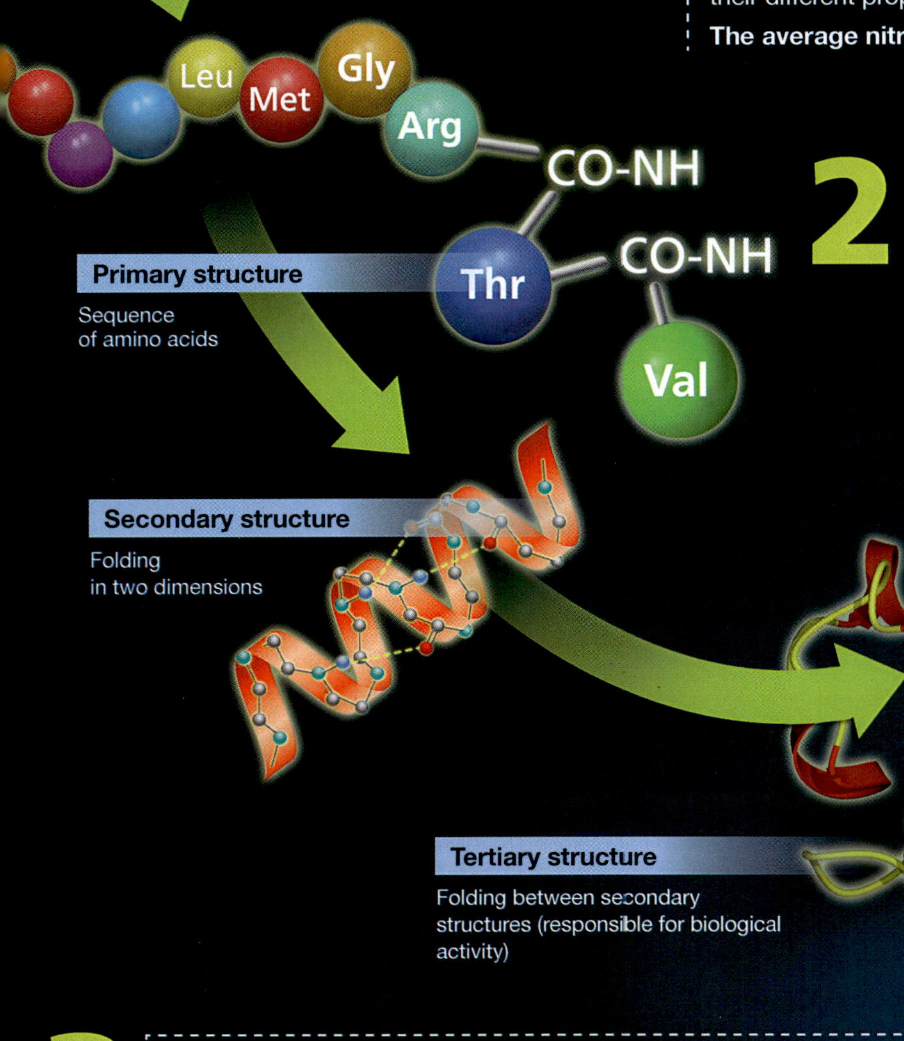

3 Classification of proteins

Simple

- **Fibrous**
  - Elastins
  - Collagen
  - Keratin
  - They give structure to the body
- **Globular**
  - Hormones
  - Enzymes
  - Antibodies
  - Transport proteins
  - They participate in different functions of the organism

Conjugated (bound to)

- **Lipids** — Lipoproteins: lipid transport, components of myelin...
- **Carbohydrates** — Glycoproteins: cell recognition, components of mucus and synovial fluid...
- **Minerals** — Haemoglobin: oxygen transport
- They participate in different functions of the organism and are part of it as structural components

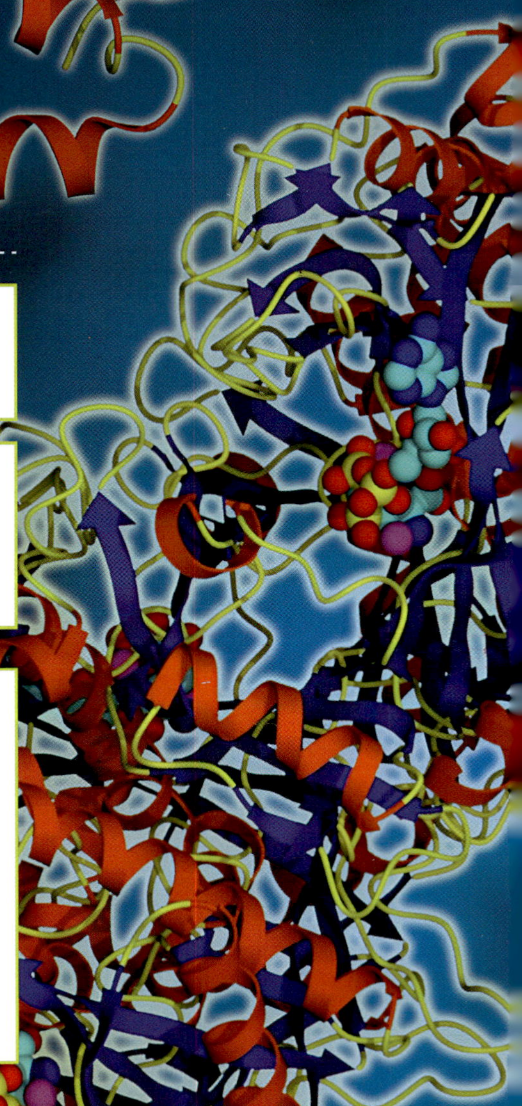

amino acids

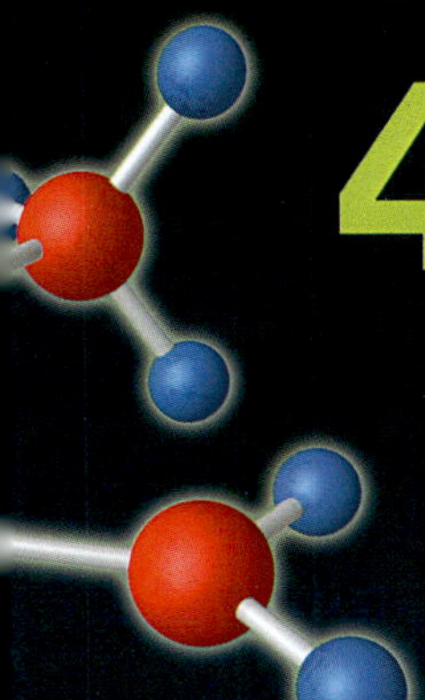

Valine

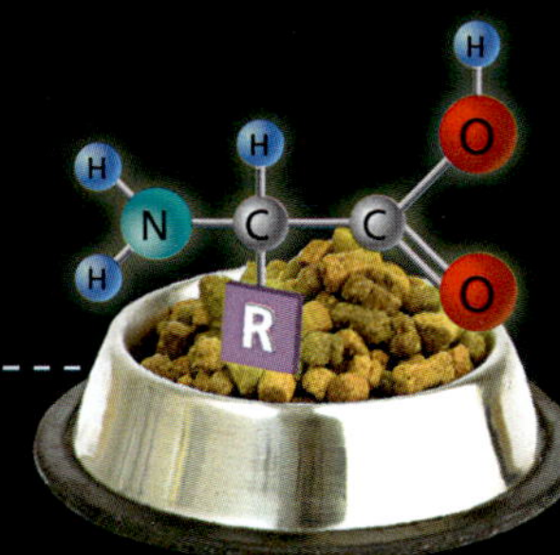

4 Essential amino acids

Since 1979, 10 amino acids have been considered essential in dogs and 11 in cats.

- ✔ Lysine
- ✔ Methionine
- ✔ Arginine
- ✔ Phenylalanine
- ✔ Tryptophan
- ✔ Histidine
- ✔ Leucine
- ✔ Isoleucine
- ✔ Valine
- ✔ Threonine

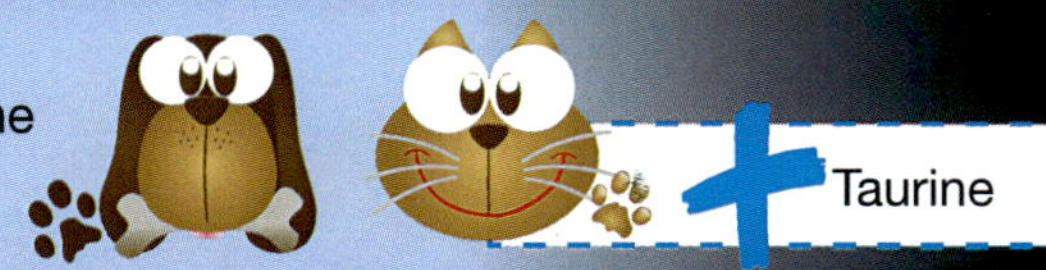

They are important and must be included in the diet since:

- ✔ They provide nitrogen for the synthesis of other compounds.
- ✔ Their carbon skeleton cannot be synthesised in sufficient amounts in the organism.

The absence of one of them leads to a decreased food intake as a neuroendocrine response to the deficiency. In the case of cats, this effect is prolonged in time, possibly because they are strict carnivores and it is therefore difficult for this imbalance to occur.

5 Non-essential/conditionally essential amino acids

Although the other amino acids are synthesised by the organism, in some cases they are considered conditionally essential depending on the animal's physiological/pathological state. This occurs with glutamine, glutamate/glutamine, cysteine and tyrosine.

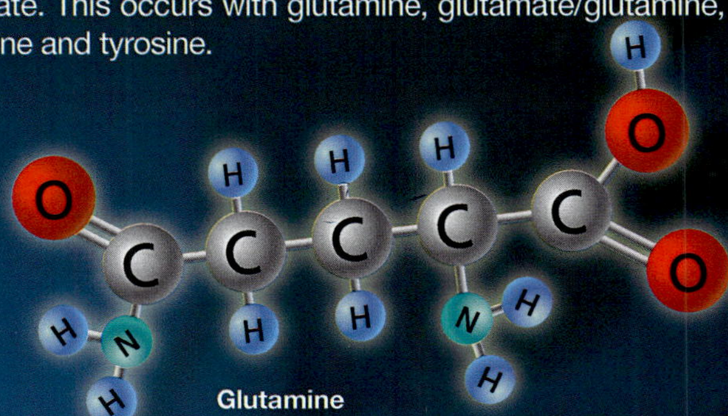

Glutamine molecule

In the case of glutamate/glutamine, its importance has been questioned since the nineties as it is a critical nutrient for cell function and it participates actively in the metabolism.

- ✔ Important neurotransmitter.
- ✔ Substrate of enterocytes.
- ✔ Participation in energy-requiring processes (e.g. immune deficiency, diarrhoea, cancer or transplants).

The needs for this amino acid are conditioned by the level and quality of the protein in the diet.
It is used as a flavouring.

6 Non-protein nitrogenous compounds

There are other components with nitrogen in their structure, but they are not proteins:

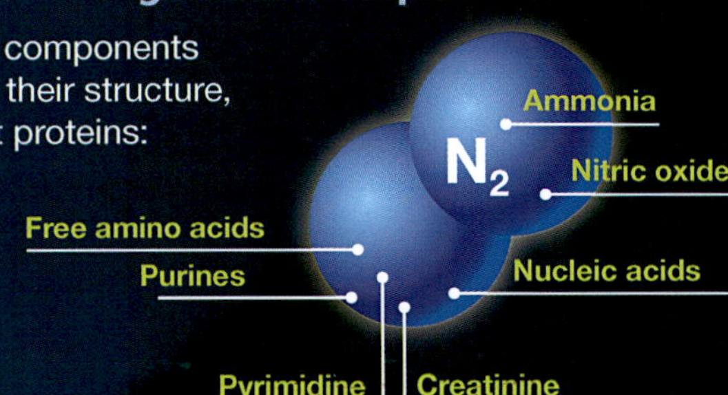

7 Functions of proteins

- ✔ Structural constituents in cartilage tissue, contractile proteins, skin and hair.
- ✔ Transport proteins in blood.
- ✔ Enzymes, hormones, neurotransmitters, cell receptors and antibodies.
- ✔ Source of energy.

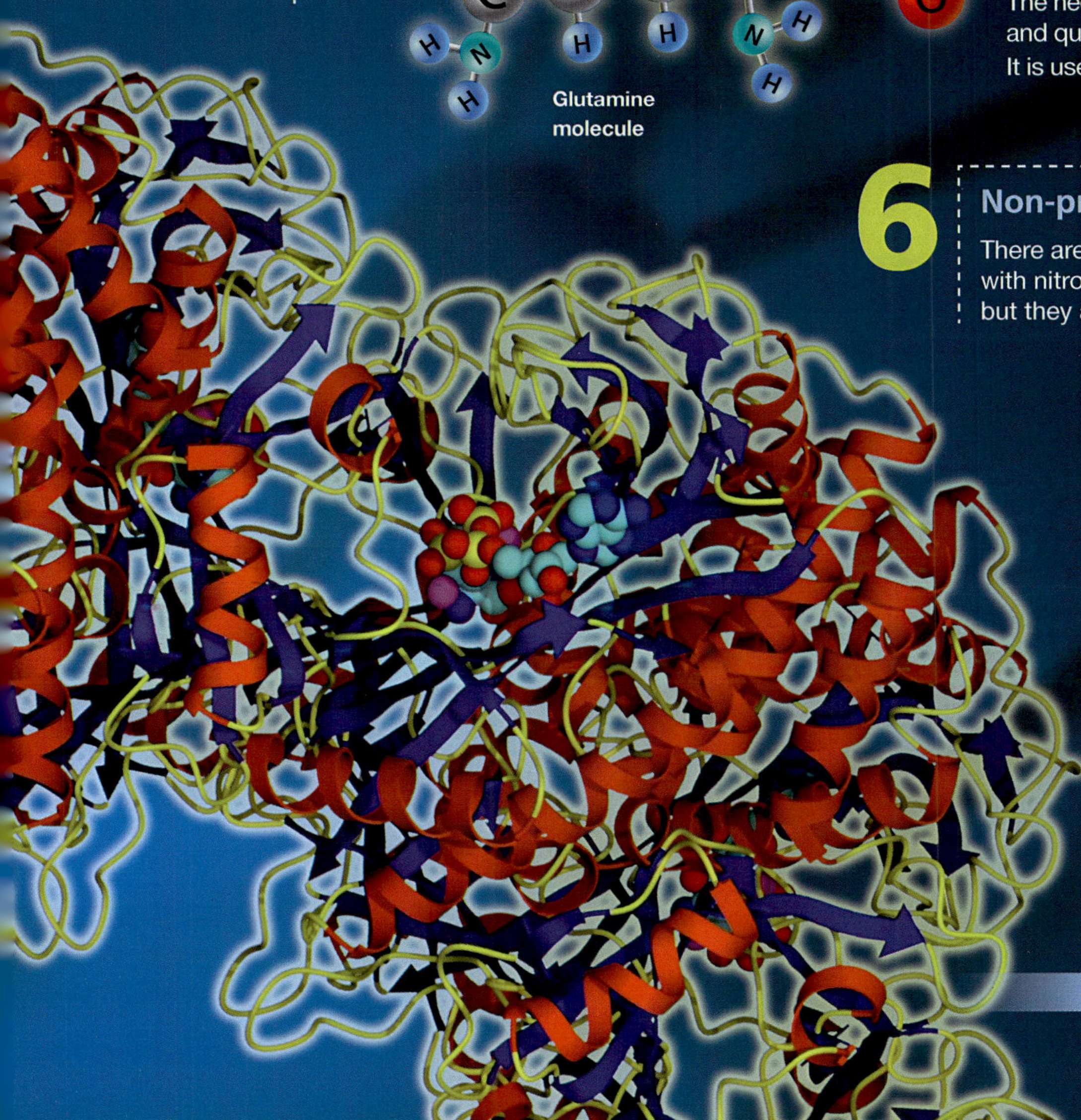

Quaternary structure

Union of several polypeptide chains

Protein

1 Protein digestion

Proteins are digested in the gastrointestinal system by the action of pepsin, HCl, endopeptidases (trypsin and quimotrypsin) and some exopeptidases of microbial origin, into simpler units, free amino acids, dipeptides and tripeptides, which are capable of being absorbed. The absorption of amino acids depends on their type; it is a process that requires energy in the form of ATP.

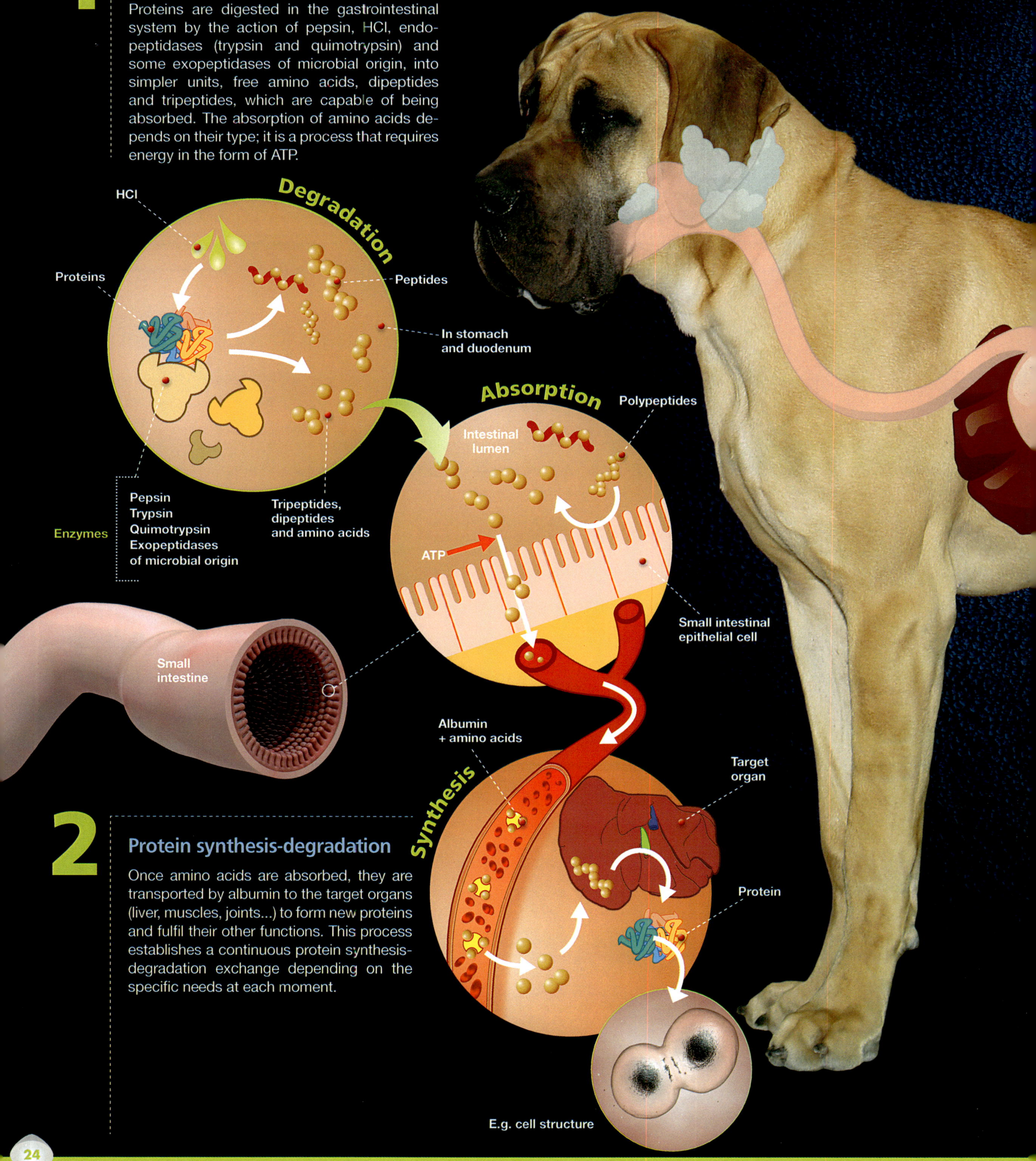

2 Protein synthesis-degradation

Once amino acids are absorbed, they are transported by albumin to the target organs (liver, muscles, joints...) to form new proteins and fulfil their other functions. This process establishes a continuous protein synthesis-degradation exchange depending on the specific needs at each moment.

metabolism

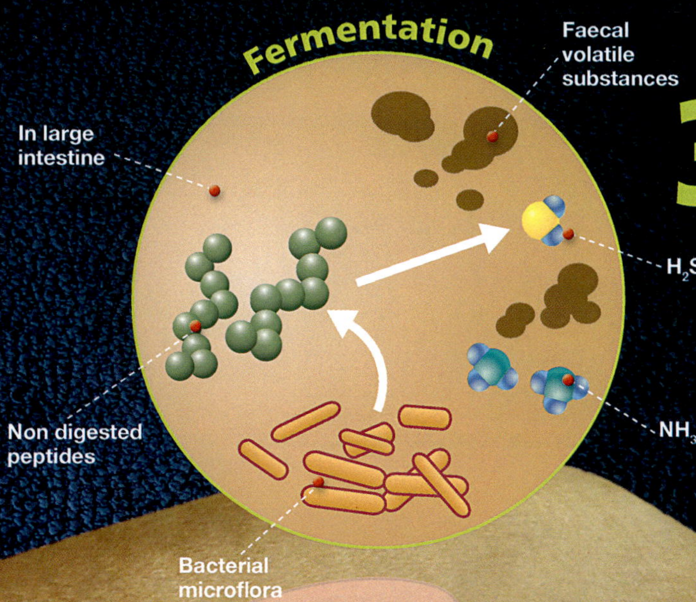

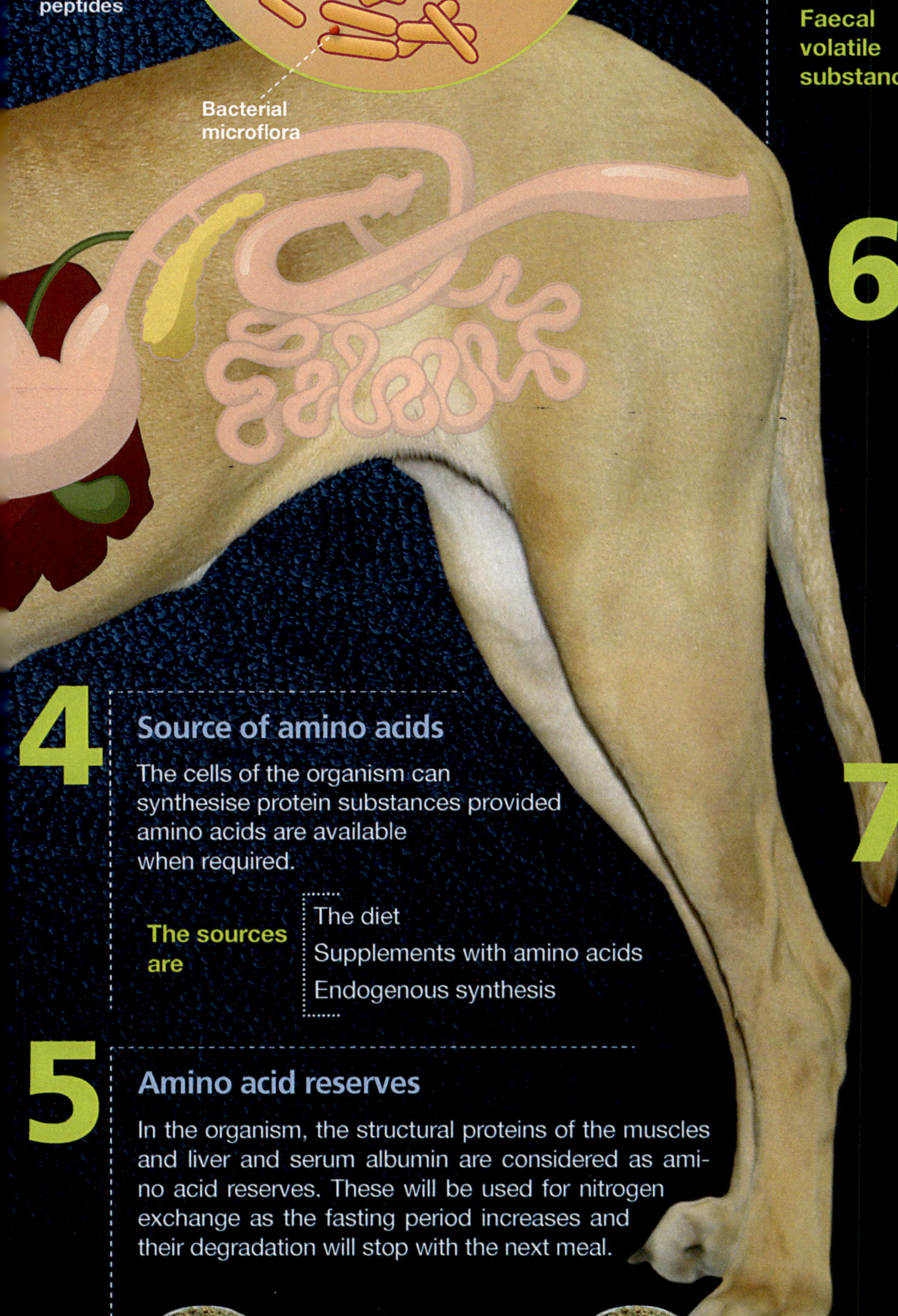

3 Microbial fermentation

The part of proteins that is not digested and absorbed progresses to the large intestine, where it undergoes a microbial fermentation process, with the formation of faecal volatile substances.
These compounds, in addition to causing bad smells, affect the digestive health of animals. Their production is affected by:

Faecal volatile substance

- Ammonia
- Amines
- Hydrogen sulfide
- Indole
- Skatole

✓ Low protein quality.
✓ High amount of dry matter and proteins ingested.
✓ Origin of the proteins source.
✓ Presence of soluble fibre and oligosaccharides.

6 Nitrogen losses

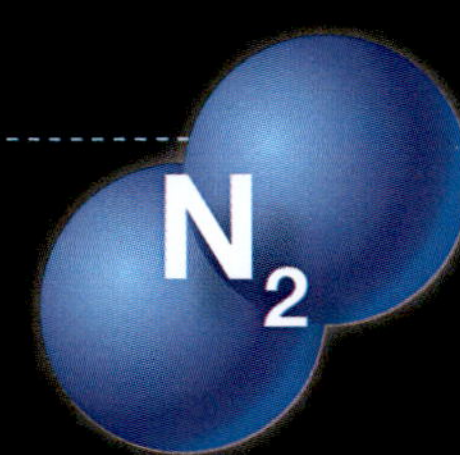

Nitrogen losses by catabolism occur throughout the whole process and must be restored through the diet.

Physiological losses

- Faeces
- Urine
- Skin flaking
- Hair

Losses in special circumstances

- Kidney failure
- Burns
- Sepsis
- Fever
- Cancer
- Cachexia
- Trauma

4 Source of amino acids

The cells of the organism can synthesise protein substances provided amino acids are available when required.

The sources are

- The diet
- Supplements with amino acids
- Endogenous synthesis

5 Amino acid reserves

In the organism, the structural proteins of the muscles and liver and serum albumin are considered as amino acid reserves. These will be used for nitrogen exchange as the fasting period increases and their degradation will stop with the next meal.

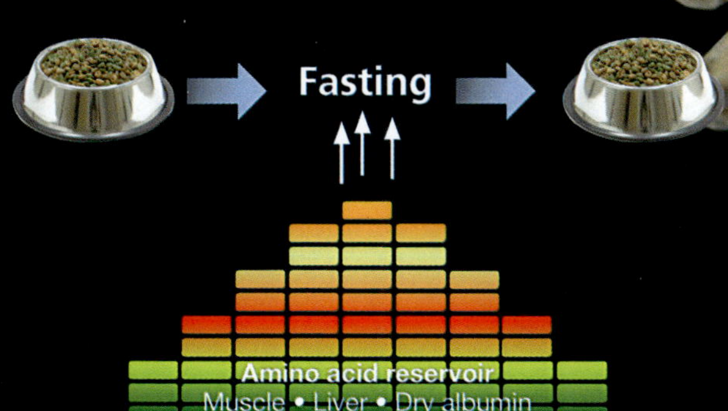

7 Nitrogen balance

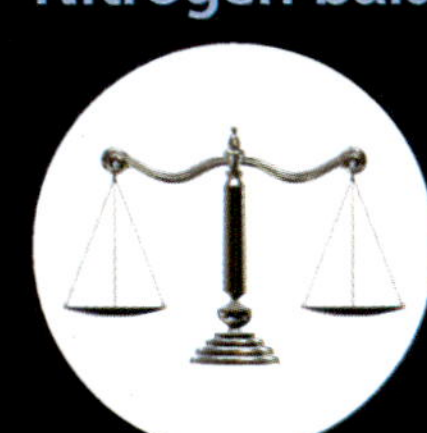

= N_2 consumed (+) – N_2 eliminated (–)

It should be considered, in general, as a reflex of the organism's protein status.

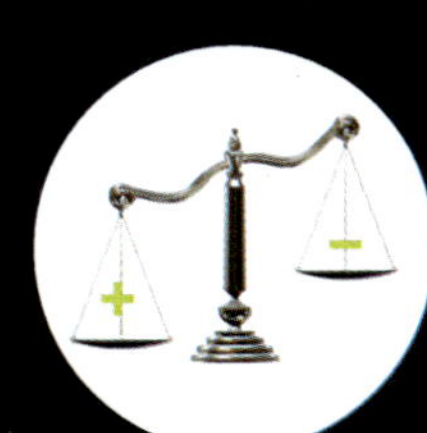

+ → Growth and gestation

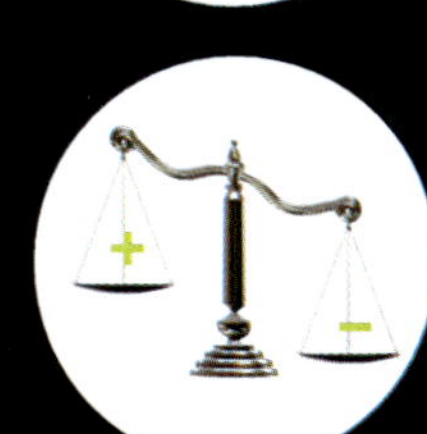

– → In lactation and some diseases

Excess of proteins

1 Amino acids as a source of energy

After the synthesis of a protein, deamination will take place with any excess amino acids and their hydrocarbon skeleton will lead to the formation of glycogen (glycogenic amino acids), fatty acids and acetyl-CoA (ketogenic amino acids) that will serve as a future source of energy. The ketogenic amino acids are leucine and lysine. The mixed amino acids (keto- and glycogenic) are isoleucine, phenylalanine, tyrosine and tryptophan. The rest of the amino acids are considered to be glycogenic.

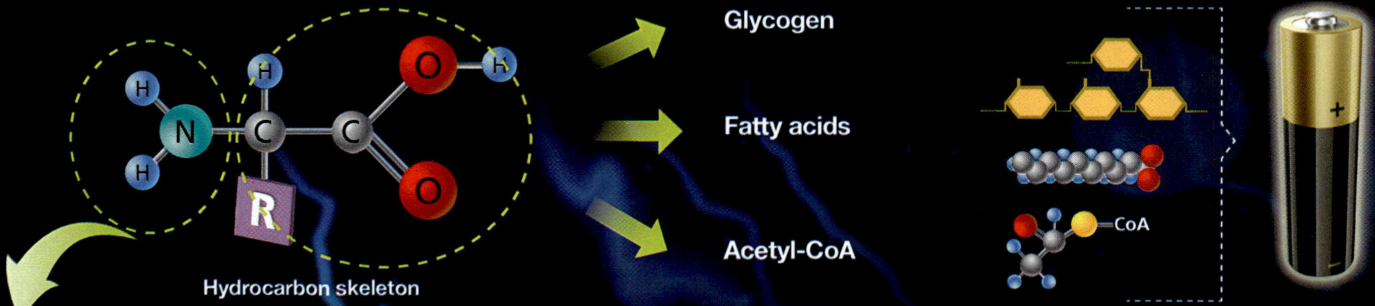

2 From nitrogen to urea

More than 90 % of the nitrogen from the degradation becomes urea

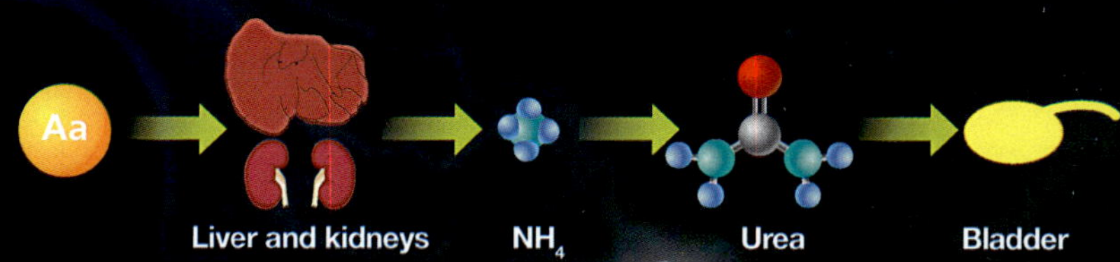

The products from the catabolism of proteins are metabolized in all tissues but primarily in the liver and kidneys to form ammonium, which is later converted into urea and eliminated through urine.

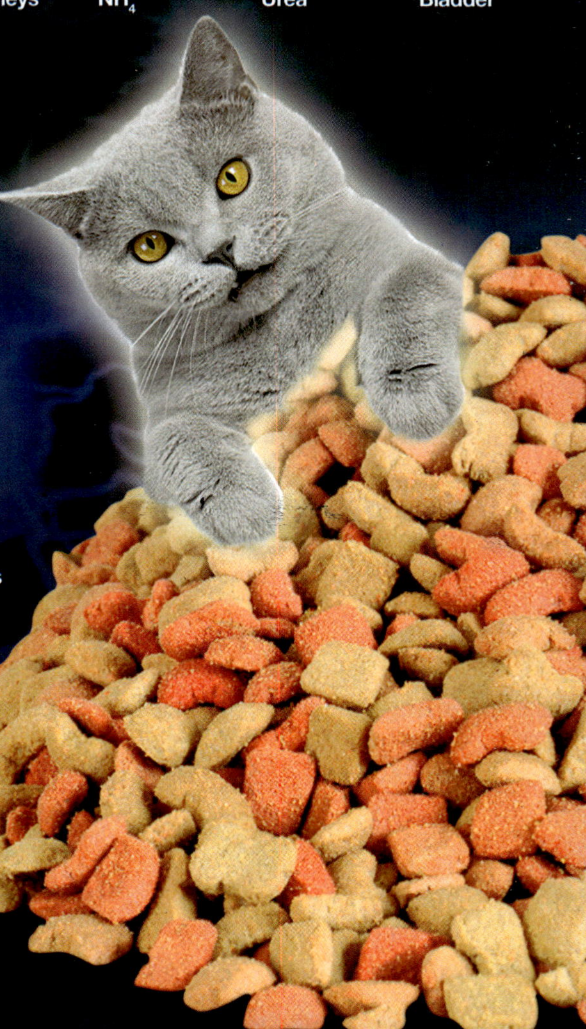

Maintenance of the nitrogen balance in the organism

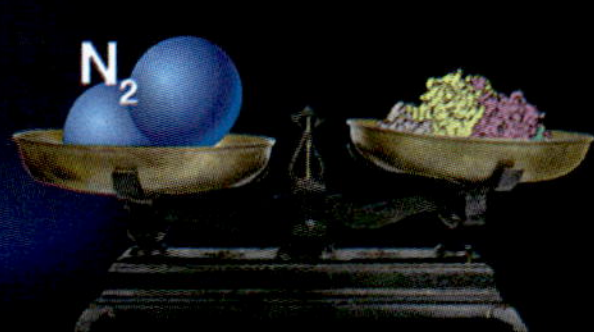

This process takes place by the following processes:

- ✓ Regulation of the enzymes responsible for the catabolism of the nitrogen in the urea cycle.
- ✓ Aminotransferase (transaminase): ALAT (GPT) and ASAT (GOT).

The four levels of changes in the urea cycle are as follows:

1. Modification of the concentration of nitrogen.
2. Regulation of the activity of the carbamoyl-phosphate-synthetase and of the N-acetyl glutamate-synthetase by means of the levels of arginine and glutamate.
3. Changes in the levels of ornitine and arginine in the liver.
4. Regulation of the enzymes of the catabolism from the mRNA. This process in dogs and cats has a poor adaptation.

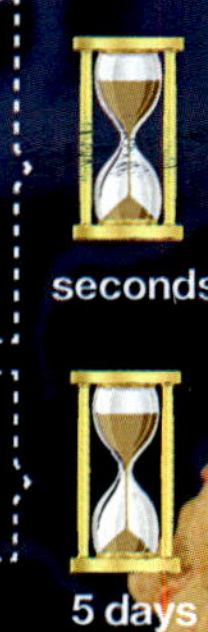

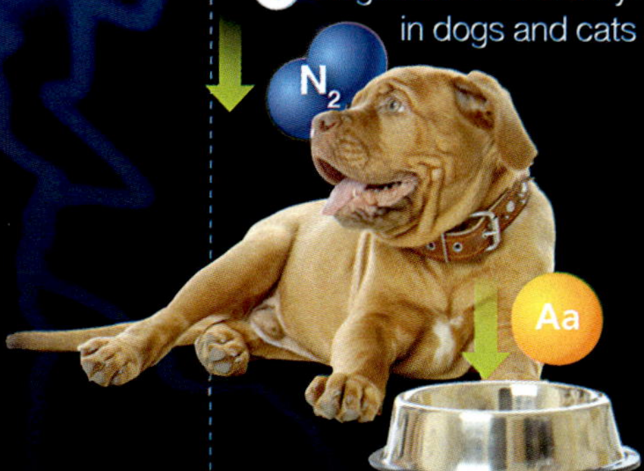

How can we reduce the accumulation of nitrogen in the body?

- ✓ Decrease the amount of proteins ingested (although the quality is more important than the quantity).
- ✓ Reduced ingestion of non-essential amino acids.
- ✓ Substitution of certain ketogenic amino acids with synthesis analogues.

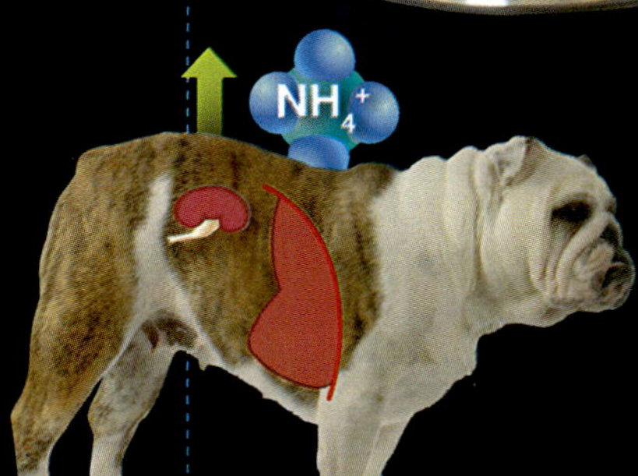

Episodes of hyperammonemia

Episodes of hyperammonemia usually take place with renal and hepatic pathologies. An excess of proteins in these patients must be considered as potentially toxic. This is very dangerous for animals in sub-clinical conditions, for example, in advanced age or geriatric animals (>5-7 years), given that it favors the progression of the pathology.

Another pathology associated with the metabolism of nitrogen is the accumulation of uric acid crystals in joints and in the urinary bladder that are produced during the catabolism of purines.

The urea cycle

The urea cycle is a principal function of the body that it is responsible for the elimination of any excess ammonium (a toxic compound) in the form of urea. The complete cycle takes places in the hepatocytes.

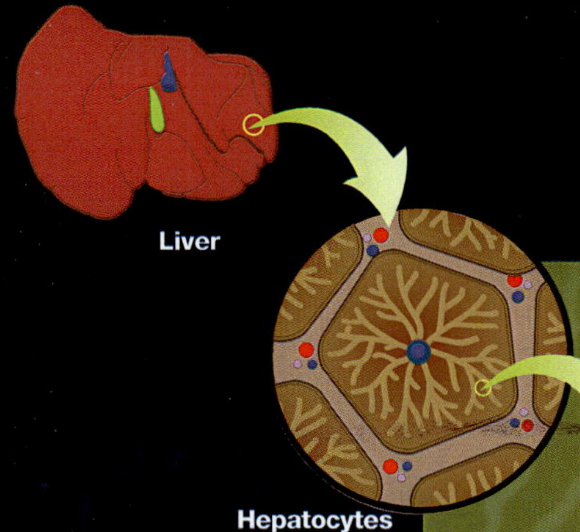

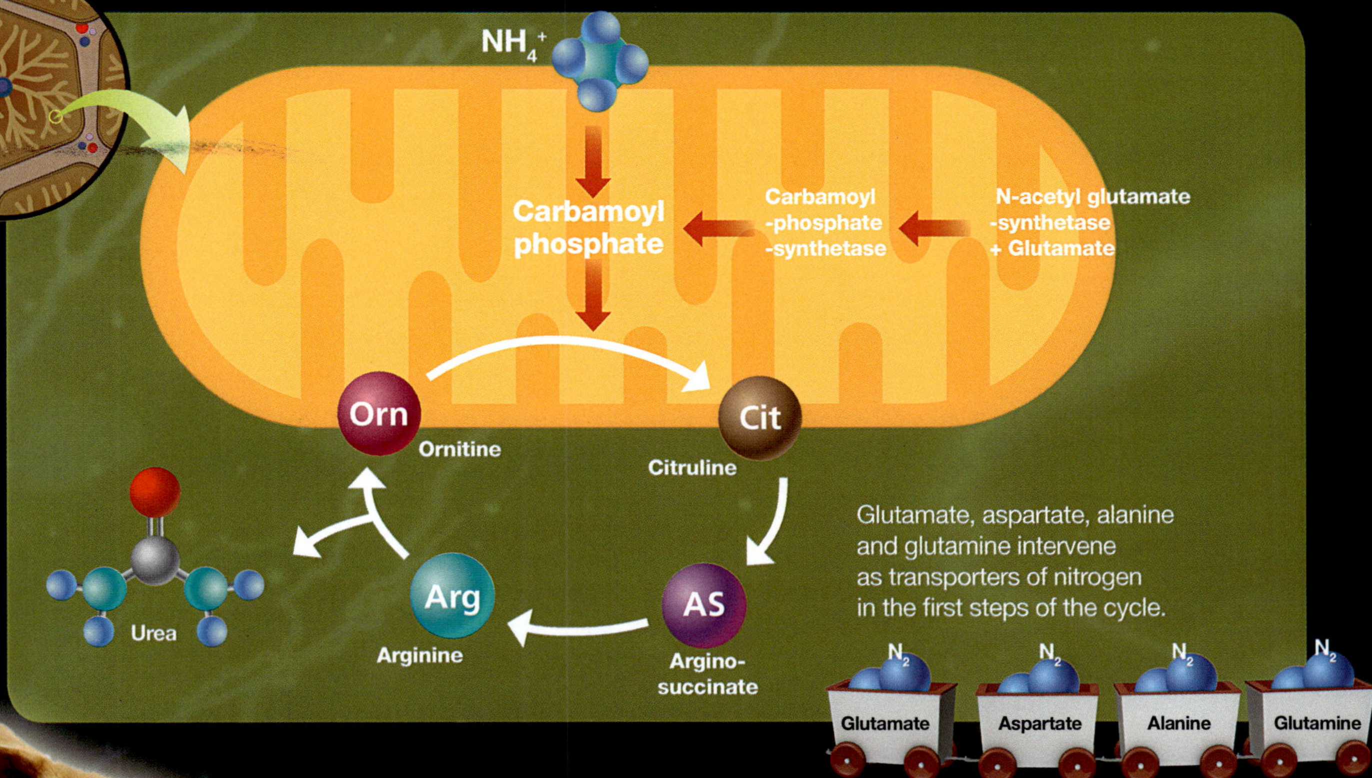

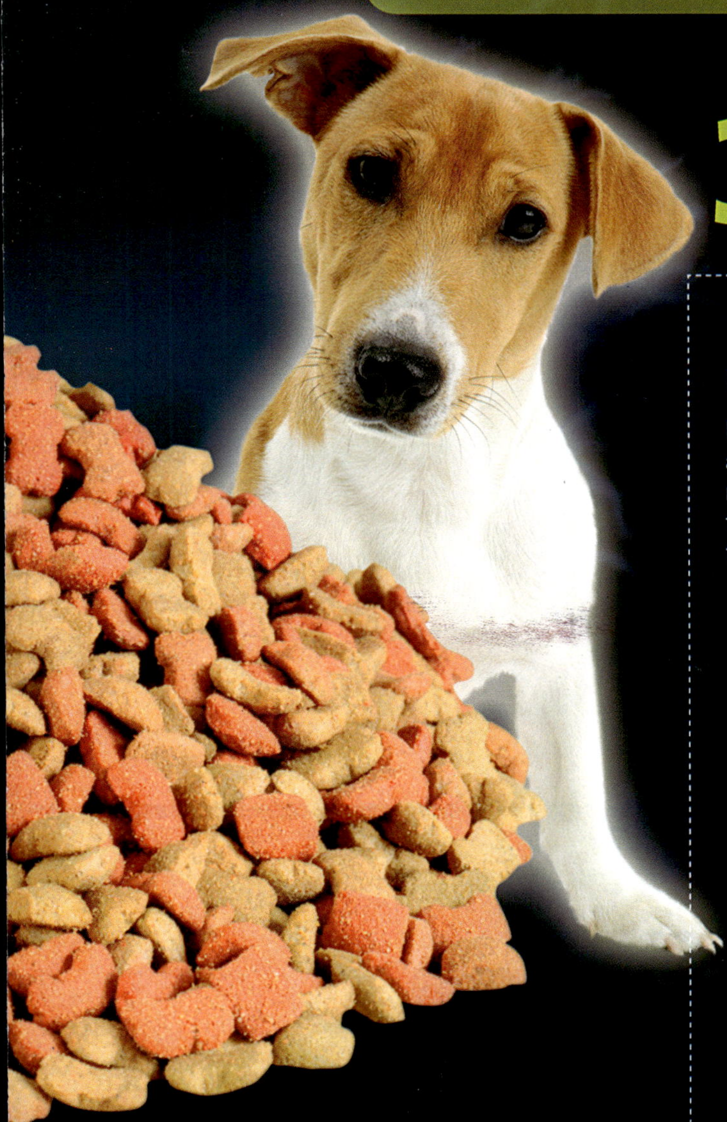

3 What problems are caused by an excess of amino acids?

Generally, an excess of amino acids does not cause any toxic episodes. That said, there are a few exceptions:

Excess of methionine

Its low cost and its role as the first limiting amino acid do not justify its undiscriminated use as preventative as cases of intoxication due to its excessive consumption in cats and dogs have been reported.

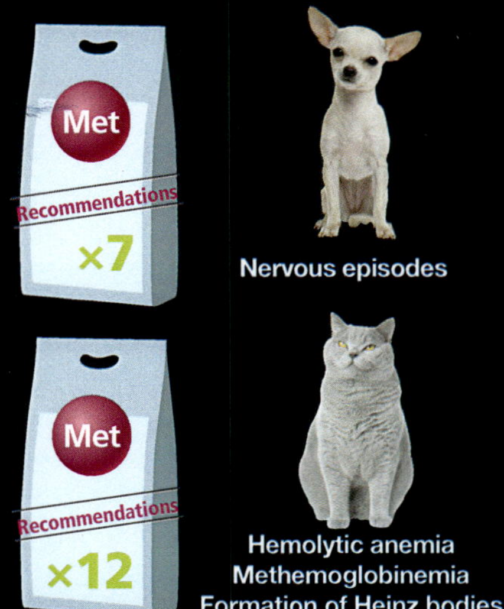

Excess of lysine

It acts as an antagonist of arginine and the clinical signs of excessive ingestion are associated with its deficiency:

- ✓ Increased nitrogen in plasma.
- ✓ Vomiting.
- ✓ Orotic aciduria with formation of crystals.

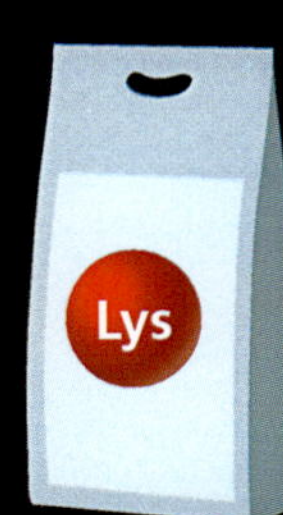

Its maximum dose is between 5-10 g/1,000 kcal ME.

To be taken into account:

Some Dalmatians have a autosomal recessive genetic defect in the activity of the urate-oxidase enzyme, which causes problems in the conversion of uric acid into allantoin. This predisposes dogs of this breed to the formation of uric acid crystals. Prevention is simple and, among other options, consists of decreasing the ingestion of protein and purine-rich ingredients (fish and animal organs).

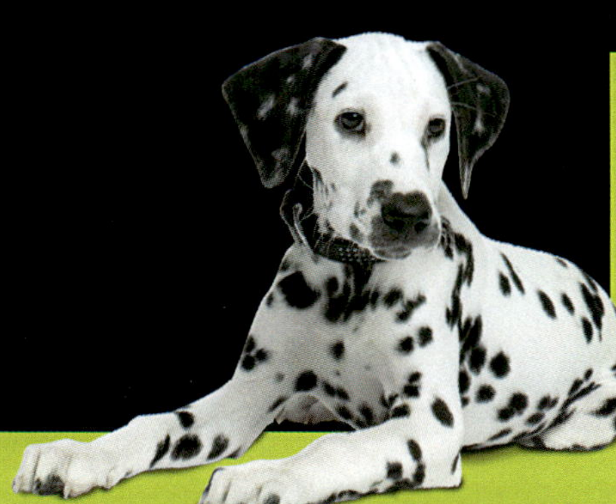

Requirements for

1 Amino acid requirements

Essential amino acids can only be obtained by ingesting proteins found in foods. For this reason, it is more appropriate to discuss amino acids requirements and not protein requirements.

Therefore, the amount of protein/amino acids that should be included in an animal's daily food rations directly depends on the amount of dry material that the animal has to consume. This consumption simultaneously depends on the physiological state of the animal (adult on maintenance, growing puppy, lactating female...).

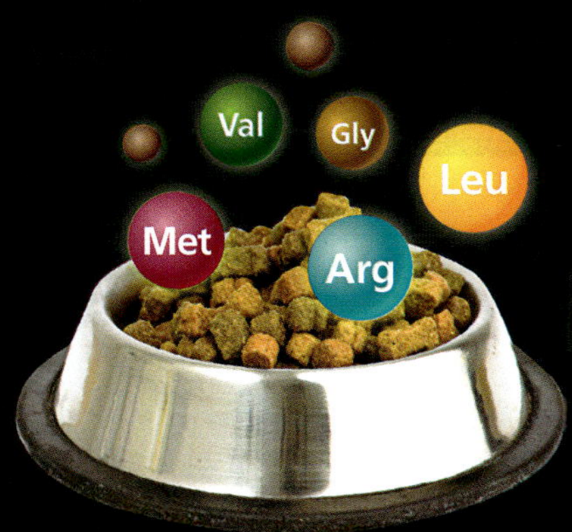

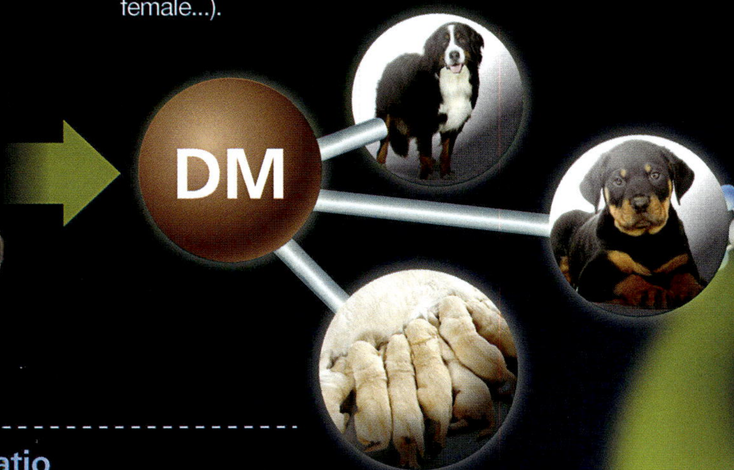

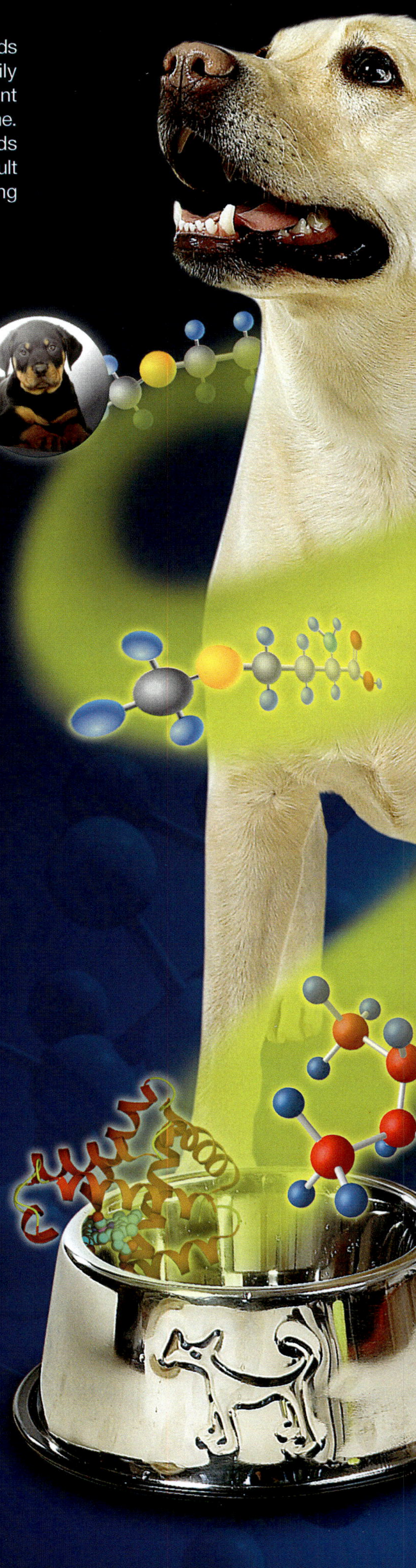

2 Protein/energetic density ratio

In healthy animals, given that their ingestion depends on their energy requirements, the concentration of proteins in their food will be proportional to the energetic density of the food ration: high energy foods have high levels of protein to compensate the decreased ingestion of dry material and vice versa.

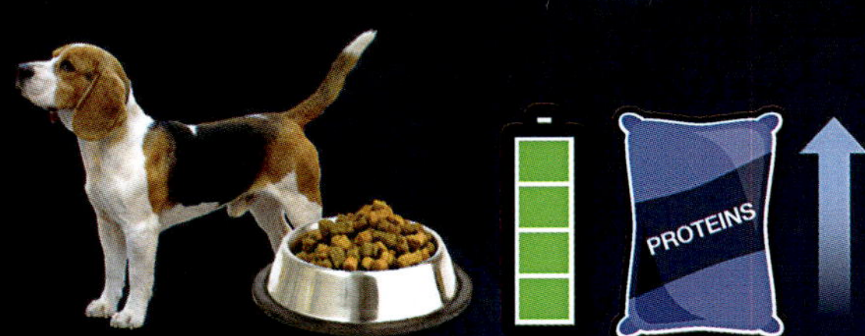

Healthy animal

Exceptions to this rule:

Management and treatment of obesity

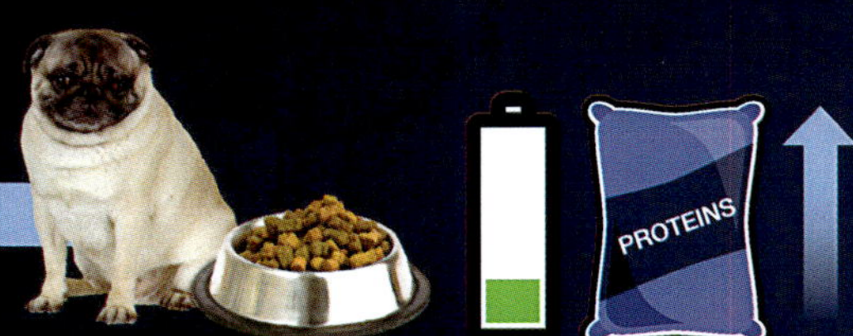

Chronic kidney failure

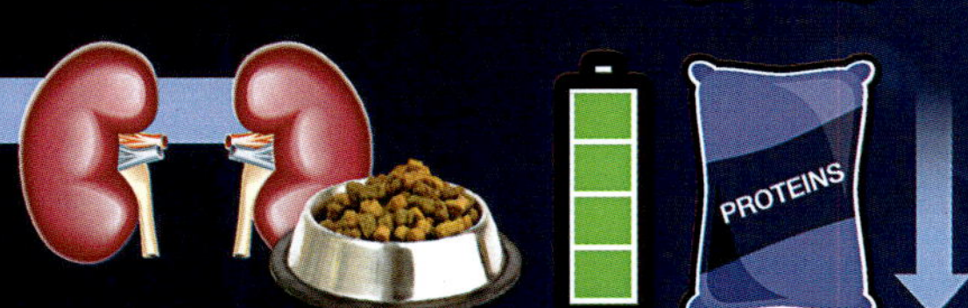

3 Amino acid antagonisms

The equilibrium of amino acids does not only depend on their correct amount and proportion, but there are also antagonisms that occur from the similarities in their chemical structure. This means that the excess of one amino acid may determine that the needs of another amino acid with a similar structure are increased.
Dogs are highly sensitive to these antagonisms, especially when their food rations are low in protein. Here are some examples:

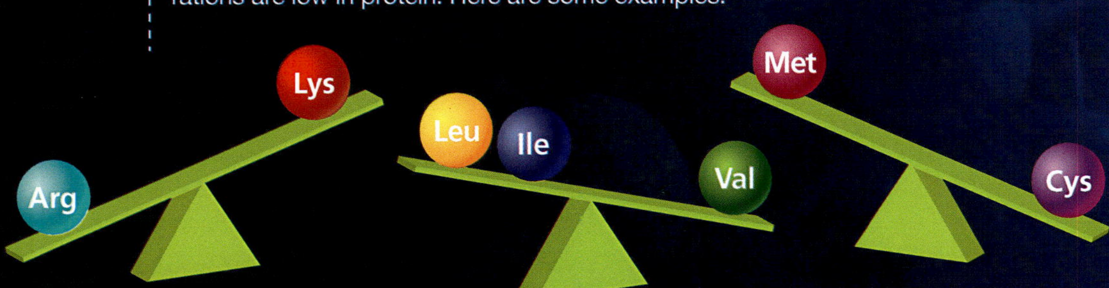

proteins and amino acids (I)

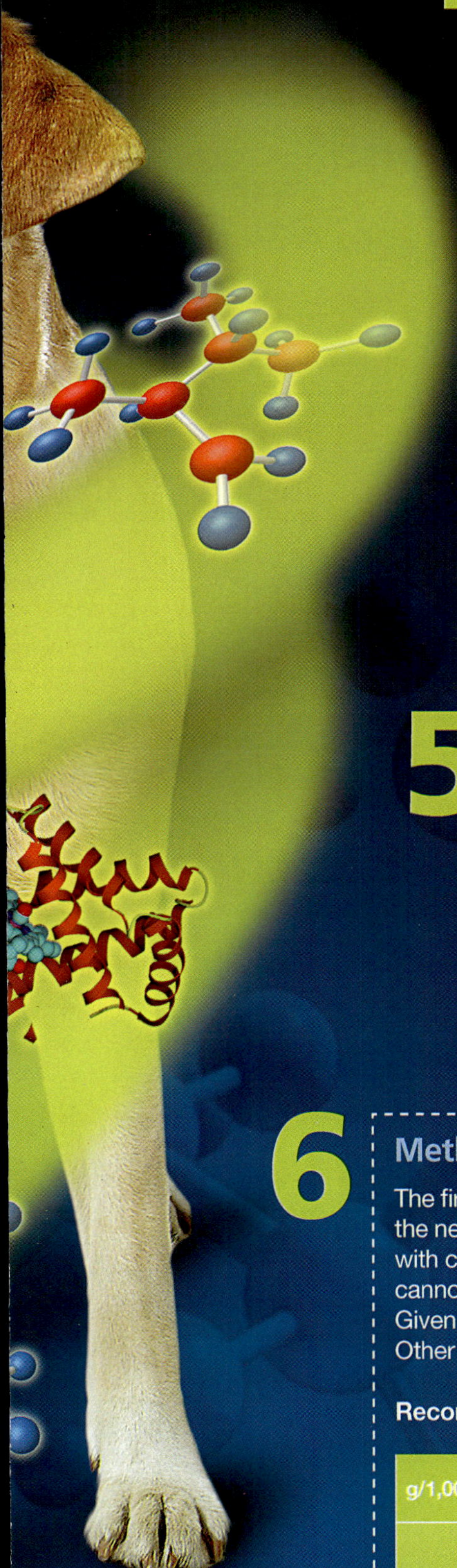

4 Ideal protein

The concept of ideal protein defines the ideal profile of amino acids to optimize the organism's different functions, using **lysine** as a reference. This ensures that the amino acid profile of a food is optimal. For dogs and cats, the ideal profile is that which appears in the table. As we can see, the requirements of cats are 30 % greater (on average) than those of dogs.

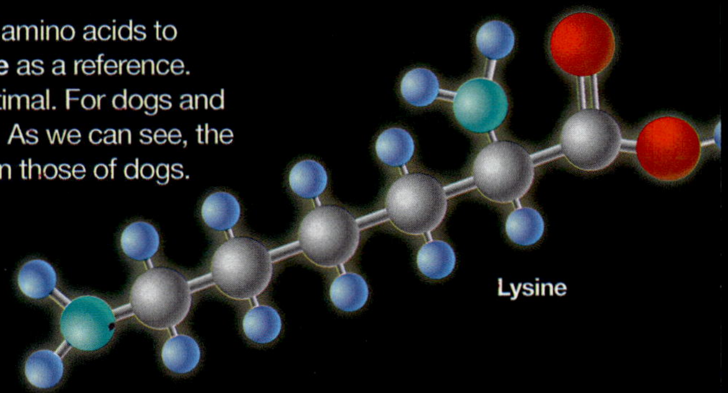

Amino acids		
Lys Lysine	1.00	1.00
Met Cys Methionine + cysteine	0.64	1.00
Arg Arginine	0.71	1.12
Phe Tyr Phenylalanine + tyrosine	1.00	1.12
Trp Tryptophan	0.22	0.19
His Histidine	0.29	0.38
Leu Leucine	1.00	1.50
Ile Isoleucine	0.57	0.63
Val Valine	0.75	0.75
Thr Threonine	0.67	0.87

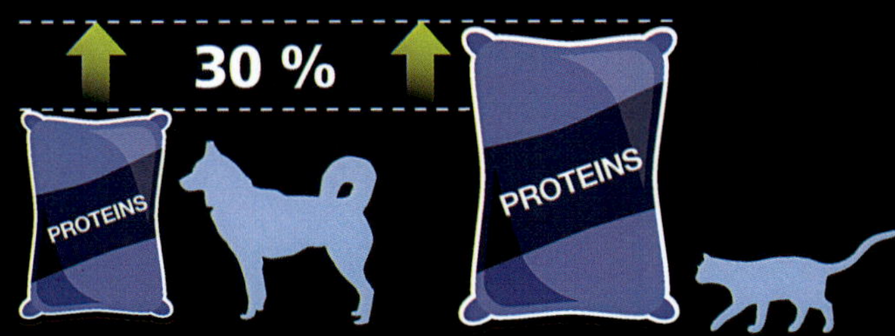

5 Minimal protein requirements

Recommendations for high quality proteins		
Minimal protein requirements in adult animals	20 g/1,000 kcal ME	40 g/1,000 kcal ME
Recommendations that include a safety margin	25 g/1,000 kcal ME	50 g/1,000 kcal ME
AAFCO and FEDIAF guidelines	45 g/1,000 kcal ME (occasionally, +40 %)	62.5 g/1,000 kcal ME (occasionally, +40 %)

The differences in data are significant, which could be due to the differences in the quality of different proteins.

6 Methionine is the first limiting amino acid

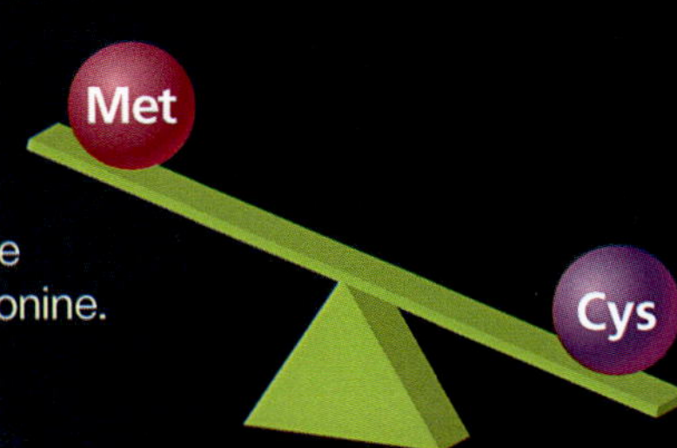

The first limiting amino acid in adult dogs and cats is methionine and covering the needs of this amino acid are mandatory. Methionine is considered together with cysteine for their contribution of sulfur; it must be kept in mind that methionine cannot be synthesized from cysteine, but cysteine can be synthesized from methionine. Given its low cost, it is added as synthesis DL-methionine in food rations. Other important amino acids are arginine and lysine.

Recommendations:

g/1,000 kcal ME	Arg	His	Ile	Met + Cys	Leu	Lys	Phe + Tyr	Thr	Trp	Val
	0.88	0.48	0.95	1.63	1.70	0.88	1.85	1.08	0.35	1.23
	1.93	0.65	1.08	0.85	2.55	0.85	3.83	1.30	0.33	1.28

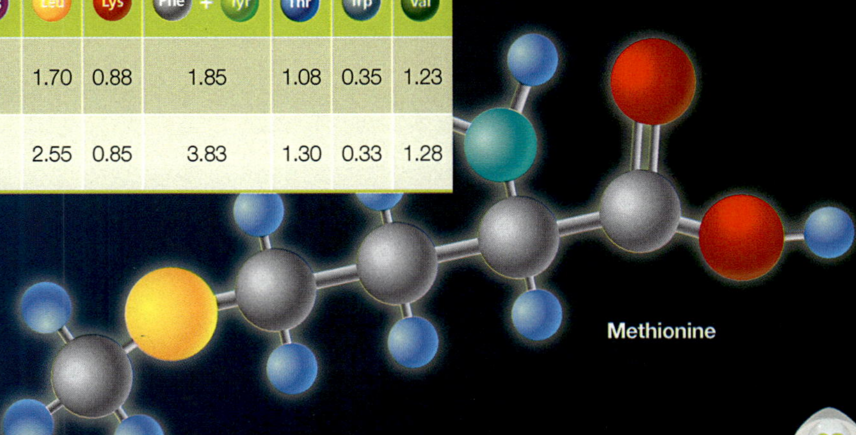

Requirements for

1 Arginine

Arginine is an essential amino acid at all ages, especially during periods of growth.

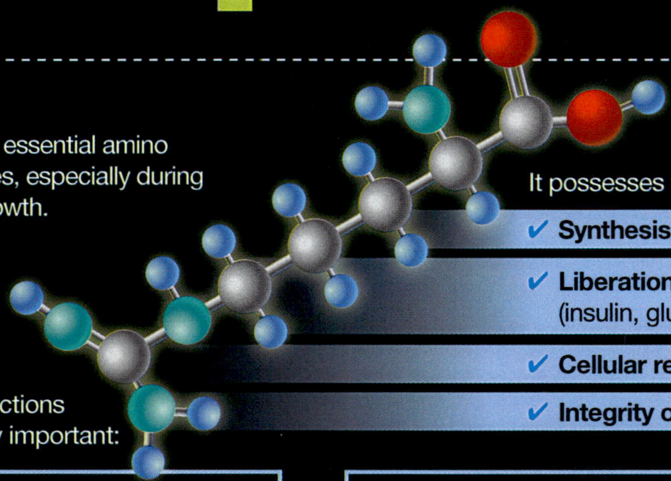

It possesses various functions:

- ✔ **Synthesis of other proteins**
- ✔ **Liberation of certain hormones** (insulin, glucagon, gastrin)
- ✔ **Cellular replication**
- ✔ **Integrity of the crystalline lens**

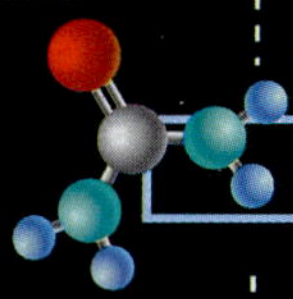

Two of its functions are especially important:

- ✔ **Intermediary in the urea cycle**
- ✔ **Precursor of nitric oxide**

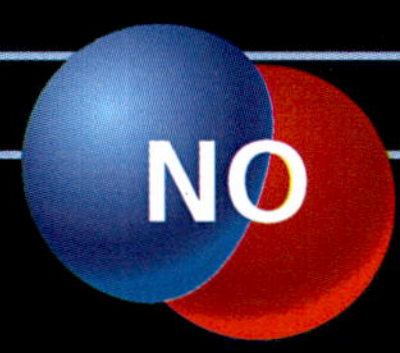

It can be substituted by ornitine and citrulline (transformed into arginine in the kidneys) but these amino acids are not found in high concentrations in pet food.

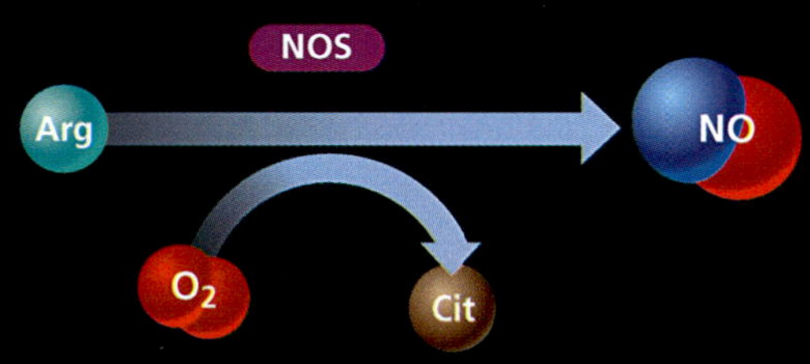

The NO acts as:

An endocrine regulator over the dilation of the smooth musculature of vessels and bronchi.

Antimicrobial agent.

Its use as a therapeutic agent in cardiovascular pathologies is currently being studied.

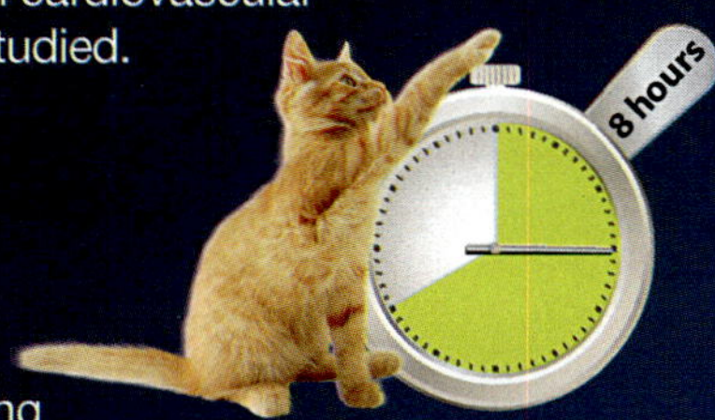

Both species are sensitive to deficiencies of arginine, but cats are more so: they develop episodes of hyperammonemia after 8 hours of deprivation.
Felines have a low activity of the enzymes responsible for the metabolic steps including **ornitine** → **citruline** → **arginine** and they are not able to replace their concentrations.
In general, the concentration of arginine in food is sufficient. That said, given its importance as an intermediary in the urea cycle, an increase of 0.01 g in dogs and 0.02 g in cats is recommended for each one point increase of the NRC recommendations from 2006 for protein (as a % of the DM, in a diet of 4,000 kcal ME/kg DM), regardless of age.

2 Other essential amino acids

✔ There is no data for the rest of the essential amino acids about the dose-response given that the majority of commercial pet foods cover their needs.

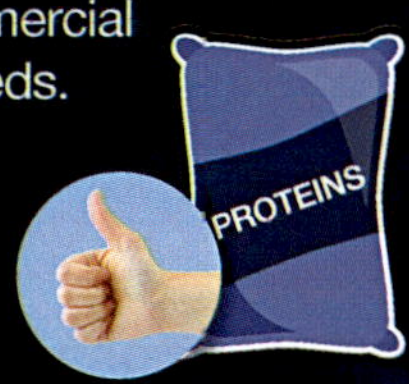

✔ Although not necessary, we can increase the recommended dose of phenylalanine/tyrosine up to four times its value to improve the black color of the animal's hair (avoiding that it turn reddish).

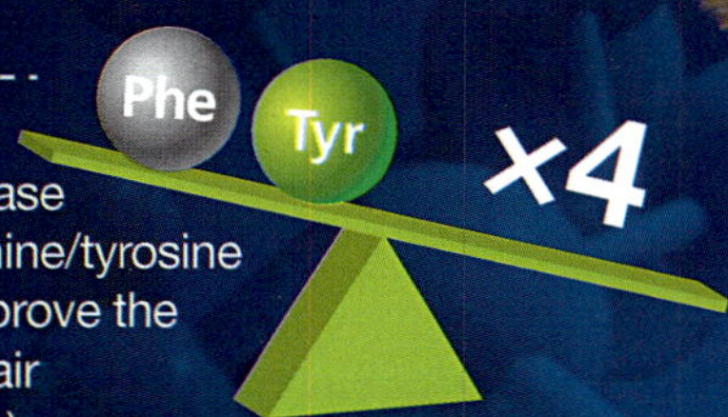

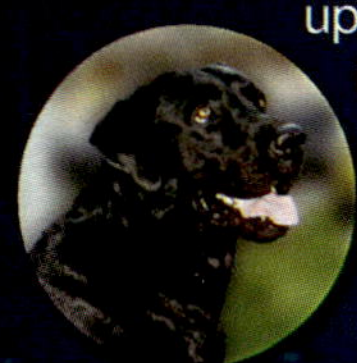

✔ If high levels of grain are used or when the quality of the protein is very low (collagen), lysine and tryptophan are the first limiting amino acids.

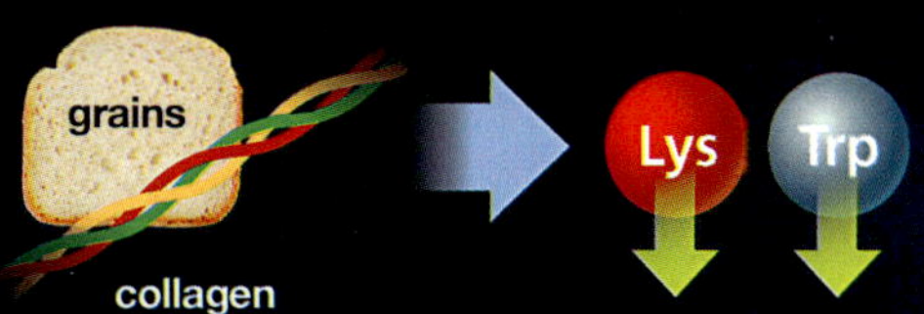

✔ Dogs, unlike cats, have the capacity to select the food ration that covers (and even surpasses up to five times) their requirements for protein.

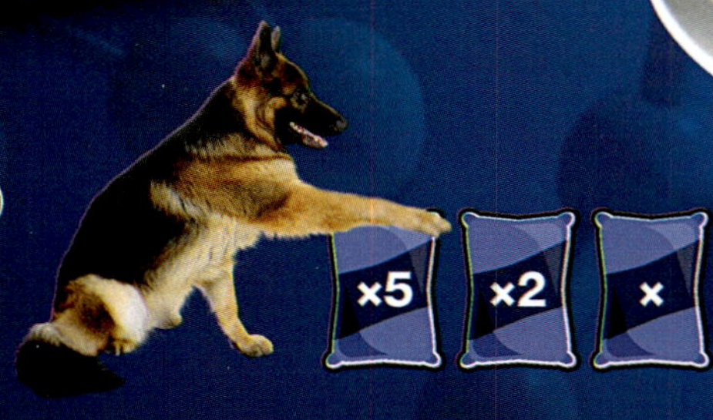

proteins and amino acids (II)

3 Why do cats need higher levels of proteins?

For cats, ensuring that their minimal needs for protein are met daily is especially important as this species has a limited capacity to adapt their metabolism to low protein foods.
The need for high levels of proteins and amino acids in the food portions for cats is related with the following:

- ✔ The incapacity to efficiently adapt the enzyme levels that participate in the catabolism of the amino acids, of the urea cycle, and of the gluconeogenesis to the food rations that are low in protein.
- ✔ The scarce capacity to retain and preserve nitrogen and essential amino acids.
- ✔ The continuous use of proteins as an energy source or to produce glucose due to the high activity of the hepatic enzymes responsible for both of the aforementioned processes.
- ✔ The elevated daily losses of endogenous urinary nitrogen: greater than 1.2 g/day.
- ✔ Poor efficiency in the use of protein.
- ✔ Lack of sensitivity to the antagonisms between amino acids.

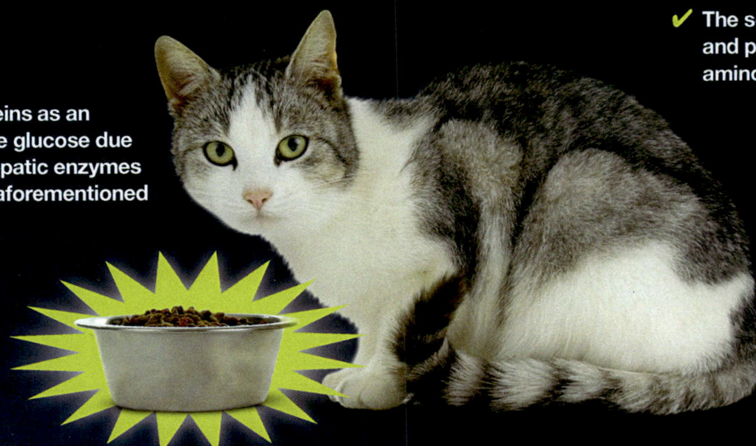

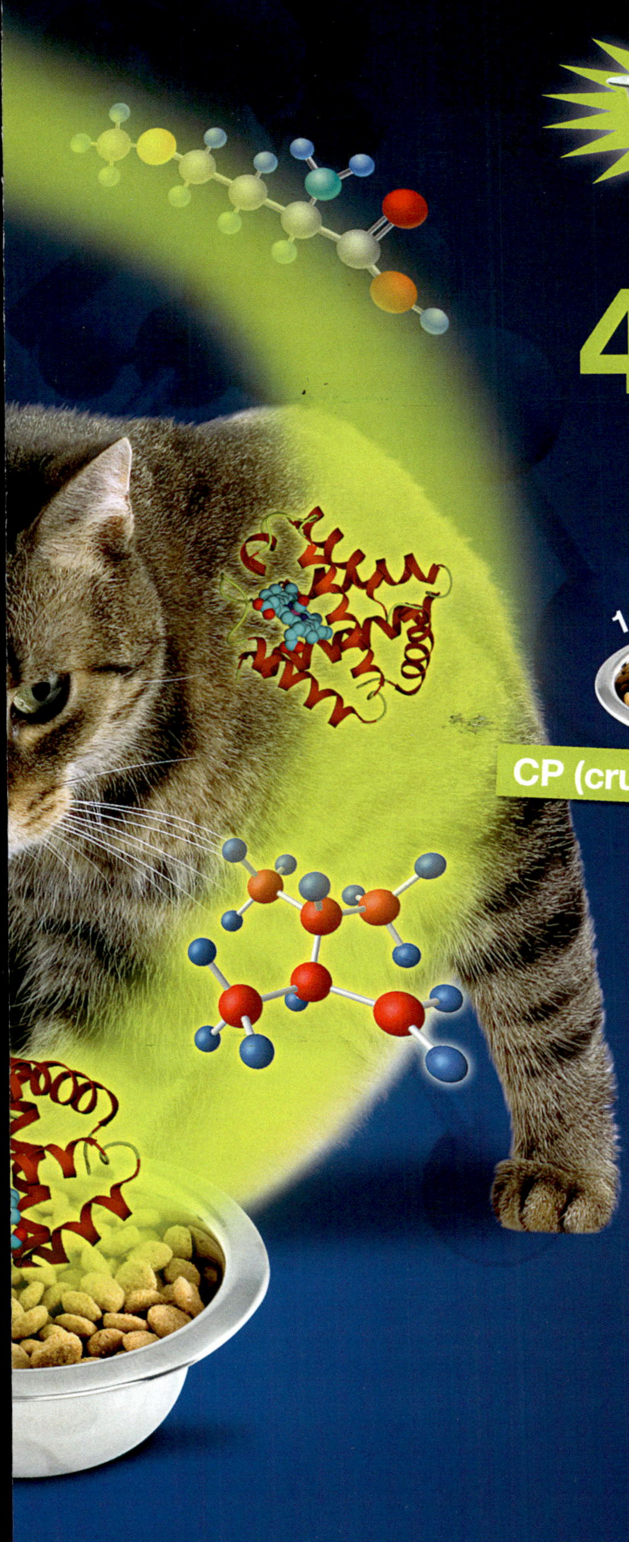

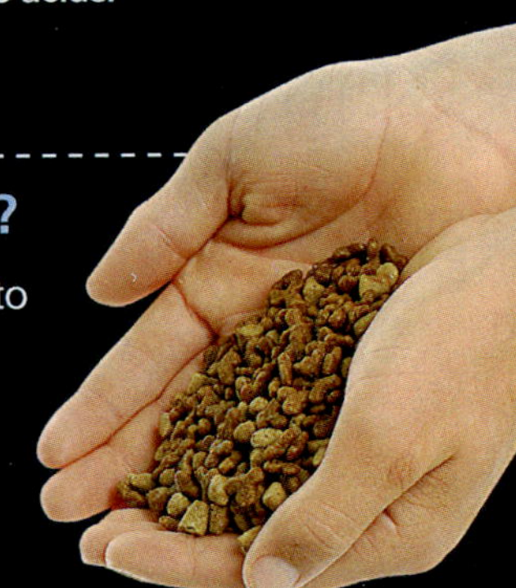

4 Why is more protein offered than that required?

Sometimes in commercial foods, these levels are increased to up to seven times their value. If we analyze the content of these foods, we see that there is an enormous variation, with levels that oscillate between **15** and **60 %** of the **DM** (in a food with an energetic concentration of 4,000 kcal/kg DM).
This is a normal practice in the manufacturing of pet foods for three reasons:

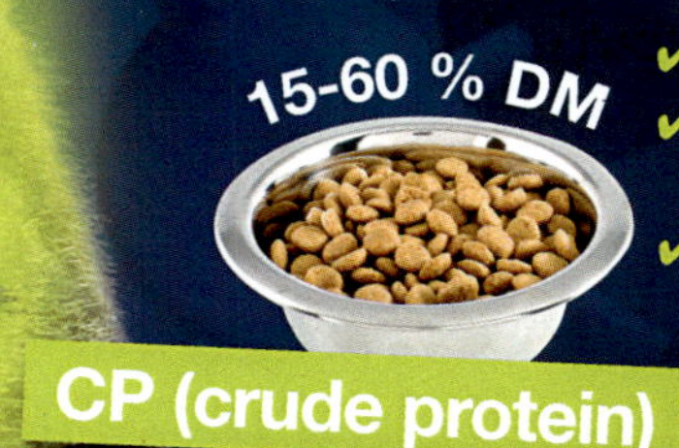

- ✔ Cats are strictly a carnivorous species.
- ✔ Dogs are omnivores but attempts are made to associate them with carnivore feeding behavior.
- ✔ Dog owners associate that a food that is rich in protein is of greater quality as it helps to create more muscle mass and improve the overall appearance of the animal.

5 Evaluation of the protein status

From a practical point of view, to know in an objective manner whether an animal is being correctly fed, the following can be evaluated:

- ✔ The muscle mass index.
- ✔ The concentration of albumin in serum.

If greater precision is desired, the following can be determined:

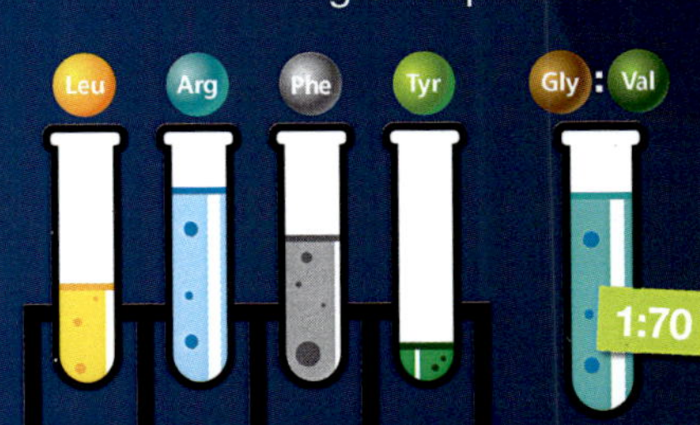

- ✔ The levels of essential amino acids in plasma.
- ✔ The ratio of the amino acids glycine:valine as an index of protein malnutrition.
  (The levels of these two amino acids are only affected when an animal is fed a low protein diet. In adult dogs that have been fed with complete and balanced commercial diets for maintenance, the glycine:valine ratio is 1:70).

To be taken into account:

Cats, as strict carnivores, have certain nitrogen metabolism pathways minimized as they are unnecessary.

An essential amino acid taurine

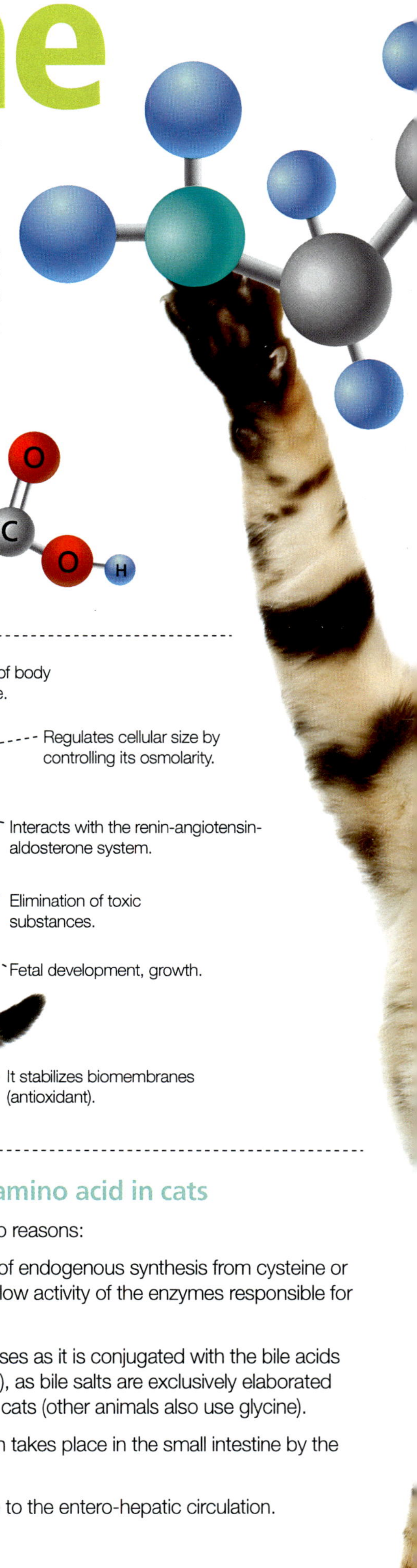

1 Chemical structure

Taurine is a β-amino acid with a sulfonic group that substitutes the carboxylic group. It is a derivative of cysteine with a thiol group.

It is not incorporated into the proteins due to its structure, but as a free amino acid, it forms part of the tissues and liquids of the body in superior animals: brain, retina, myocardium, liver, muscle, platelets, leukocytes and in milk and bile. It is also present in high concentrations in algae. Superior plants and bacteria contain trace elements of this β-aminosulfonic acid and therefore, strict vegetarians present taurine deficiencies.

Taurine

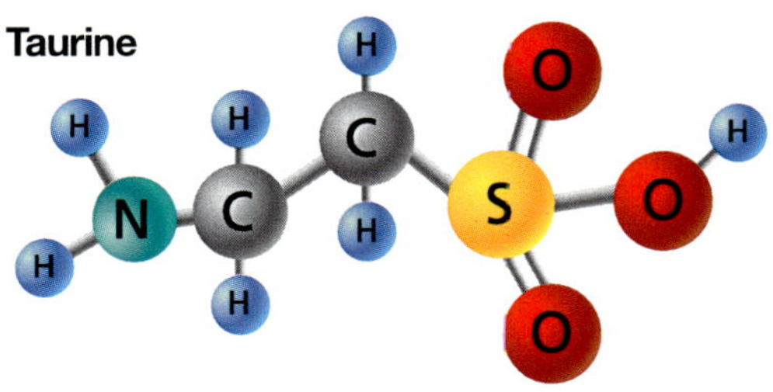

Cysteine

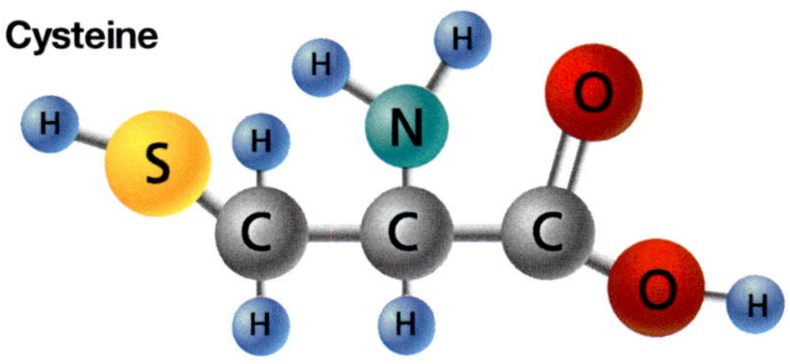

2 Functions in the organism

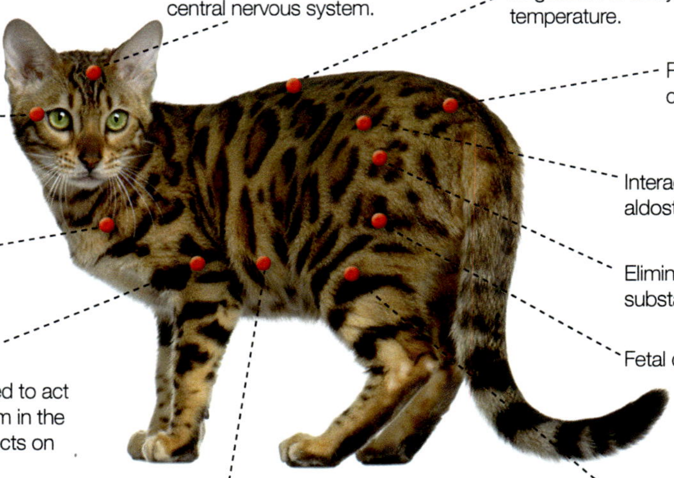

3 Non-essential amino acids in healthy dogs

Dogs obtain taurine from sulfur-containing amino acids (methionine and cysteine) in their food rations.

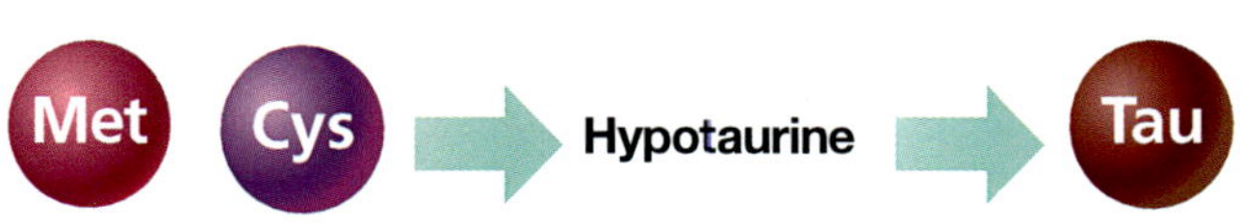

However, it becomes of interest when the animals' food rations include high levels of fats and in cases of certain cardiac pathologies (dilated cardiomyopathy and valve diseases): it does not prevent these diseases but it produces improved cardiac function.

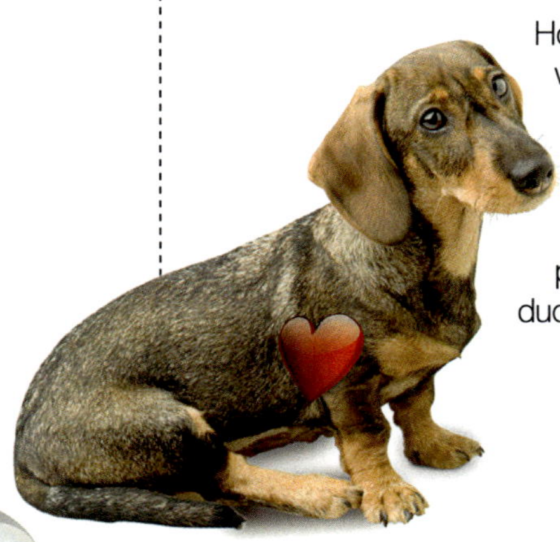

An essential amino acid in cats

It is essential for two reasons:

- ✓ Scarce capacity of endogenous synthesis from cysteine or methionine, due to low activity of the enzymes responsible for conversion.
- ✓ Significant losses as it is conjugated with the bile acids (taurocholic acid), as bile salts are exclusively elaborated with taurine in cats (other animals also use glycine).
- ✓ Degradation takes place in the small intestine by the microflora.
- ✓ Losses due to the entero-hepatic circulation.

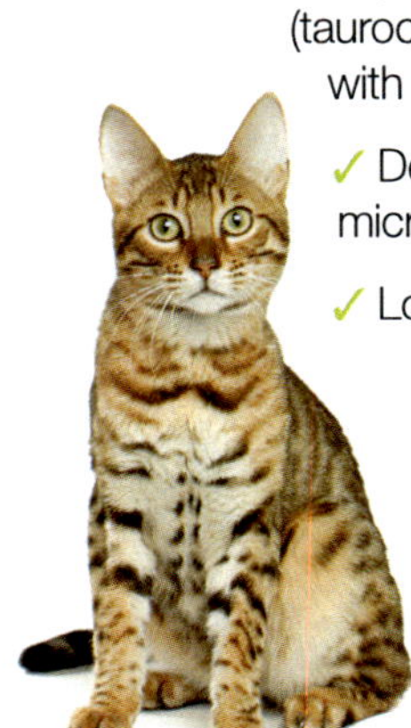

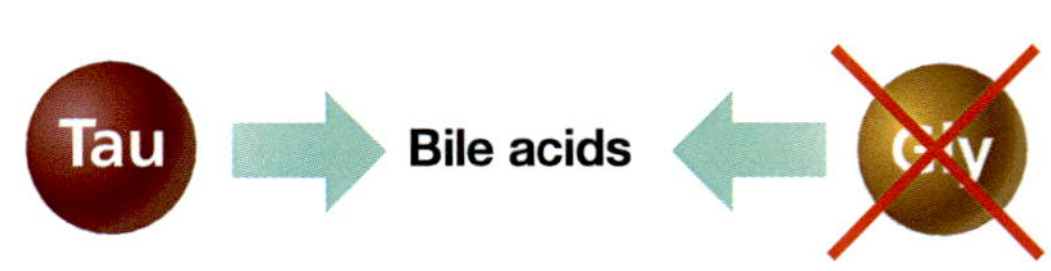

in cats:

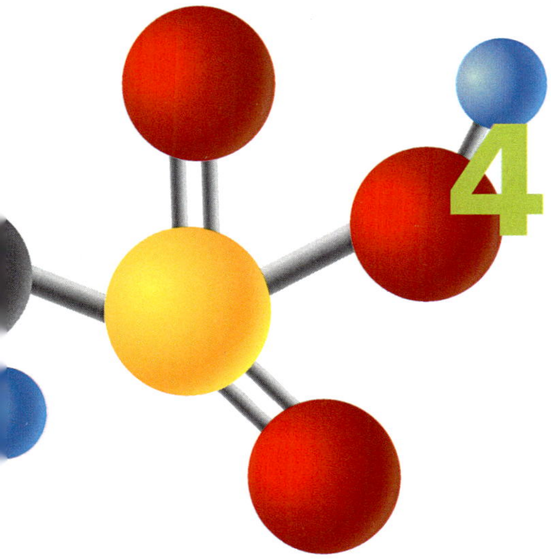

4

What conditions the requirements of this amino acid?

There are no specific recommendations for taurine. There are a series of factors that condition its daily requirements:

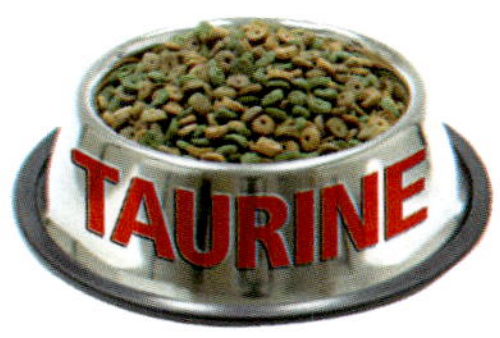

Daily requirements

- ✓ The type of protein, its quality and digestibility, as low quality proteins cause the following:
  - Favor bacterial overgrowth with cholehydrolase activity (which degrades the taurocholic acid into taurine + cholic acid).
  - Stimulate the liberation of cholecystokinin, which then stimulates the secretion of bile.
- ✓ The presence of certain types of fiber determine direct modifications in the intestine and induce changes in the microflora.
- ✓ The thermal treatments during the manufacturing process of the foods: its exact cause is unknown (possibly products created from Maillard reactions), but the processing increases the number of bacteria that are capable of degrading the taurine. For this reason, the amount of taurine in wet foods should be from 2 to 2.5 times greater.

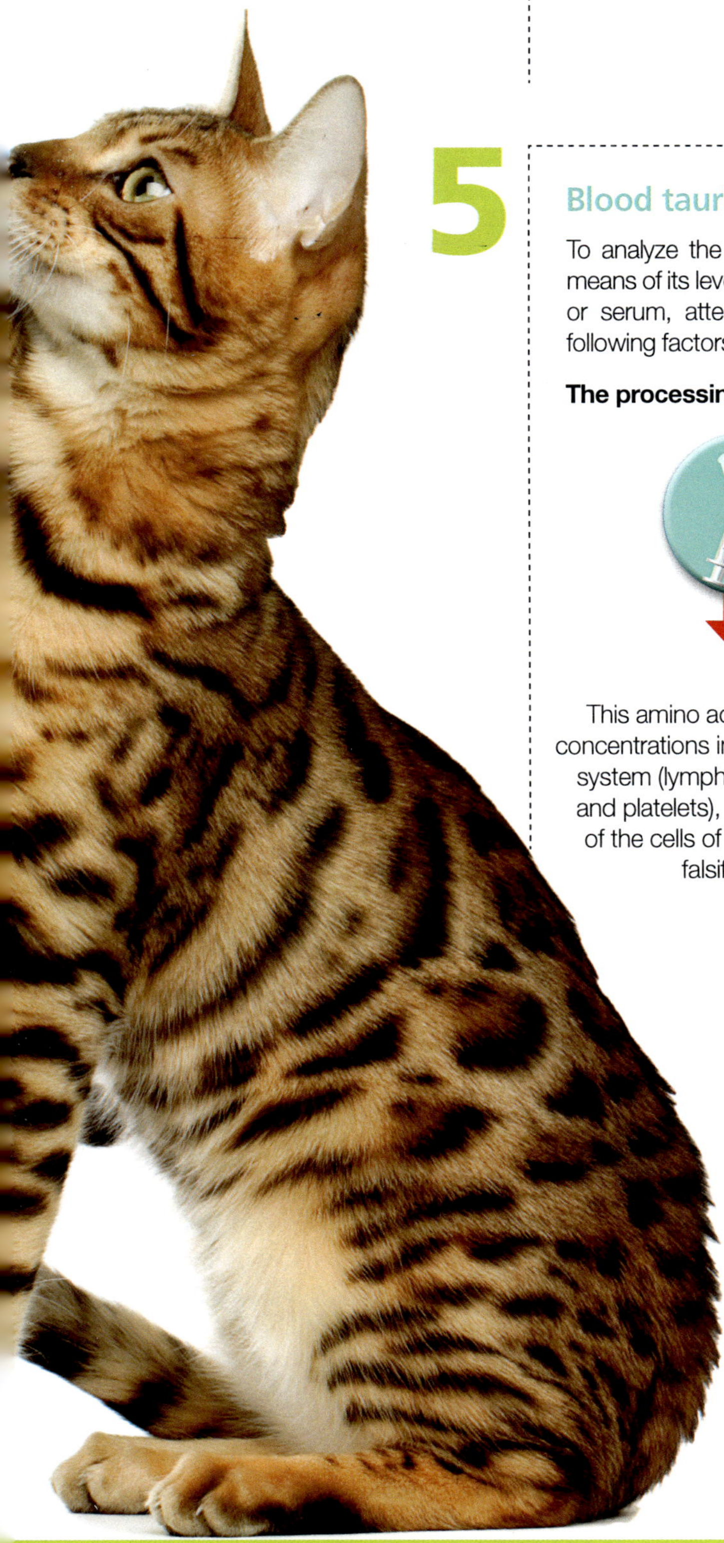

5

Blood taurine levels

To analyze the taurine in the organism by means of its level in complete blood, plasma or serum, attention must be paid to the following factors:

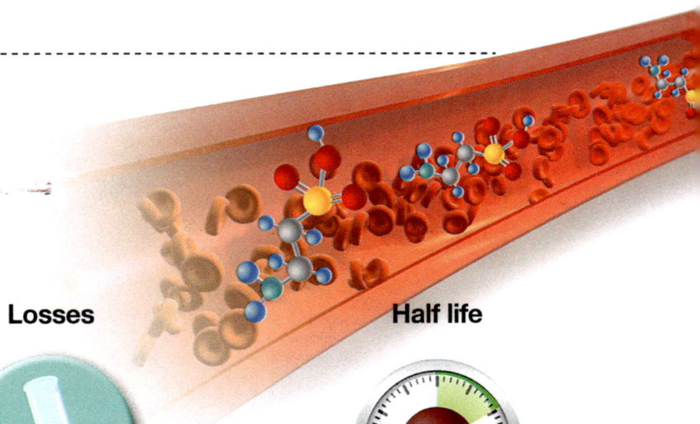

The processing of the sample

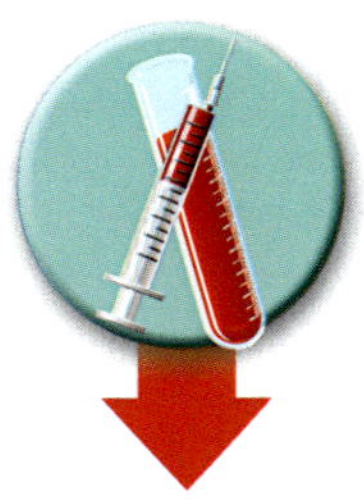

This amino acid is present in high concentrations in cells of the circulatory system (lymphocytes, granulocytes and platelets), for which the rupture of the cells of the white series can falsify the data.

Losses

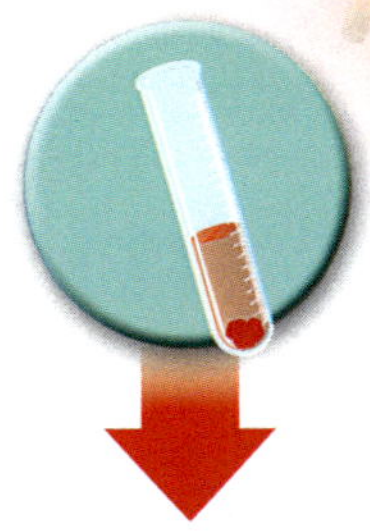

Losses are produced during the formation of a clot.

Half life

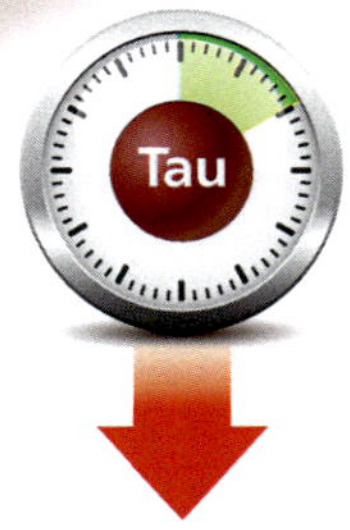

The half life of taurine in plasma is very short as it is quickly used by the tissues, especially the muscle and nerve tissue.

For these reasons, the use of complete blood is preferable for its analysis. The values in blood are as follows:

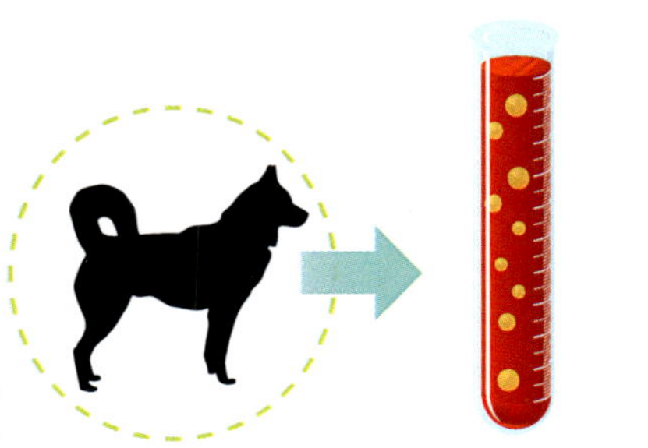

255,8-276,2 nmol/ml

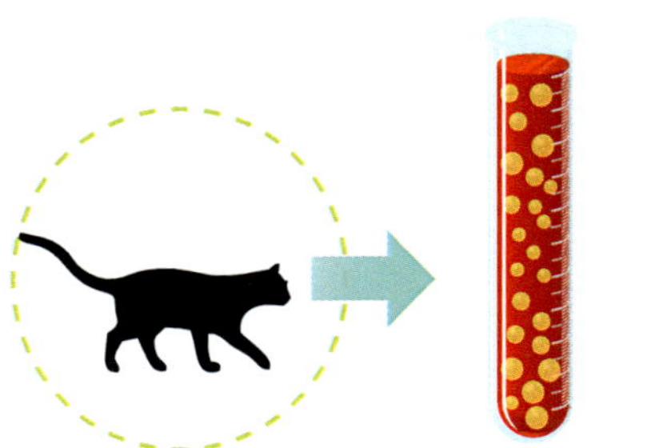

300-600 nmol/ml

Taking into account these factors, the recommendations for this amino acid in adult cats are:

Taurine (g/1,000 kcal ME)	NRC 2006	AAFCO and FEDIAF
Wet food	0.42	0.5
Dry food	0.25	0.25

Fat functions

Lipids are an extensive group of substances with structural and functional purposes. They are classified according to their union with glycerol (triglycerides, glucolipids and phospholipids) or without said alcohol (cholesterol and its esters, waxes, terpenes, sphingomyelins, cerebrosides).

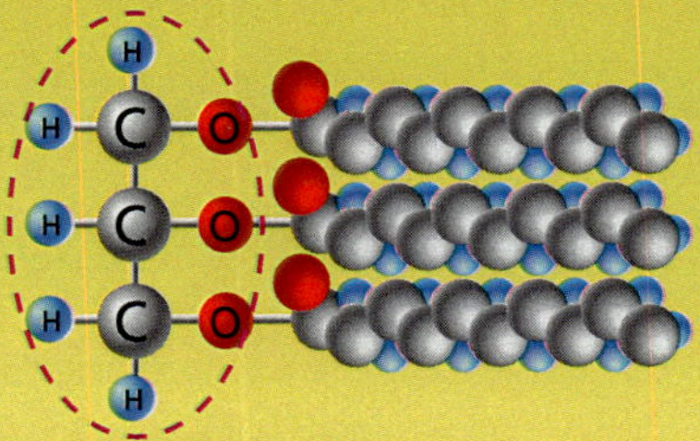

1 Functions

Fat is the primary source of energy for the body, both in its stored form as well as for its immediate use, and of the essential fatty acids (EFA). It provides 2.25 times more metabolizable energy than carbohydrates or proteins and its use efficiency is also greater. Its content in ME is 8.5 kcal/g.

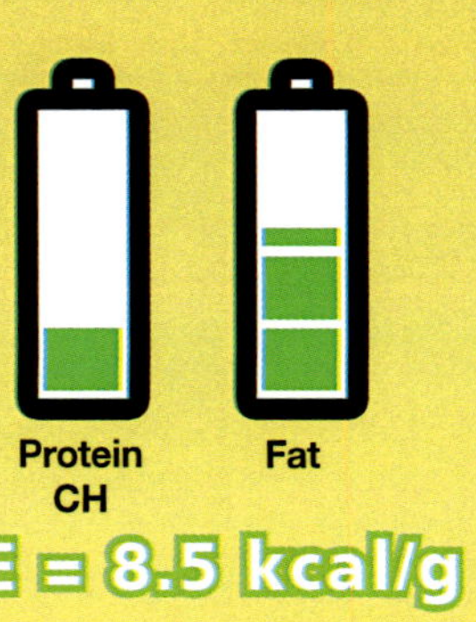

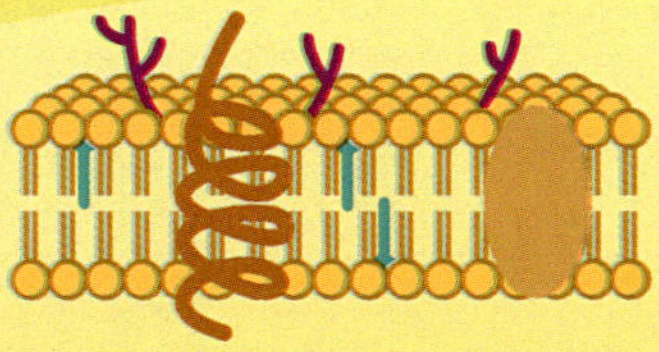

Other functions are:

- ✓ Structural in the cellular membranes.
- ✓ Regulators of cellular function, such as prostaglandins and eicosanoids.
- ✓ Transportation and absorption of liposoluble vitamins. The fat content in foods should be 1-2 %, regardless of its profile in fatty acids (FA), for these vitamins to be correctly absorbed.
- ✓ They provide palatability and texture to the food rations.

2 Lipids in food rations

They are a mixture of the two categories of fatty acids, saturated and unsaturated. The EFA are long-chain polyunsaturated fatty acids with a cis configuration, although the trans configuration is not incompatible with the activity as an EFA. They originate from the stored animal or plant fats.

The composition in EFA varies depending on the source. A simple and easy-to-remember nomenclature has been used in the following table based on the comparison between a specific EFA and the different sources. There is no proportion regarding the content among the other EFAs of one same fat.

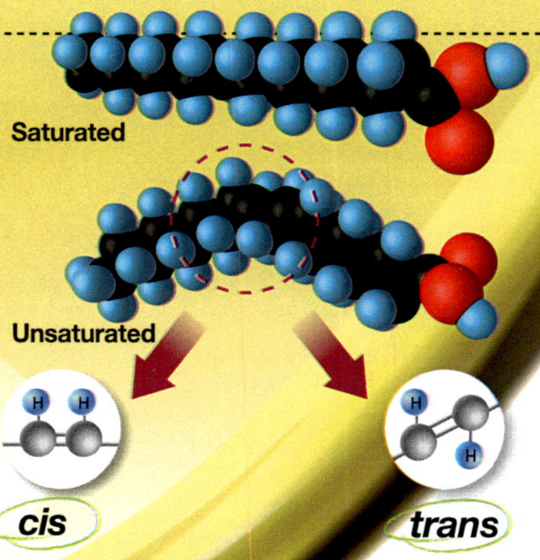

			Content in EFA* from different sources of fat							
Acid			Tallow	Lard	Fowl	Fish	Sunflower	Soy	Corn	Olive
Saturated:unsaturated ratio			12.8	3.47	1.47	0.51	0.22	0.24	0.21	1.55
LA	18:2n-6**	Linoleic	M	L	L	S	XL	XL	XL	L
ALA	18:3n-3	α-linolenic	M	M	M	L	S	XL	L	M
AA	20:4n-6	Arachidonic	XL	S	M	L	S	S	S	S
EPA	20:5n-3	Eicosapentaenoic	S	S	S	XL	S	S	S	S
DHA	22:6n-3	Docosahexaenoic	S	S	S	XL	S	S	S	S

* The values S to XL do not correspond with real values (g EFA/100 g of fat). S represents the lowest value and XL is the highest.

** The FA are named according to the number of carbon atoms and depending on the position of the double bonds from the methyl group (ω or n family) or of the carboxyl (Δ family). Both names are correct, but according to its biological properties, we will name them according to the ω family, A:Bn-E, where A is the number of carbon atoms, B is the number of double bonds that it possesses and E is the position of the first double bond regarding the methyl group.

Generally, it is understood that the fats and oils from plant original are primarily unsaturated. In fat from animal origin, there is a mixture of saturated (predominant) and unsaturated and their EFA profile is conditioned by the animal species, the fat profile of the food ration ingested and its metabolism (for example, in ruminant animals, the microflora produces a hydrogenation of the unsaturated fatty acids before their absorption).

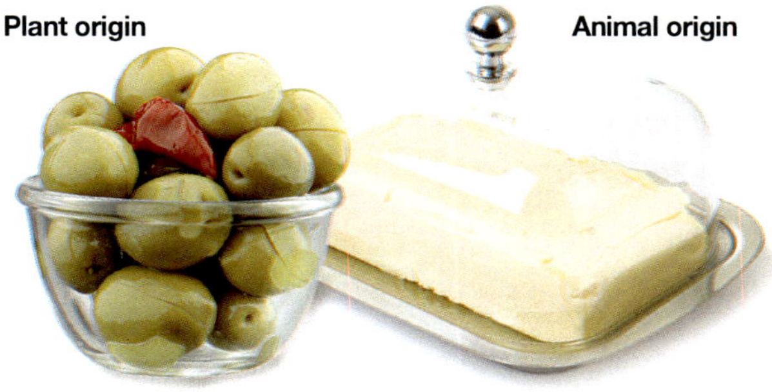

and metabolism

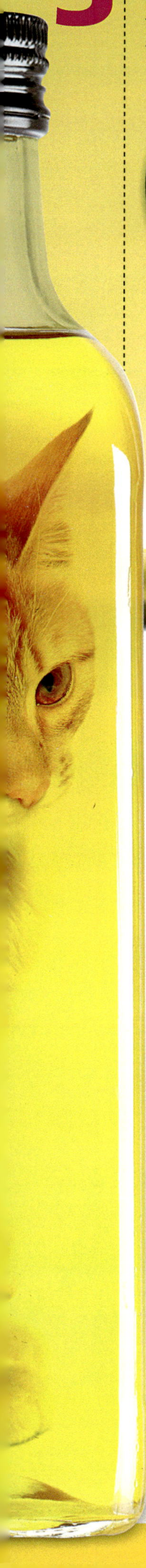

3 Metabolism of fats

Digestion

The digestion of fats depends on their hydrolysis by the lipases present throughout the gastrointestinal tract. These processes take place in the:

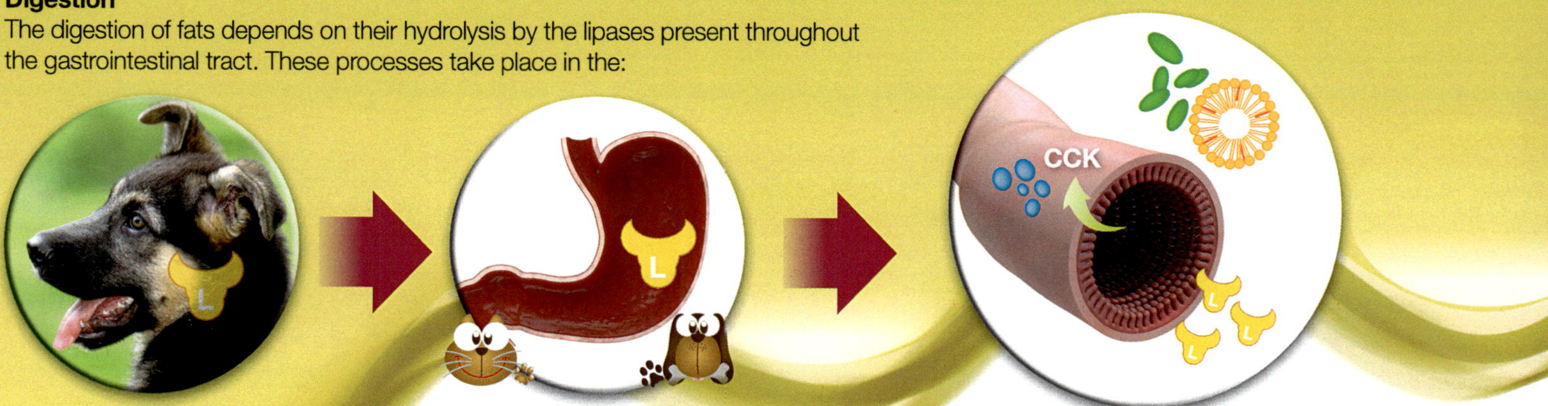

Oral cavity: lingual lipase (or oropharyngeal), whose activity is only noted in puppies.

Stomach: Gastric lipase, present in both species. Its activity is related to the lactating period. It represents the first step of the digestion of fats, as it hydrolyzes and facilitates emulsion. This pre-hydrolysis allows for digestion to be more efficient.

Small intestine: CCK is released in the duodenum due to the presence of the FA, and the formation of mixed micelles (made of FA, cholesterol and its ethers, phospholipids and acylglycerols). Bile salts and colipase allow for the creation of a substrate that is adequate for the activity of the pancreatic lipase, making the products of the hydrolysis more solubles. The pancreatic lipase simultaneously favors the activity of other lipases: carboxyl-ester-hydrolase, cholesterol-esterase and phospholipase A.

Absorption and transportation

This takes place in the small intestine, and it reaches its maximum activity in the jejunum. It is produced by passive diffusion or with carrier proteins (middle and long chain FA and cholesterol) of the lipids to the cytoplasm of the enterocytes.

Inside of the cell, FA carrier proteins will take them to the endoplasmic reticulum, where the triglycerides are re-synthesized. This process of re-esterification conditions the absorption of the fats.

During their transportation through the vascular system, the chylomicrons are degraded, releasing triglycerides. These in turn, through the activity of the lipoprotein-lipase present in the vascular endothelium, are hydrolyzed in glycerol and esterified fatty acids. This enzyme also acts on the VLDL. The residual chylomicrons (without triglycerides) reach the liver where they are metabolized.

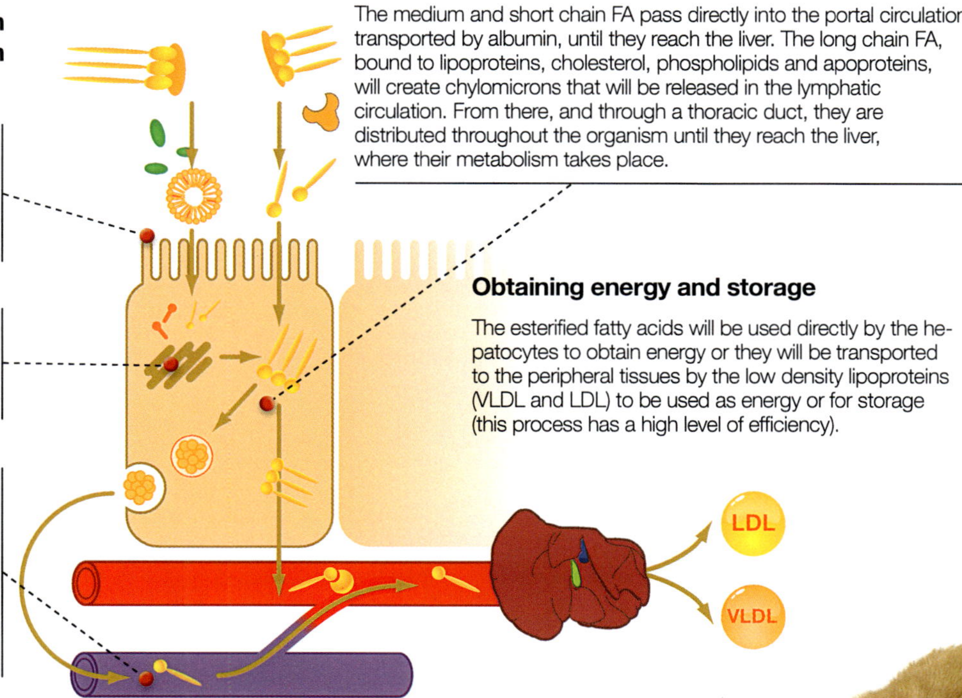

The medium and short chain FA pass directly into the portal circulation, transported by albumin, until they reach the liver. The long chain FA, bound to lipoproteins, cholesterol, phospholipids and apoproteins, will create chylomicrons that will be released in the lymphatic circulation. From there, and through a thoracic duct, they are distributed throughout the organism until they reach the liver, where their metabolism takes place.

Obtaining energy and storage

The esterified fatty acids will be used directly by the hepatocytes to obtain energy or they will be transported to the peripheral tissues by the low density lipoproteins (VLDL and LDL) to be used as energy or for storage (this process has a high level of efficiency).

Digestibility of fats

Pets digest fats with great efficiency. The apparent digestibility of a mixture of animal and plant fat in dogs is from 85 to 95 %, although there are studies that estimate up to 70 to 90 % for commercial dry foods.

The digestibility is affected by the unsaturated:saturated FA ratio and by the size of said components. When more than 50 % of the total amount of fat of the food ration is made up of unsaturated FA or the length of the chains are medium or short, the digestibility is greater (5 %). Generally, the digestibility of the saturated FA is 4 % lower compared to unsaturated FA.

In cats, in a study on the apparent digestibility of certain commercial foods, it varied between 85 and 94 %. Currently, these rates are controversial. Some authors consider that the digestibility of the fat in cats is lower than in dogs. In spite of this, and given their carnivorous nature, it is estimated that felines can utilize high levels of fat in their food rations.

The digestibility decreases in both species as age increases. The digestibility of fat in senior animals is 2 % lower than in adult animals.

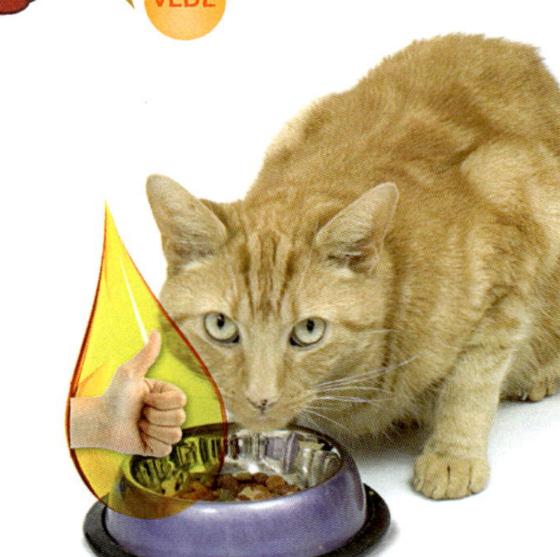

To be taken into account

Mammals are different in the predominance of the different types of lipoproteins. Dogs and cats are considered "HDL" animals, which gives them a lower sensitivity to cardiovascular accidents derived from the metabolism of fats. Also, there is no exchange of cholesterol between HDL and LDL in these two species due to the low levels of protein responsible for the exchange.

Requirements of fat

The levels of inclusion of fat in food rations for pets has been widely argued. Different nutrition studies between species have been used as references, especially those related with the EFA n-6:n-3 profiles and to the metabolism of cholesterol, and the physiological particularities of dogs and cats (for example, HDL metabolism, the acceptance of high levels or lack of Δ-6 desaturase).

Dog

In adult dogs, the NRC recommendations from 2006 indicate that the total fat should represent nearly 12 % of the ME consumed, allowing for values between 10 and 50 %. The upper limit of incorporation is 70 % of the ME, that is, 82.5 g/1,000 kcal ME, but this depends on the levels of protein. The use of these doses closer to the upper limit should be restricted to animals used for sports that undergo endurance tests. The use of high levels of fat and low protein content causes changes in the pancreas. Other undesired effects include obesity, hypercholesterolemia, or pansteatitis.

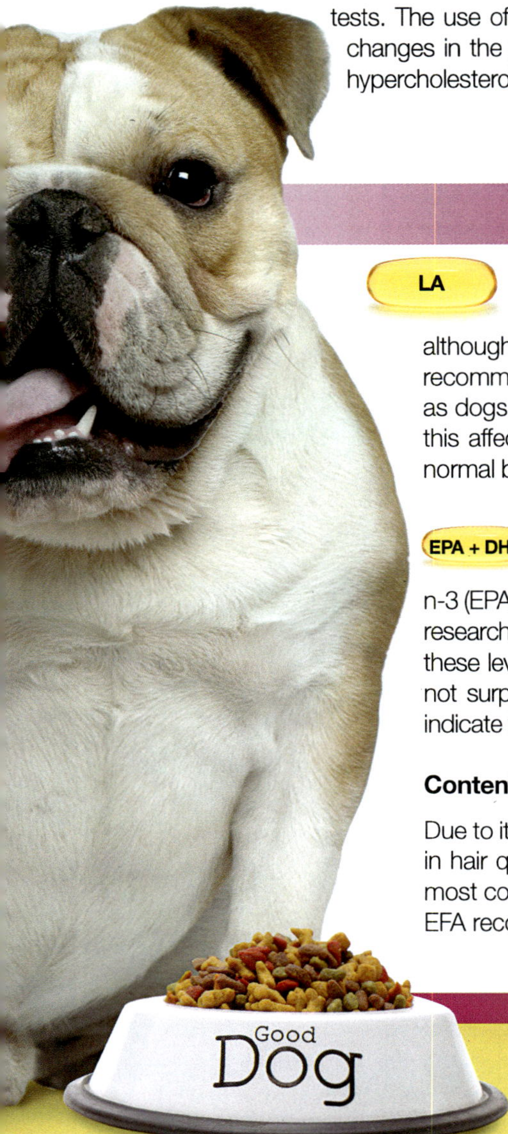

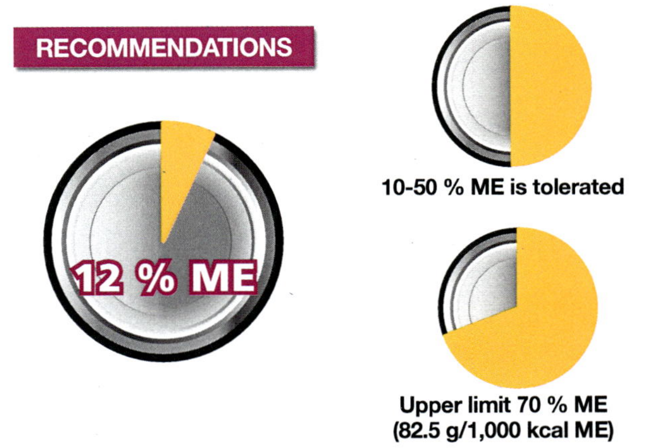

ESSENTIAL FATTY ACIDS

LA Regarding the EFA, a content of at least 2.3 % of linoleic acid of the ingested ME must be provided, although the minimum needs are close to 55 % of these recommendations. Using the higher amount is preferable as dogs can synthesize arachidonic acid (AA) from LA and this affects their minimum concentration to carry out their normal biological activity.

EPA + DHA **AA** There is no specific data on the recommendations for the EFA of the n-3 (EPA and DHA) or n-6 (AA) families. The levels found from research in human medicine are currently used. Based on these levels, the upper safety limit for EPA and DHA should not surpass 2.4 % of the ME ingested; recommendations indicate that the ideal amount is 0.1 %.

Content in foods

Due to its influence in the palatability of the food rations and in hair quality, a minimum of 5 % of the DM is included in most commercial dog foods. This amount ensures that the EFA recommendations for this species are met.

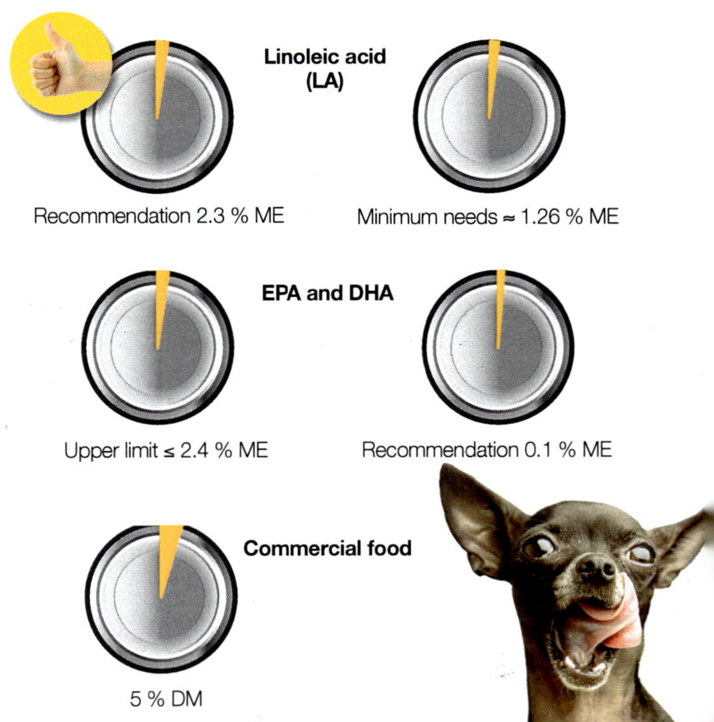

Why are essential

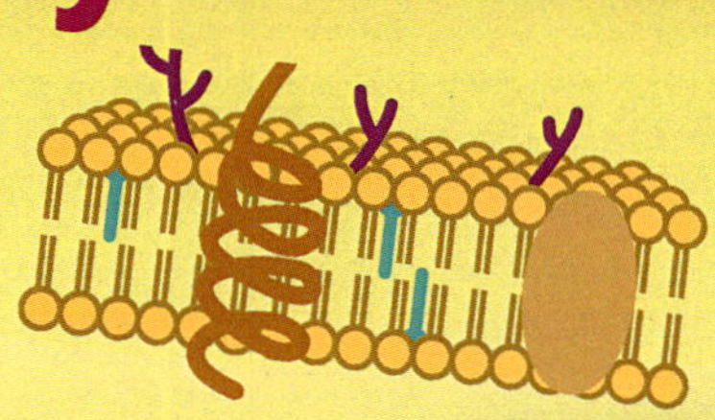

The EFA and their derivatives are important during growth and for proper functioning of an animal's body. Their functions include:

- ✓ Composition and integrity of the cellular membrane. Twenty five percent of the phospholipids of the cellular membranes have AA.
- ✓ Interaction with the membrane proteins.
- ✓ Platelet aggregation.
- ✓ Growth and development of CNS, retina, vascular system and blood flow.
- ✓ Integrity of the skin and hair by maintaining correct hydration.
- ✓ Reproduction and fertility in female cats.

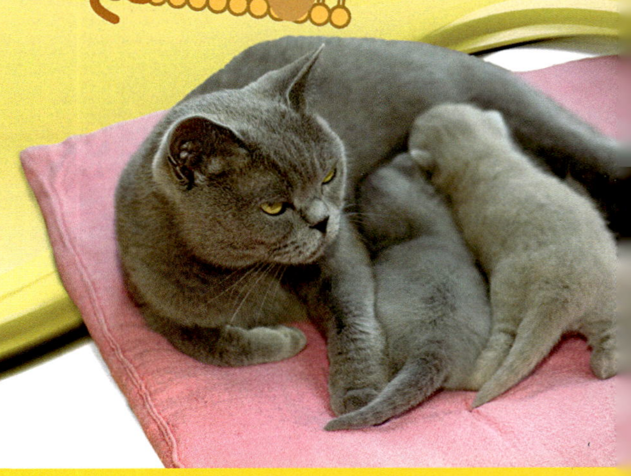

in pets

Cat

The recommendation for adult cats in maintenance care is a minimum of 19 % of the ME ingested in the form of fat. Compared with dogs, this amount is nearly 60 % greater. However, its upper limit of tolerance is similar. Cats tolerate levels that represent 67 % of the ingested ME without any problems.

The fats are also responsible for the palatability of the foods for cats, but this is also conditioned by its profile. The acceptance of medium-length chain fats is very low in this species. For example, the existence of caprylic acid (8:0, rich in palm and coconut oil), with a concentration of 0.01-0.1 % of the DM, will lead to the animal rejecting this food.

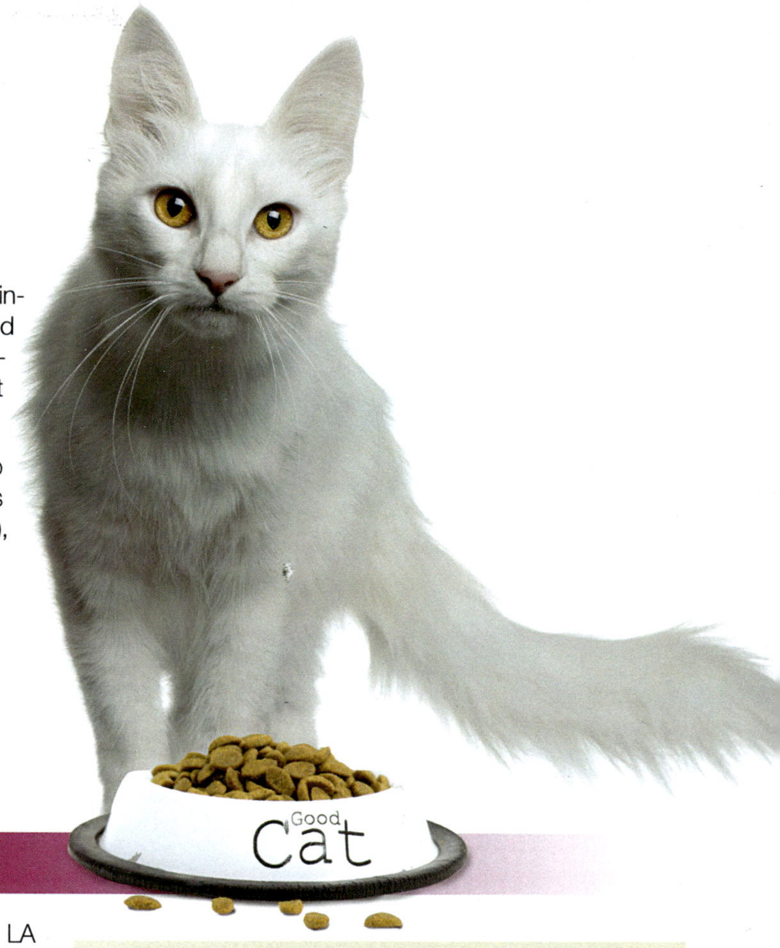

RECOMMENDATIONS

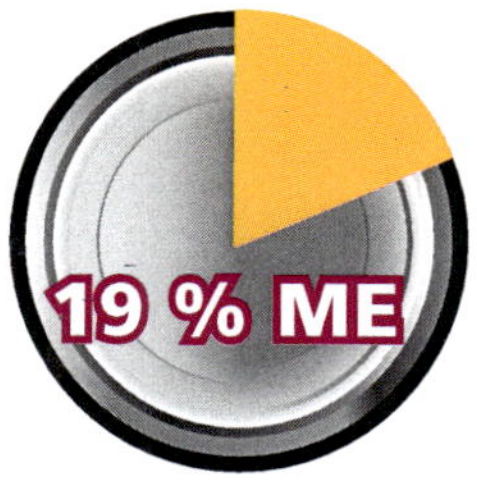

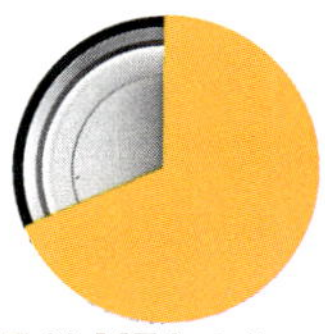

67 % ME is tolerated

ESSENTIAL FATTY ACIDS

LA The data available regarding EFA is scarce. The recommendations for LA are of 1.19 % of the ME ingested. The requirements of cats are lower when we compare them with those of dogs, close to 50 % of their value, as LA is not used to synthesize long chain EFA.

1.19 % ME

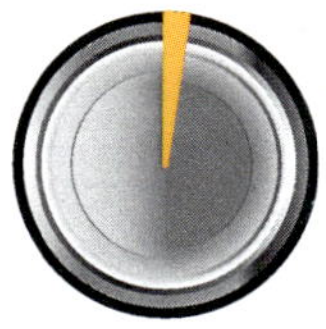

Linoleic acid (LA)

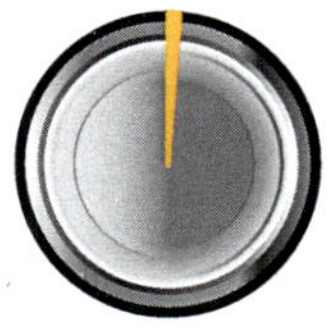

Needs ≈ 0.6 % ME

AA

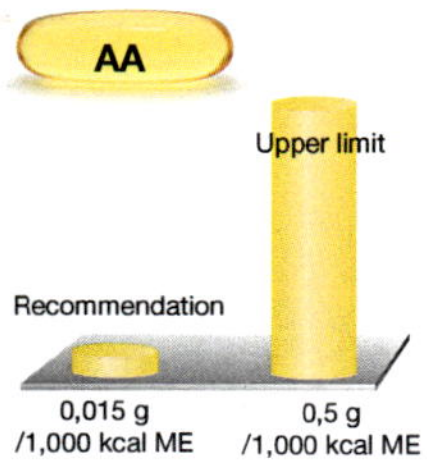

EPA + DHA

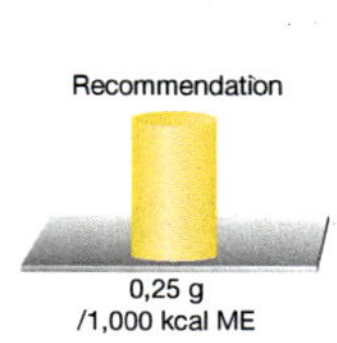

The same applies to AA and EPA/DHA where little information is available. It has been estimated that 0.015 g of AA/1,000 kcal ME is sufficient, although in the presence of EFA from the n-3 family, its amount must be increased, without surpassing the upper limit (0.5 g/1,000 kcal ME). In the case of EPA+DHA, 0.25 g/1,000 kcal ME is recommended.

8-13 % DM (25 % DM)

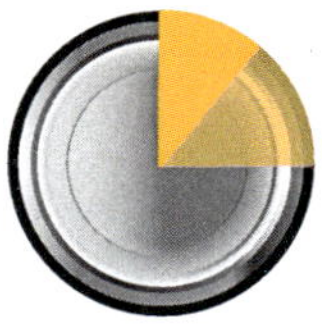

Content in foods

Commercial cat foods include levels of 8 to 13 % of the DM, reaching 25 % at times, depending on the category of the food. The preferences of cats are closer to this value than 10 %.

Recommendations in fats and EFA in dogs and cats
The FEDIAF recommendations regarding total fats, LA and AA are similar

NRC 2006 (g/1,000 kcal ME)	Dogs	Cats
Total fat	13.8	22.5
LA (linoleic acid)	2.8	1.4
ALA (α-linolenic acid)	0.11	Not used
AA (arachidonic acid)	Not needed	0.015
EPA + DHA	0.11	0.025
EPA:DHA	50-60:40-50	20:80
n-6:n-3*	5-4:1	

* Based on studies on cardiovascular health in human medicine.

Vit. E When the levels of polyunsaturated EFA are high in food rations, especially of the n-3 family, increasing vitamin E from 0.6 to 1.8 mg is recommended (depending on the type of fatty acid) for each g of EFA ingested to stabilize the cellular membranes as well as the concentration of antioxidants authorized in the foods due to how easily they oxidate.

fatty acids important?

- ✓ Production of eicosanoids, for example: prostaglandin, leukotriene, thromboxane, lipoxin and prostacyclin.
- ✓ Humoral and cellular inflammatory response (related with the previous point). Some of these factors, derivatives of DHA and EPA, are called resolvins (Rv) and protectins (Pn).

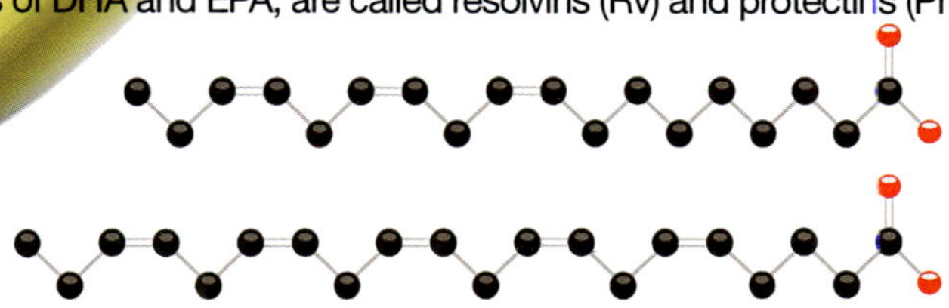

Two series have been identified: E and D from the EPA and DHA, respectively. For example, RvE1 acts by reducing inflammation and produces interleukin 12 (IL-12); RvD blocks the tumor necrosis factor (TNFα) and controls the migration of leukocytes to the focal point of inflammation.

Due to their protective activity on the CNS, neurons and retina, the name docosanoids has been proposed for the derivatives of DHA. In human medicine, they are used in the treatment of the consequences of cerebral infarctions and senile dementia.

Conclusion

- ✓ The LA is essential in dogs and cats.
- ✓ The EPA, DHA and DPA (docosapentaenoic acid) are conditional essential acids in both species during periods of growth.
- ✓ AA is essential in felines.

To be taken into account:

The de novo synthesis of saturated and monounsaturated FA (16:1n-7 and 18:1n-9) from glucose and the amino acids is a process that takes place in almost all mammals when their food rations contain high proportions of base nutrients. In spite of the aforementioned, the synthesis of FA is not sufficient to cover their needs and therefore, they must be included in their diets.

Carbohydrates

1 General characteristics

Carbohydrates include sugars, starches, non-starch polysaccharides, and dietary fiber (fiber will be explained later on). They comes from plant cells, where storage functions are carried out. Some of them are associated with the cellular wall as structural components of plants. They primarily come from grains, tubers, and to a lesser extent, from legumes. They are added to dry extruded foods for their palatability (in dogs) and for their technological characteristics: they are responsible for the texture, structure and form of the food. Together with fat, they are the primary source of energy for omnivore animals.

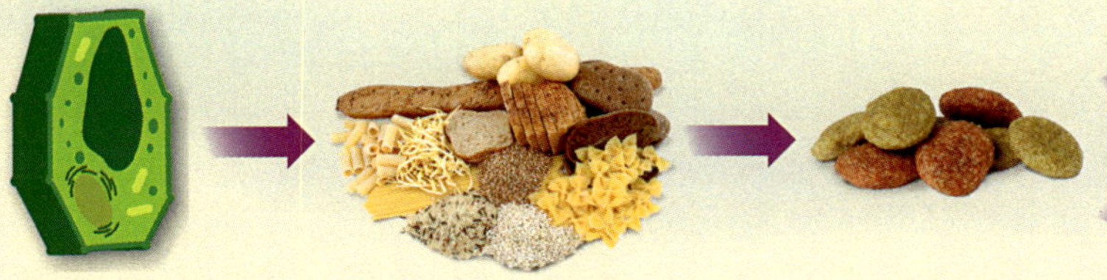

They have a great capacity to uptake water due to their chemical structure:

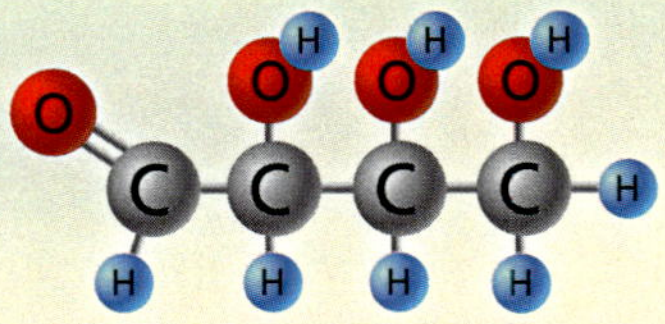

$C_n(H_2O)_n$

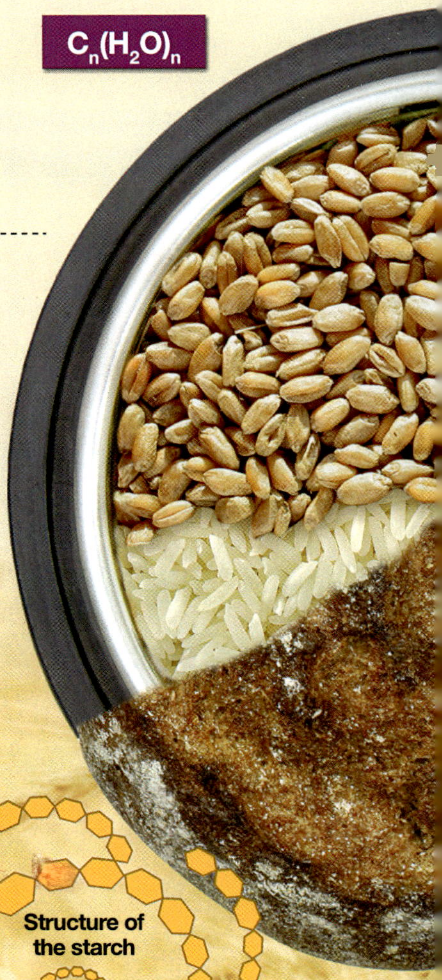

2 Classification of carbohydrates

Carbohydrates can be classified depending on the following:

- ✓ Chemical structure.
- ✓ Number of carbon atoms (triose, pentose...).
- ✓ Units that they integrate (mono-, di-, oligo- and polysaccharides).
- ✓ Resistance to endogenous enzymatic attacks (β-glycosidic bonds in the fibers).
- ✓ Granular structure of their starches and their digestion (digestible and resistant).
- ✓ Origin: plant (the majority) or animal (lactose and glycogen, glycosaminoglycans).
- ✓ Beneficial effect for the body (prebiotics and symbiotics, for example: fructooligosaccharides).

From a nutrition point of view, we are interested in classifying starches according to their digestive capacity and the velocity of the process.

Type of starch		Digestion in small intestine	Example
Digestible	Fast	Fast and complete.	Cooked grains and tubers. Extruded foods.
	Slow	Slow and complete.	Chopped raw grains.
Resistant	Unaccessible	It is released during chewing and salivation. Slow and incomplete in pets.	Whole grain seeds.
	Resistant	Not produced. They ferment in the large intestine.	Raw roots and tubers, plantain, legumes.
	Retrograde or re-crystallized	Not produced. They ferment in the large intestine.	Cold potato puree, bread, corn flakes.
	Modified (bound to phosphates)	There is no information available; supposedly, their availability in pets is good due to the low starch content (<2.5 %). Their use is technological.	Frozen foods, canned soups, baby foods.

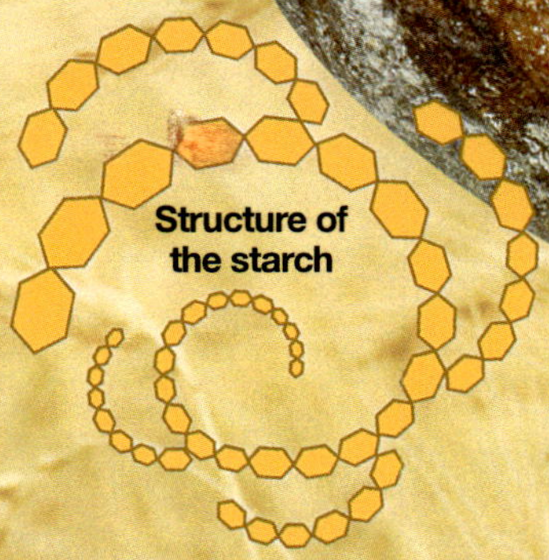

3 Functions

Their principal function is to provide units of glucose to the organism that will serve for the following purposes:

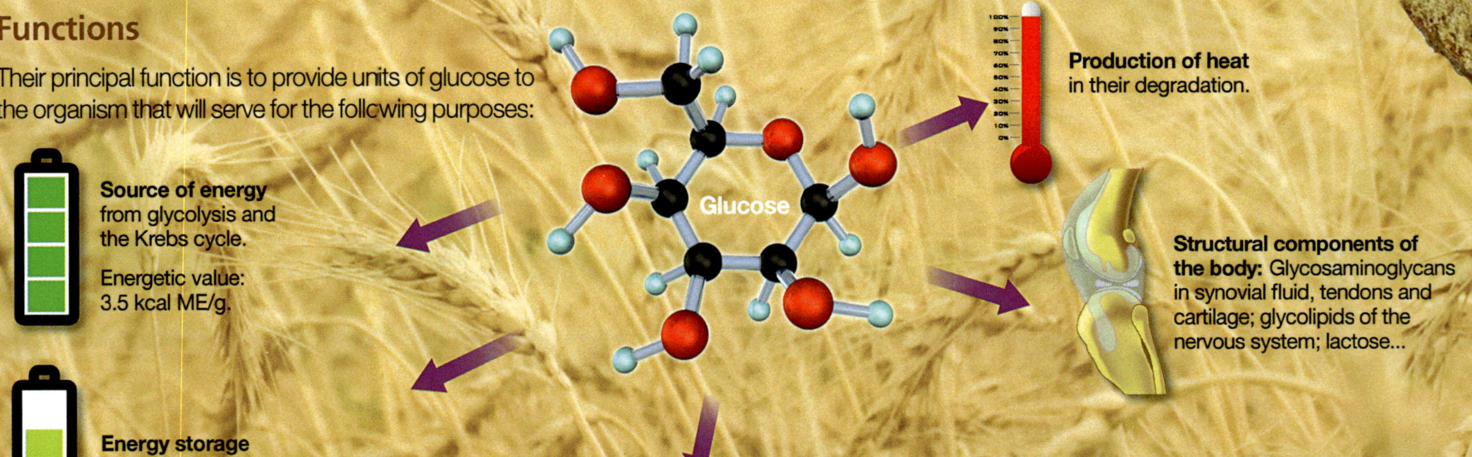

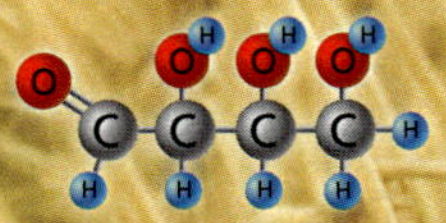

Carbohydrates also affect the intraluminal osmotic pressure, the absorption of water and of some minerals as well as bacterial growth in the small intestine.

4 Glycosaminoglycans

Glycosaminoglycans are polysaccharides associated with proteins. They form part of the skin, tendons, cartilage and some interstitial fluids (synovial). The two primary glycosaminoglycans are:

Chondroitin sulfate (glucuronic acid + N-acetylgalactosamine)

Hyaluronic acid (glucuronic acid + N-acetylglucosamine)

Their use in degenerative joint diseases is broad, although there is certain controversy regarding their efficiency as a consequence of the nature of the product, its bioavailability, its concentration in tissues and due to the lack of a standard of quality.

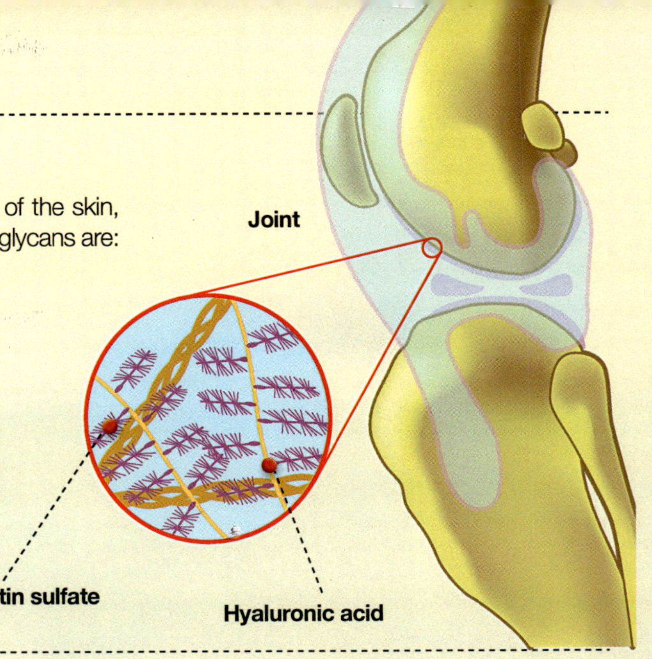

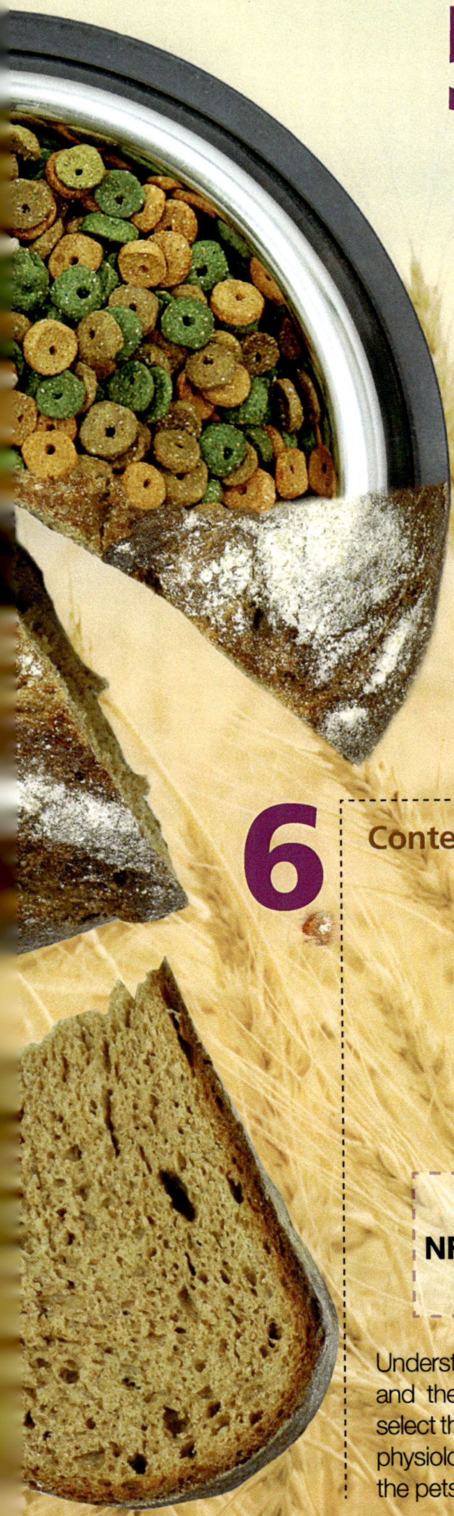

5 Carbohydrate requirements

The body, to maintain the equilibrium of this nutrient, can obtain glucose from the food rations, from glycogen, from glycogenic amino acids and/or from fat by means of gluconeogenesis (exclusively in the liver and kidneys). This mechanism is very efficient in dogs.

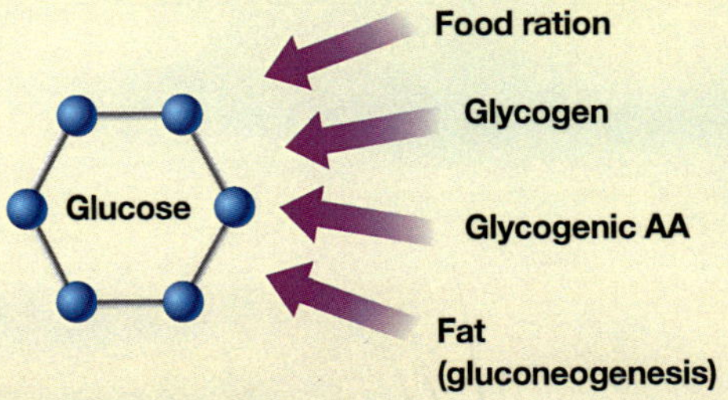

In cats, the importance of glucose in their metabolism is due to the fact that they are constantly in a state of gluconeogenesis (they preferentially use amino acids and fats as their primary sources of energy). For this reason, glucose must be provided in their food rations, in spite of the fact that their use is slower (their postprandial glycemia is longer) when compared with dogs.

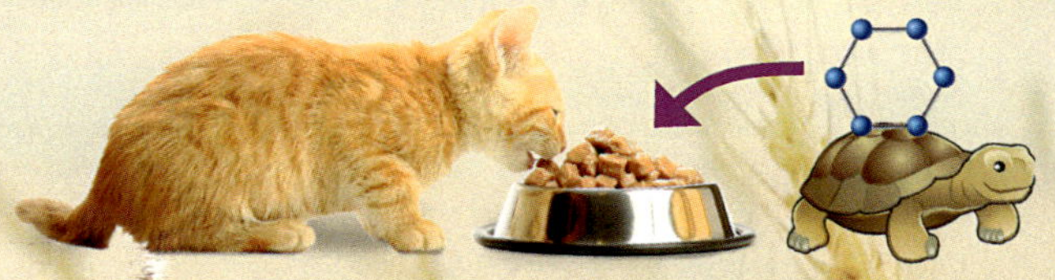

If we surpass the 40 % (as DM) of digestible carbohydrates in cat food, metabolic (hyperglycemia) and digestive changes may appear: diarrhea, gas, bloating, flatulence and abdominal pain.

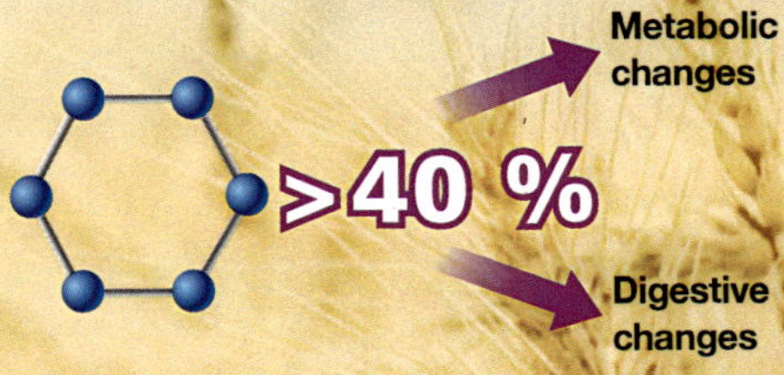

6 Content of carbohydrates in foods

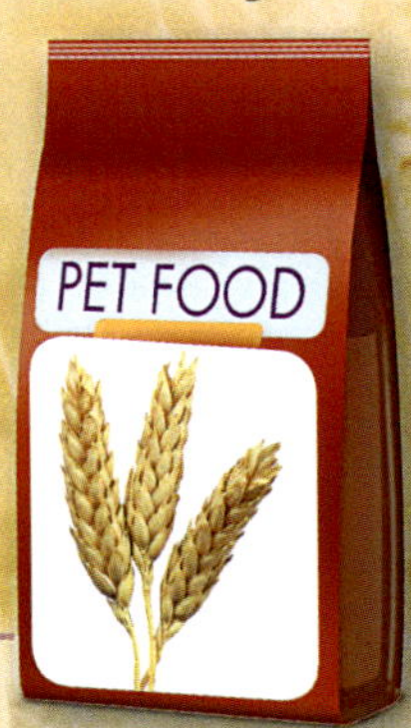

NFE = 30-40 % (60 %) DM
E = 4,000 kcal/kg DM

Understanding the content in hydrates, starch and their glycemic index (GI) allows for us to select the type of food that best suits the species, physiological condition and any pathologies of the pets.

Generally, commercial dog and cat foods include 30-40 % (up to 60 %) of the DM as nitrogen free extracts –NFE– (in a food with an energy concentration of 4,000 kcal/kg DM). Regarding raw materials, the content in starches is also variable depending on the source:

Ingredient	Approximate content (g/kg DM)
Barley, wheat, corn, rice	500, 590, 650, 810
Oats, rye	400, 500
Legumes	350
Potato	650
Corn or rice bran	250
Wheat bran	140

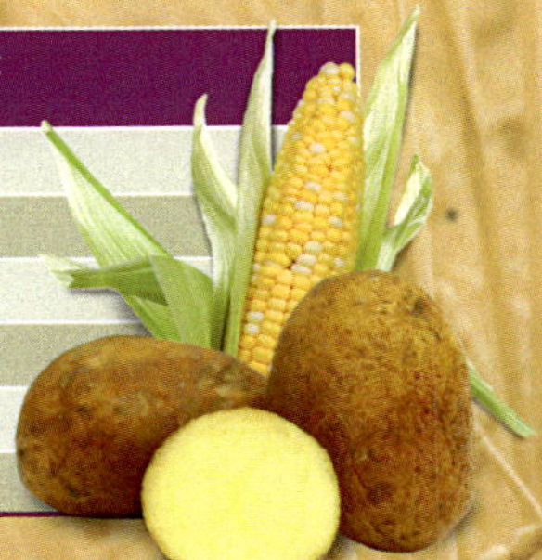

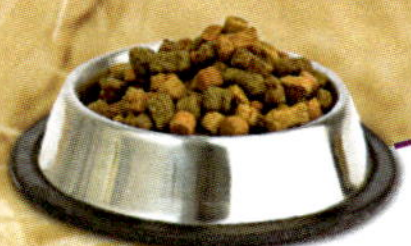

Min = 50-62.5 g of CH/1,000 kcal ME (20-25 % of the DM in 4,000 kcal ME/kg DM)

To be taken into account:

There are no specific requirements for carbohydrates in our two pet species. However, there are certain tissues and situations where the provision of glucose is mandatory: CNS, red blood cells, crystalline lens and retina, growth, lactation, and gestation. Therefore, the incorporation of a minimum of 50-62.5 g of carbohydrates/1,000 kcal ME (20-25 % of the DM in a food of 4,000 kcal ME/kg DM) in foods is recommended. They will appear as nitrogen free extracts (NFE) on the label. In some cases, the starch content is also indicated (this is interesting for animals with certain pathologies such as diabetes).

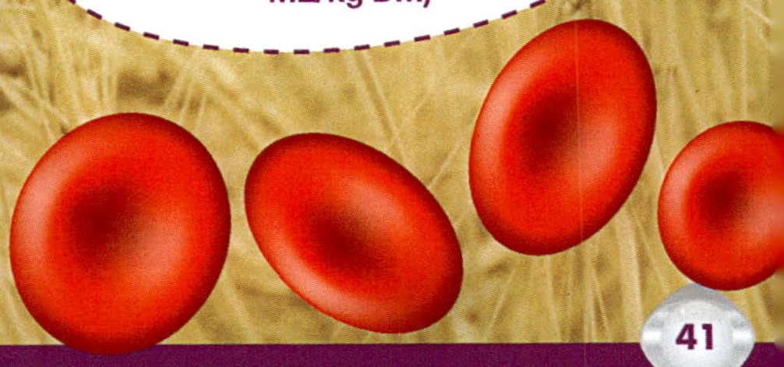

Metabolism of the

1 Intestinal digestion

In pets, digestion starts in the small intestine, given that the participation in the oral cavity (that lacks salivary amylase) and in the stomach is scarce. The majority of carbohydrates are digested in the jejunum by the animal's enzymes. The pancreas and the brush-border enterocytes participate.

They present a high digestibility, with an 84 % as an average, with values above 95 % when dealing with extruded foods. The monosaccharides from the diet are directly absorbed (the absorption is 100 % for both species), while the pancreatic α-amylase degrades the α-1,4 and α-1,6 bonds of the polysaccharides into simpler units. On their behalf, the maltase, lactase, sucrase and isomaltase enzymes, secreted by the enterocytes, degrade said disaccharides.

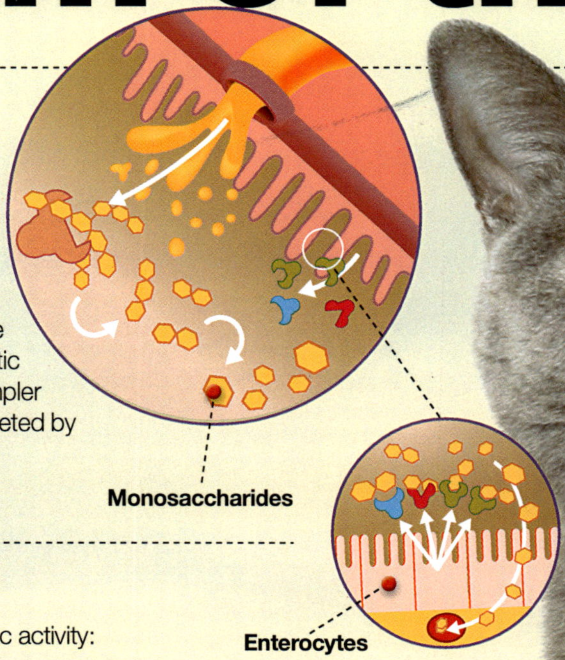

2 Intestinal enzymatic activity

There are certain particularities regarding the development and intestinal enzymatic activity:

1. **The activity (Unit/g protein) of these enzymes is maximum in the jejunum and the ileum, with an optimal pH of 5 (lactase) or 6 (maltase and sucrase), average in the colon and lower in the duodenum.**

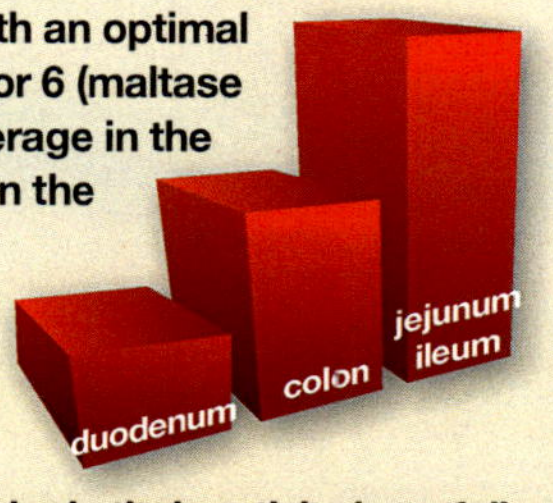

2. **The increasing order in their activity is as follows:**

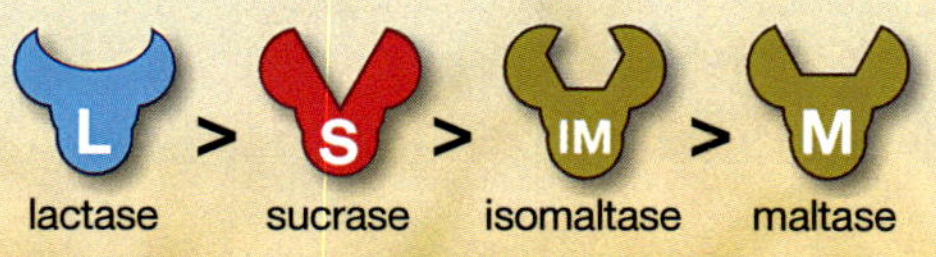

3. **In adult dogs and cats (>1 year), the activity and concentration of the amylase, maltase, sucrase and isomaltase is greater than in newborns. There is no difference between adults and kittens in cats regarding the concentration of sucrase.**

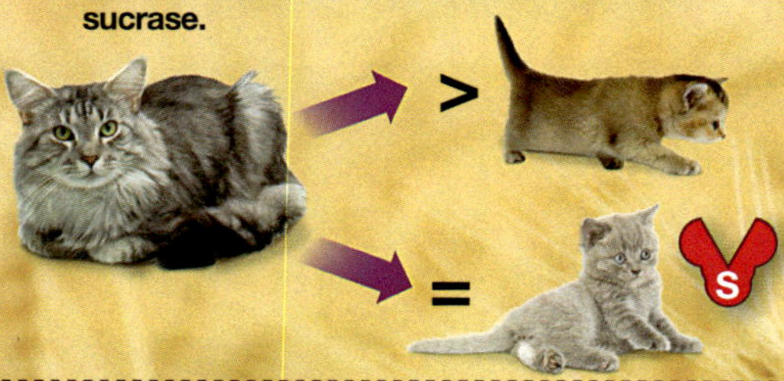

4. **The activity of the canine disaccharidase is approximately 30 % greater than that of felines.**

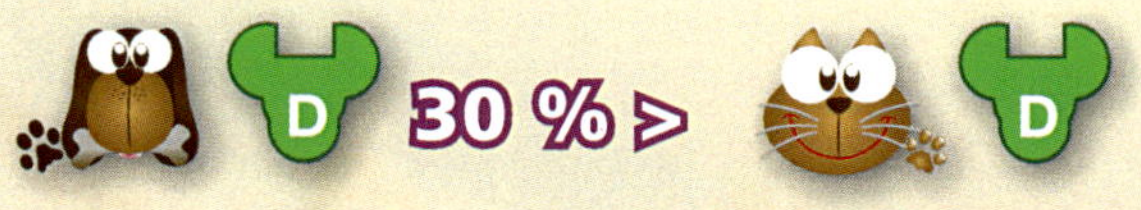

5. **Dogs modify their concentrations in sucrase and α-amylase depending on the type of food: as the proportion of disaccharides or starch increases, the activity increases.**

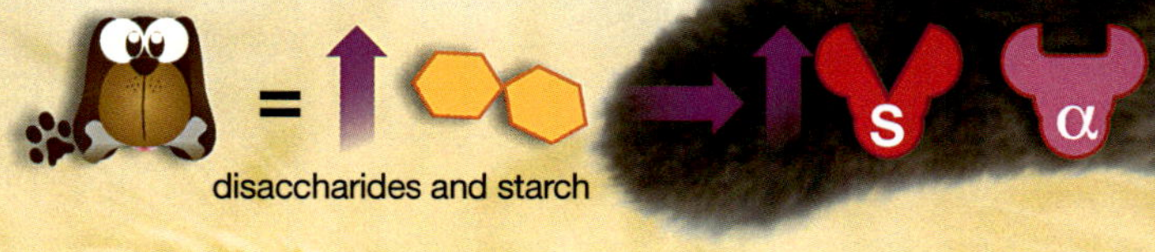

6. **Compared with dogs, cats only produce 5 % of the pancreatic amylase.**

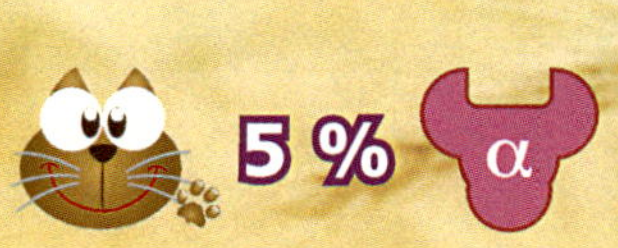

7. **In the feline intestines, the activity of the trehalase is very low (it degrades the carbohydrates of the exoskeleton of insects and of mushrooms).**

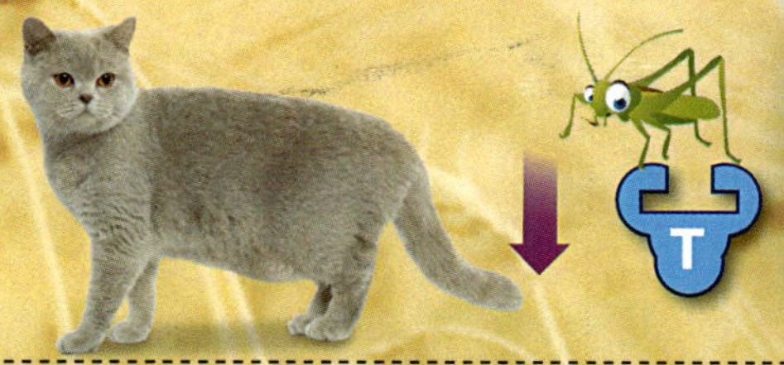

3 Source of energy and storage

The central organ for the metabolism of glucose is the liver. The synthesis, storage, transformation and liberation of glucose to the rest of the organism all take place in the liver. The insulin and glucagon hormones control these processes. The normal glucose level in plasm in healthy animals is: 70-120 mg/dl.

Once absorbed, the monosaccharides are distributed in the tissues where they will be used as a source of energy (the complete oxidation of a mole of glucose produces 38 moles of ATP) or it will be stored as glycogen, in the liver and muscles, or as long chain fatty acids in adipose tissue. In periods of fasting, under the influence of the glucagon, glycogenolysis and glyconeogenesis take place. This process is critical to maintain the homeostasis of the CNS.

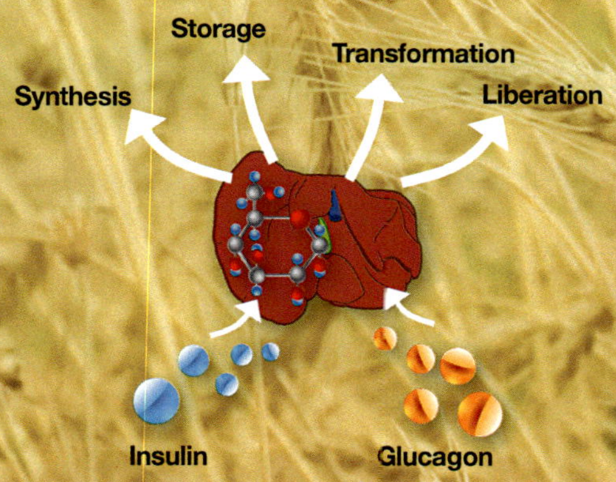

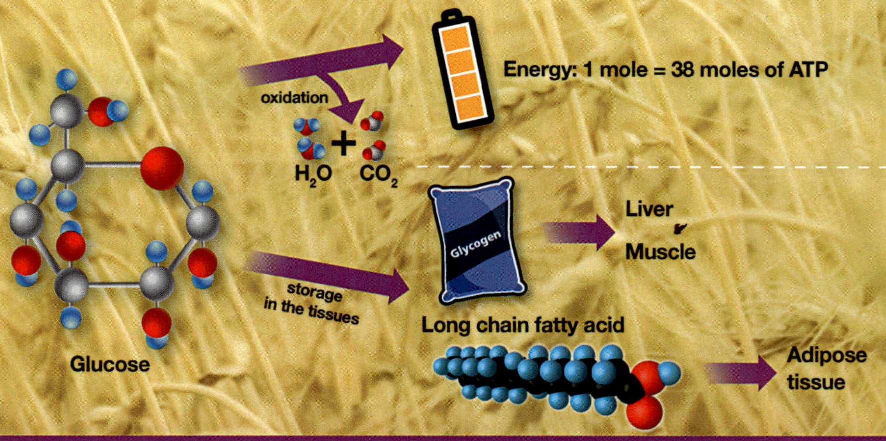

carbohydrates

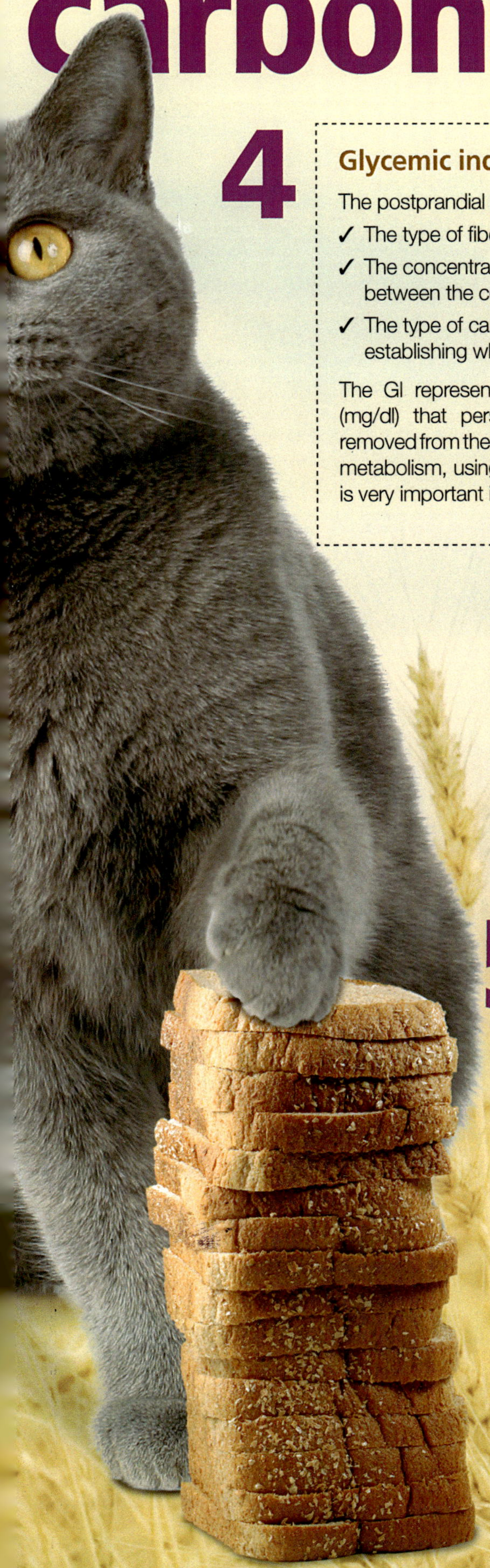

4 Glycemic index

The postprandial glycemia can be affected by:

- ✓ The type of fiber present in the food ration.
- ✓ The concentration of starch (there is a linear correlation between the content in starch and the glycemia).
- ✓ The type of carbohydrates in the food ration, establishing what is known as the glycemic index (GI).

The GI represents the quantity of postprandial glucose (mg/dl) that persists over time (minutes) before being removed from the circulation to participate in the intermediary metabolism, using glucose as a reference. Knowing the GI is very important in diabetic patients and working dogs.

It allows for us to classify the carbohydrates following this index as follows:

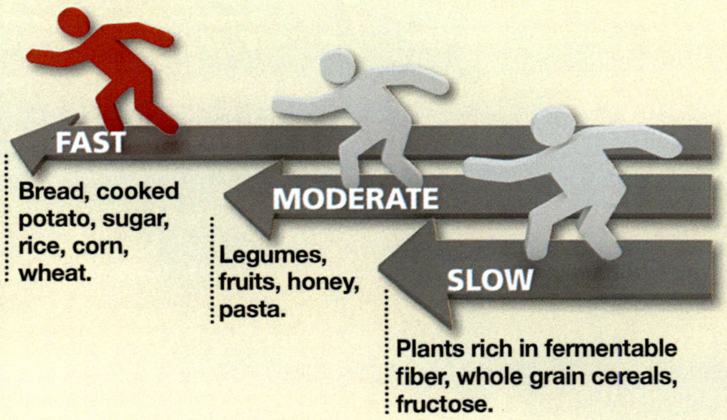

It is known that the amylose/amylopectin ratio affects the GI: a greater proportion of amylopectin leads to a greater GI. **↑% amylopectin → ↑GI**

In the case of grains (a majority ingredient in pet foods), if we classify them in increasing order according to their GI, it would be as follows:

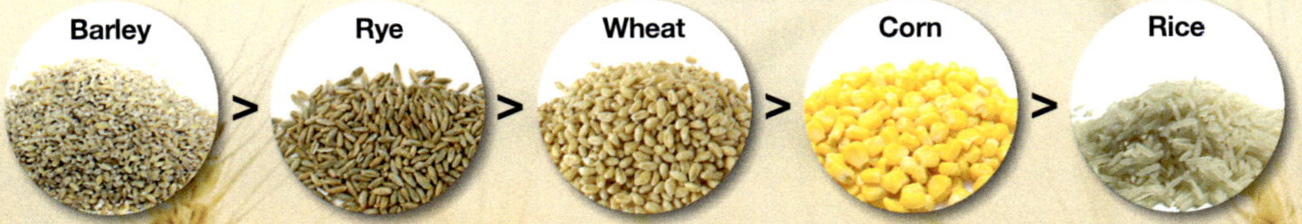

5 Prebiotics

The non-starch polysaccharides, the resistant starch and fiber, will be fermented by the microflora present in the colon. Some are beneficial to the organism because they are part of the microflora substrate and the cells of the colon. They are called prebiotics.

Most of these prebiotics are polymers of more than nine units of sugar:

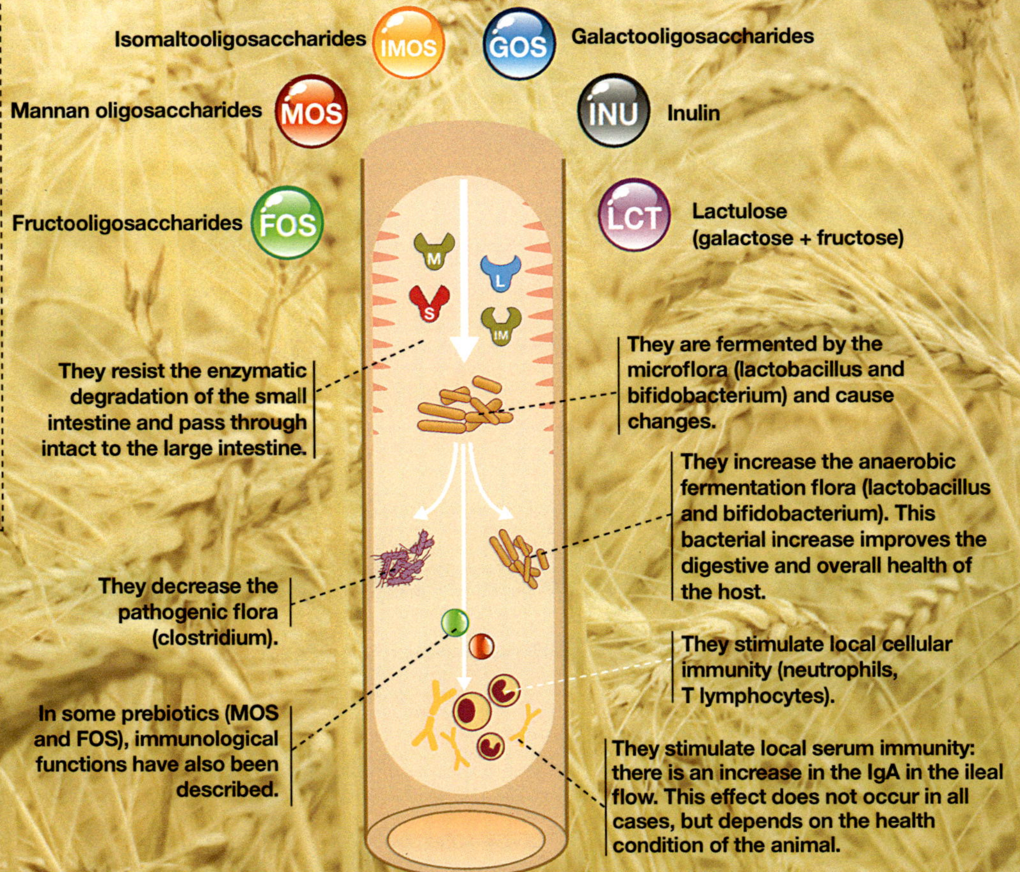

In the absence of more studies on the use of prebiotics in pets, their use in food rations for adult dogs is limited:

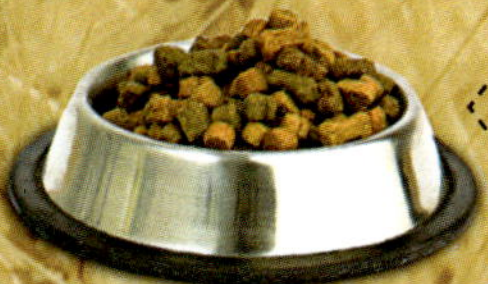

- **0.5 %** (MOS, XOS*)
- **2-4 %** (FOS)
- **<7 %** of the DM (inulin)
- **0.5-3 g** FOS/day

*Xylooligosaccharides

Fiber

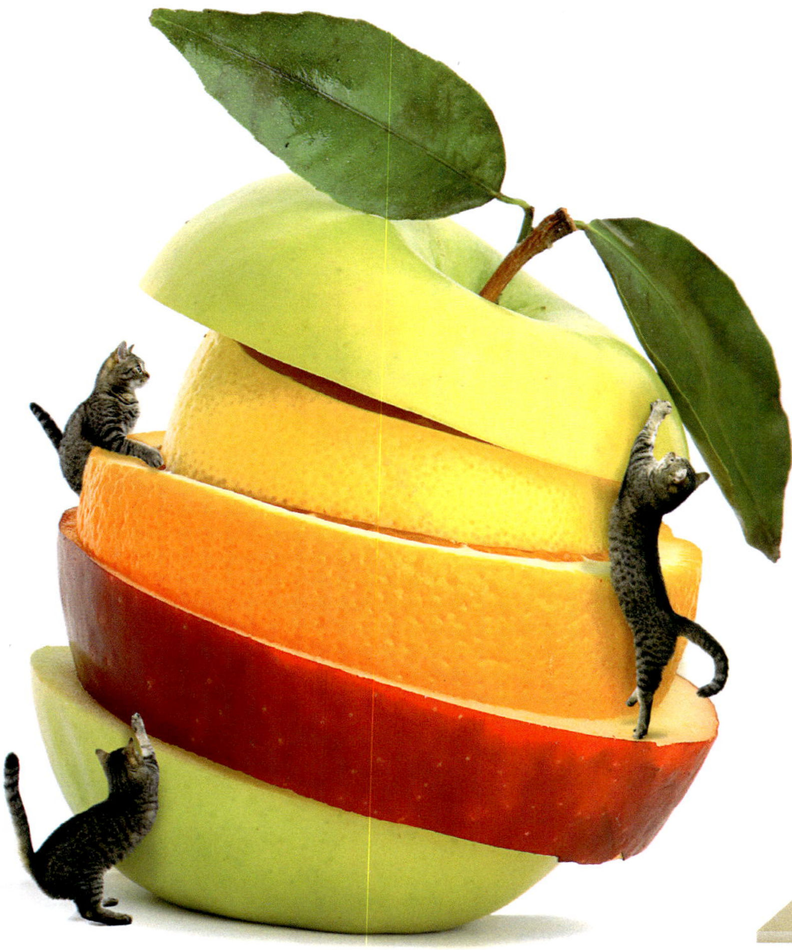

1 General characteristics

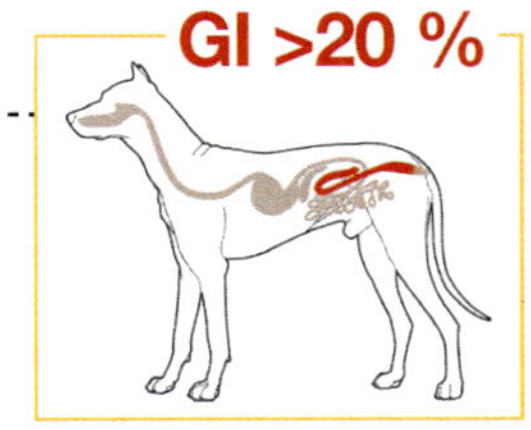

Fiber is one of the most complicated nutrients to classify and thus lacks any official definition. There is little information regarding dogs and cats as their anatomy allows for little intestinal fermentation (the large intestine represents less than 20 % of the total digestive apparatus and cecal fermentation is extremely scarce).

That said, dogs have shown to be more efficient than cats in the use of fermented carbohydrates. The digestibility of the hemicellulose and cellulose is 47 and 18 %, respectively. However, the digestibility of a mixture of fermentable (pectin)/non-fermentable fiber (cellulose) increases linearly as the concentration of pectin increases.

Fermentation has contributed to digestive health and the quality of life and life expectancy of pets. Longevity and well-being are likely the most important factors for owners. The use of fiber prevents the presentation and development of certain pathologies such as diabetes mellitus, colon carcinoma, diarrhea, constipation, and irritable bowel syndrome.

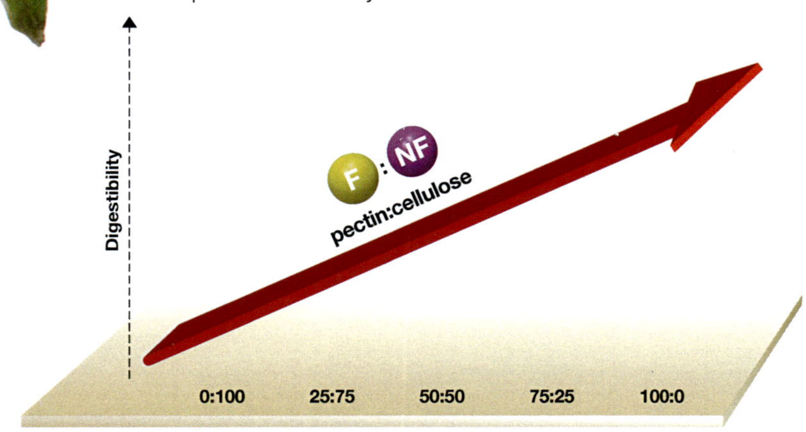

3 Functions of the fiber

Its actions within the organism include physical-chemical and physiological effects:

✔ Delay in gastric emptying (GET) and modification of the intestinal transit time (ITT)

These effects are a consequence of the fiber content or its viscosity and do not affect the motility of the stomach or the duodenum, however they do affect the muscular contractions of the proximal colon.

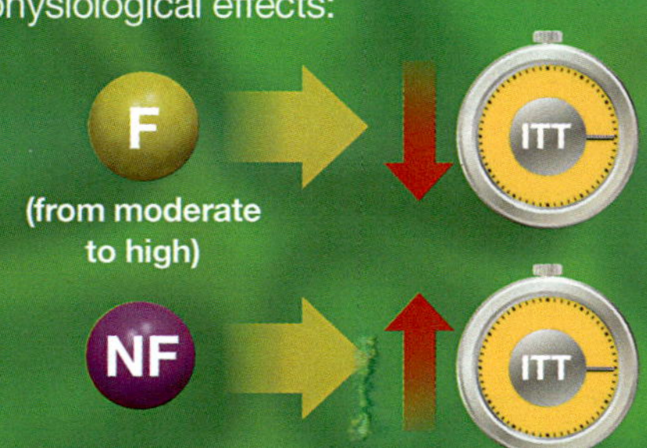

✔ Responsible for the form and effective volume of the feces

This is due to its capacity to retain water and due to the presence of microflora.

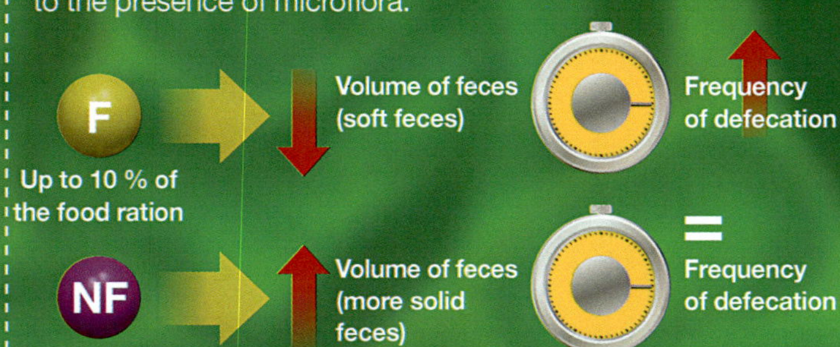

Cats are more susceptible to these changes: the incorporation of 9.5 % of fermentable fiber in their food rations causes digestive changes in the small intestine (bacterial overgrowth, reduced pancreatic exocrine activity due to the decrease in the pH and interference of the activity of the pancreatic enzymes due to increased viscosity), while in dogs, these effects can be observed with values over 10-12.5 %.

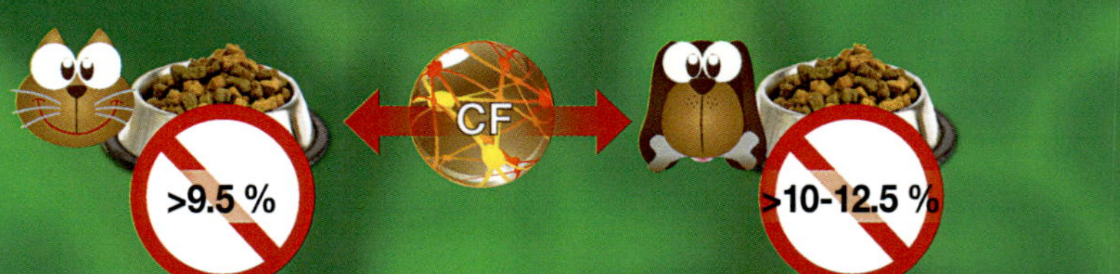

✔ They affect the bioavailability of minerals

Depending on the type and proportion of fiber, it can be increased or decreased, affecting each mineral differently. The incorporation of insoluble fiber decreases the digestibility of the organic material, protein, and ash. The availability of certain minerals –calcium, phosphorus, potassium, zinc, iron and magnesium– is increased with fermentable fiber to maximum levels of 20 g/1,000 kcal ME.

Above these values, losses are produced through feces.

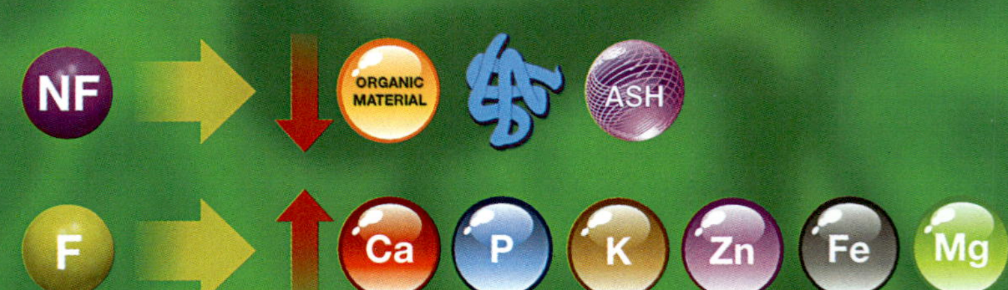

2 Classification of fiber

Fiber includes certain plant-based hydrocarbon compounds, primarily of the cellular wall, which cannot be digested by digestive enzymes:

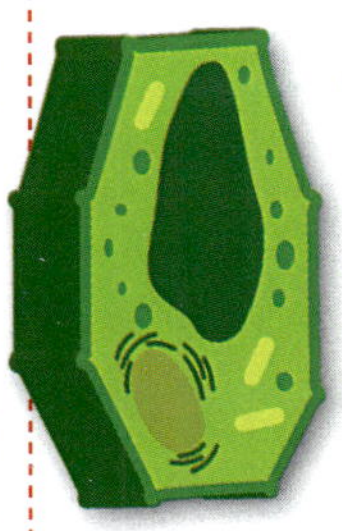

- Non-starch polysaccharides.
- Pectin.
- Hemicellulose.
- Cellulose.
- Lignin (not a carbohydrate).

Its classification depends on the following:

- Its structure.
- Solubility in water.
- Viscosity.
- Digestibility.
- Analysis technique.

According to that described, we can talk about:

- Crude fiber.
- Neutral and acidic fiber.
- Total dietary fiber.
- Soluble/insoluble.
- Fermentable/non-fermentable.

Due to the similarity of its characteristics and functions at the digestive level, we classify fiber into two large groups.
The following table summarizes the properties of the different fractions of the fiber.

F **Fermentable/soluble/viscose**

NF **Non-fermentable/insoluble/non-viscose**

Fraction	Fermentation	Solubility	Viscosity	Example
Fructans, galactans, mannans and mucilage	Fast	Soluble	High	Apple, citrus, broccoli, guar gum
Pectin	Fast/moderate	Soluble	High	Beet pulp
Hemicellulose	Moderate/slow	Insoluble	Medium	Bran
Cellulose	Slow	Insoluble	Low	Cellulose

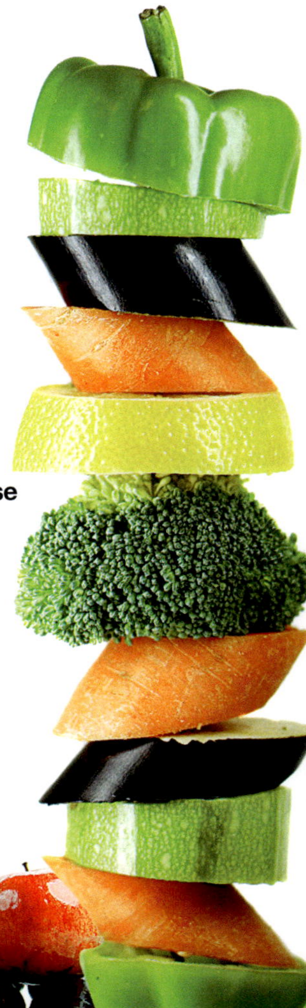

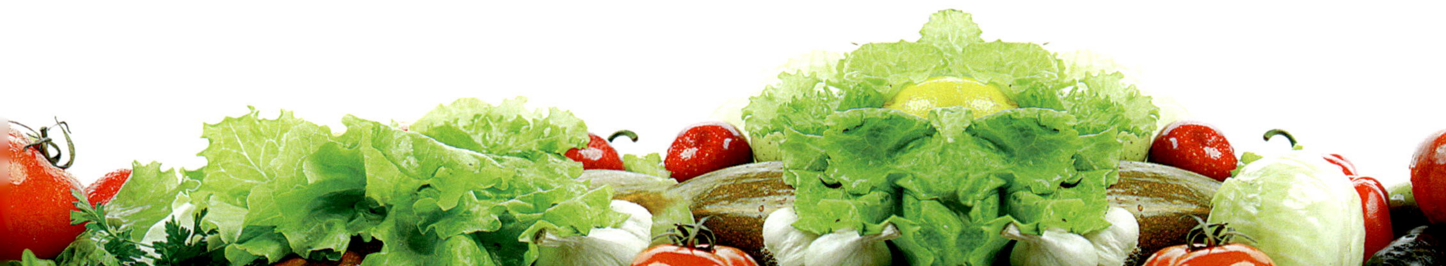

✔ Decrease in the digestibility of the nutrients

Although it has been observed that the ileal digestibility is not affected.

✔ Glycemia control

It has been observed that the gastric emptying time and the intestinal transit speed modify the levels of glucose and postprandial insulin.

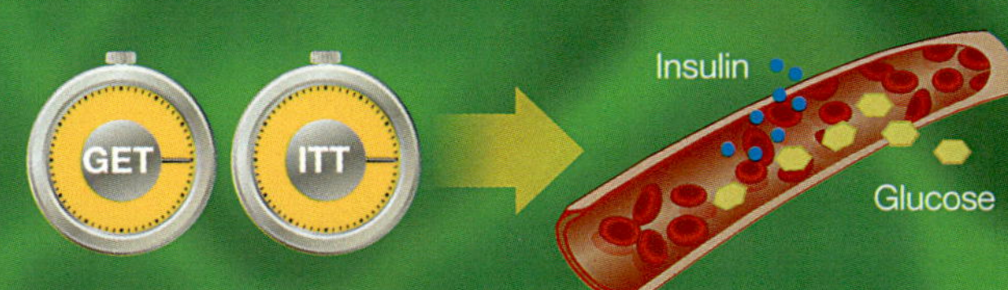

✔ Control of cholesterol in blood

This process is related to low levels of insulin (due to its activity that affects the metabolism of fats) as well as to losses of cholesterol and bile salts absorbed by the fiber that is later eliminated through the feces. The losses in bile salts increase as the fiber's capacity to ferment increases.

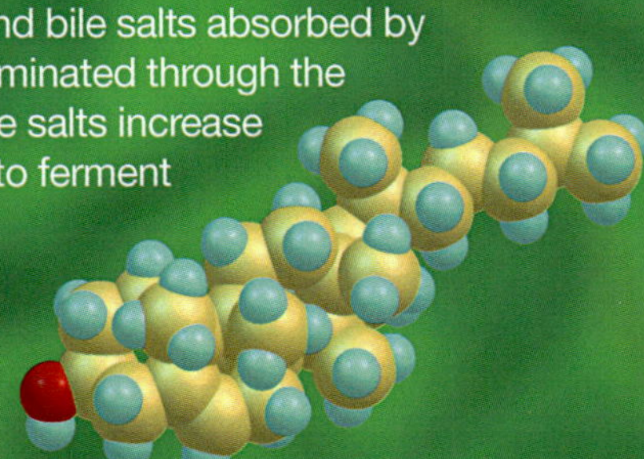

✔ Scarce energetic contribution (less than 5 % of the needs for maintenance)

The average energetic value for fermentable carbohydrates in dogs and cats has been estimated to be 1-2.4 kcal ME/g.

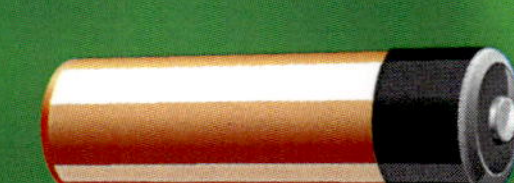

1-2.4 kcal ME/g

✔ Maintenance of body weight

It dilutes the food ration and controls the ingestion of food, satiety, and appetite. This point is very important in the management of obese patients.

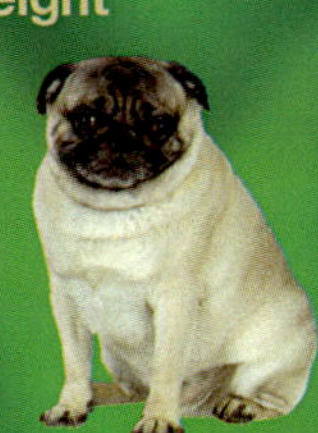

✔ Maintenance of the morphology and intestinal function, especially in the large intestine

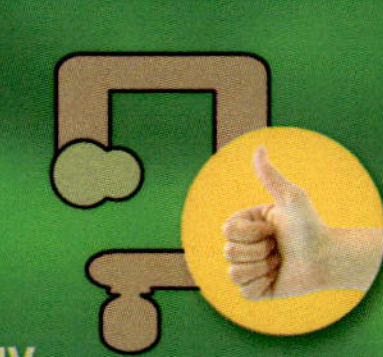

✔ It participates in the metabolism of nitrogen

Fermentation determines an increase in the number of bacteria which, in turn, use ammoniac, a product of the hydrolysis of the urea (the urea is released in the colon by circulation), in order to reproduce (synthesis of protein and nucleic acids).

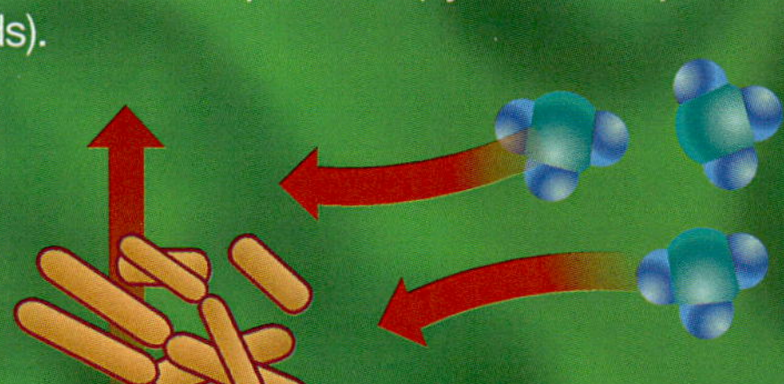

✔ Prebiotic effect on the distribution and health of the microbial population in the colon (oligosaccharides)

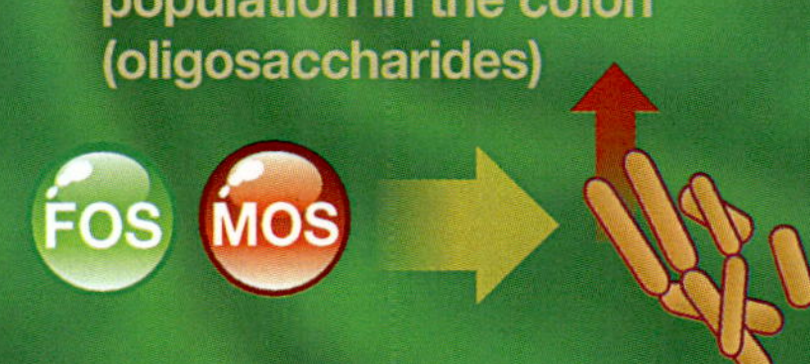

✔ Prevention of pathogenic bacterial overgrowth

The decrease in the luminal pH, due to the formation of volatile short chain fatty acids, favors the growth of anaerobics (lactobacillus and bifidobacterium) and has an antibacterial effect on the pathogenic flora (*C. perfringens*).

Metabolism for fiber

1 Metabolic pathways

Fiber is broken down in anearobic conditions by the digestive microflora (bacteria, yeast and protozoa) to obtain energy.
These microorganisms have the capacity to break the α-1,4 and β-1,4 bonds present in the different types of fiber, and to use the monosaccharides.
Each type of fiber is made of different monosaccharides:

- ✔ Cellulose: glucose.
- ✔ Hemicellulose: glucose, galactose, mannose, xylose, arabinose, and uronic acids.
- ✔ Pectin: galacturonic acid, galactose, arabinose and rhamnose.

Without providing excessive details, pectin, hemicellulose, and pentosans use uronic acid and phosphate pentose pathways to obtain glucose. Pyruvate is then obtained through glycolysis. Cellulose uses this pathway directly. By breaking down pyruvate, and depending on the metabolic pathway followed, different fatty acids are obtained that serve as a substrate for the host organism.

The metabolic pathways of acetyl CoA, acetoacetyl CoA, lactate and oxaloacetate produce acetic acid, butyric acid and propionic acid, respectively. Between 90 and 95 % of these acids are absorbed.

Acetic and propionic acids are used by the striated muscle and by the hepatic cells as a source of energy, while the colonocytes use butyric acid as a source of energy (better than glucose or amino acids).

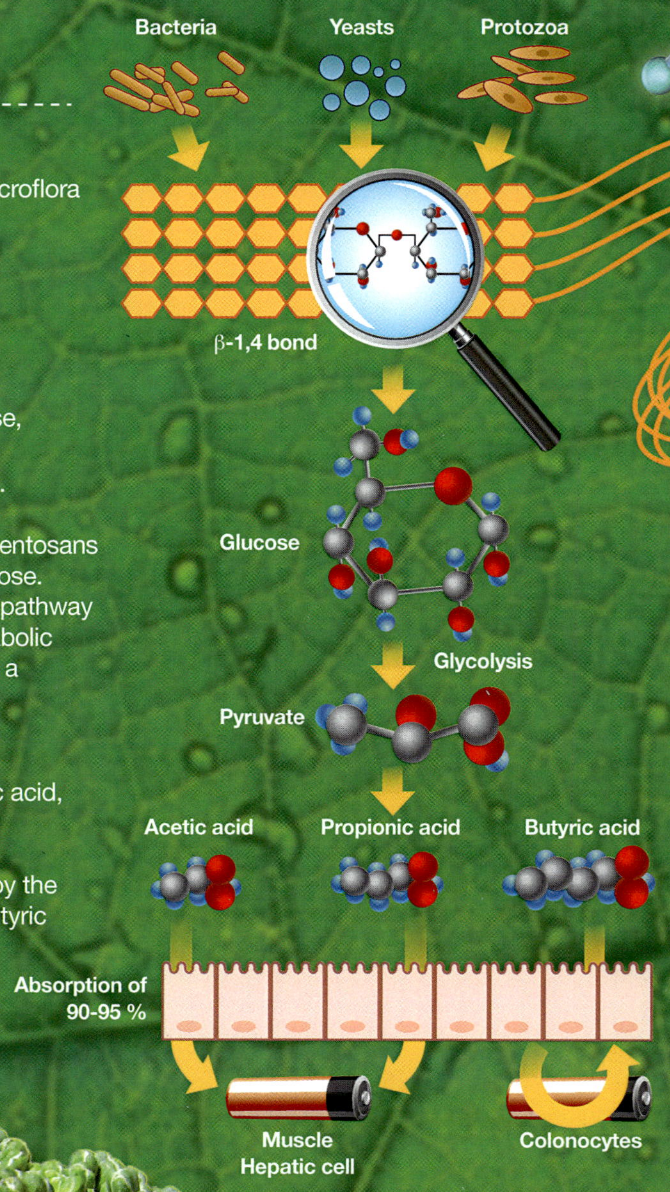

Clinical application

The clinical importance of fiber resides in those patients where the digestive physiology is affected or whose nutrition needs must be controlled or restricted. Its use should follow certain limitations: percentage of use, fermentable/non-fermentable ratio and viscosity. The use of one type of fiber or another will be determined by the physiological effect desired.

Function	Fermentable fiber (soluble)	Non-fermentable fiber (insoluble)
Gastric emptying	Delayed	Delayed. No effect
Intestinal transit velocity	Increased	Decreased
Intestinal transit time	Decreased	Increased
Digestibility of nutrients	Decreases protein	Decreases dry material and protein
Bioavailability of minerals	Increased	Decreases ash
Moisture in feces	Increased	Increased
Volume of feces	Increased	Increased
No. of defecations	Increased in cats. No effect in dogs.	Increased
Production of volatile fatty acids (VFA)	Increased	Slightly increased
Trophic effect in the colon	Increased	No effect
Prebiotic effect	Yes	No
Glycemia control	Yes	No

and requirements

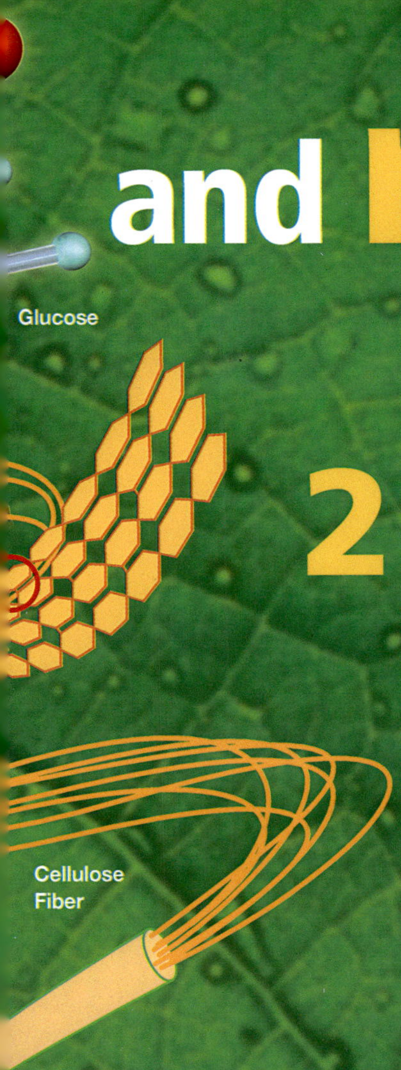

They depend on various factors:
- ✓ Animal species.
- ✓ Type of fiber.
- ✓ Quantity of food (as DM) consumed.
- ✓ Energetic density of the food ration.
- ✓ Daily energy requirements.

2 Fiber requirements in pets

Specific optimal or maximum levels have not been established for the incorporation of fiber to improve health without affecting digestibility, although a few examples are available of the upper safety limits:

Type of fiber (g/kg DM)		
Cellulose	94	100
Cellulose:pectin (3:1)	83	83
Fructooligosaccharides	40	7.5
Guar gum	34	Not available
Inullin	70	Not available
Tomato juice	87	Not available
Mannan-oligosaccharides	5.9	Not available
Pectin	34	Not available
Beet pulp	75	Not available
Wheat bran	128	100

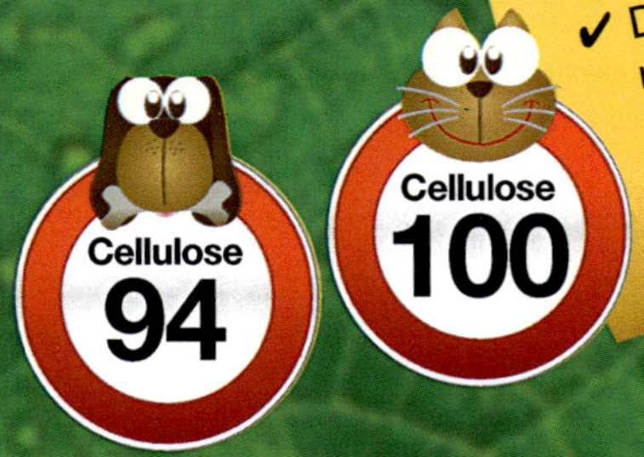

The question about the adequate fermentable (soluble)/non-fermentable (insoluble) ratio and the viscosity to ensure good quality feces and not affect the digestibility of the nutrients is also considered.

In healthy adult animals, the incorporation of 37-50 g of dietary fiber/1,000 kcal ME (15-20 % of the DM in a food of 4,000 kcal ME/kg DM) is an adequate value, with a 17-20 % of fermentable fiber. Examples of this type of "ideal" fiber are: beet pulp or bran from grains.

Ingredients or mixtures of pectin, hemicellulose, and cellulose are currently used that provide moderate fermentation.

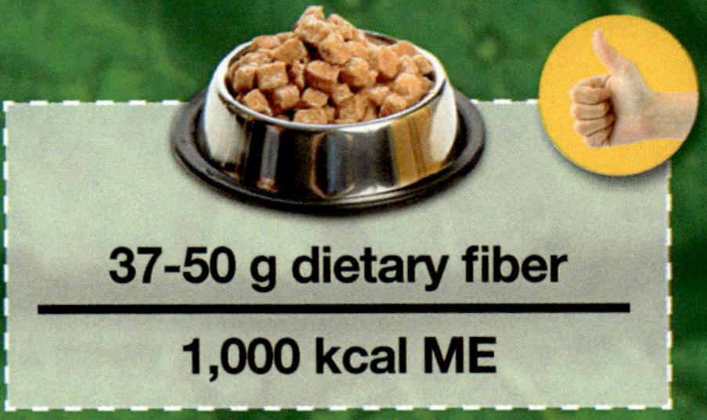

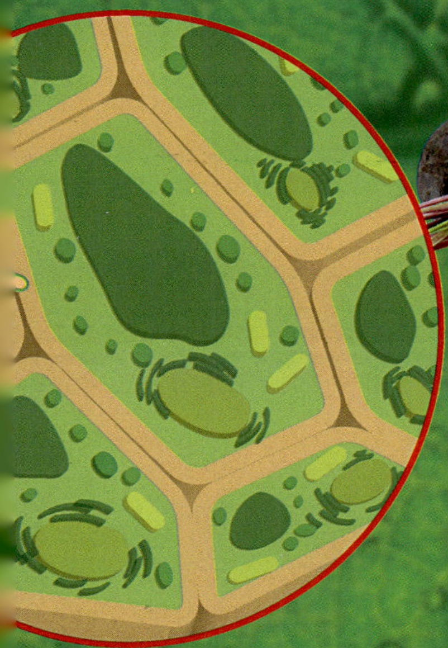

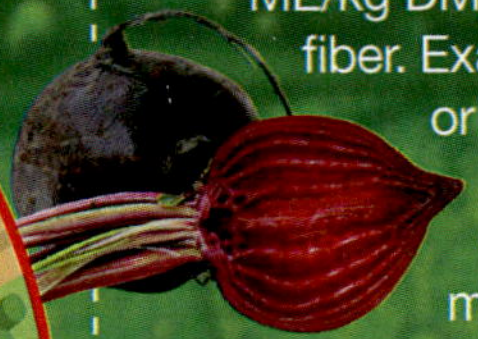

Most of the dry foods usually include levels of crude fiber (CF), hemicellulose, and cellulose, from 2.5 % to 4.5 % of the DM (food of 4,000 kcal ME/kg DM), with higher amounts in specific foods for the treatment of obesity, diabetes, digestive cancer, or chronic kidney failure. This expression changes over time given that the CF underestimates the real content in non-digestible carbohydrates: CF includes 5 to 20 % of the total fiber found in the food.

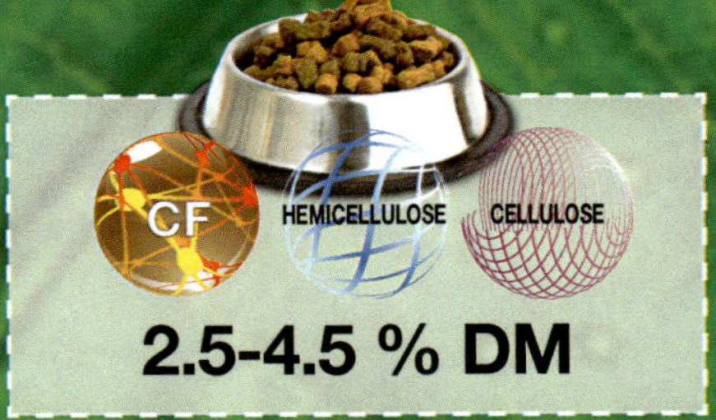

Using the term **total dietary fiber** (TDF) is more correct, specifying its characteristics, due to its implications in the digestive physiology and overall health. A few examples:

Ingredient	CF (%)*	TDF (%)*	Solubility	Fermentation	Viscosity
Peanut shell	57	w76	Insoluble	Slow	No
Cellulose	80	98	Insoluble	Slow	No
Guar gum or gum arabic	0	80-90	Soluble	Fast	Yes
Apple (pectin)	0	95	Soluble	Fast	Yes
Citrus pulp	12	77	Soluble	Fast	Yes
Beet pulp	20	66	Insoluble	Moderate	No
Rice bran	44	13	Insoluble	Moderate	No
Soy bran	20	83	Soluble	Fast	No
Wheat bran	10	43	Insoluble	Moderate	No

* As an ingredient; TDF: total dietary fiber.

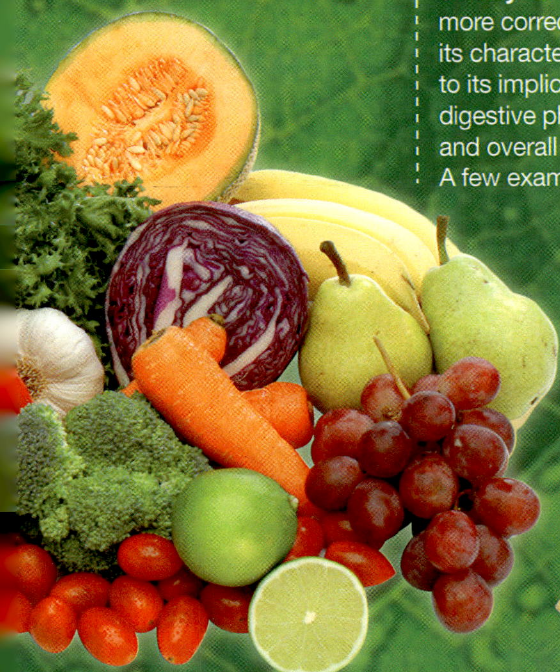

The extrusion process reduces the molecule size of the fiber and redistributes the insoluble/soluble ratio so that the solubility of the substrates increases, which in turn increases the ileal digestibility, and the production of short chain VFA (SCFA) is reduced.

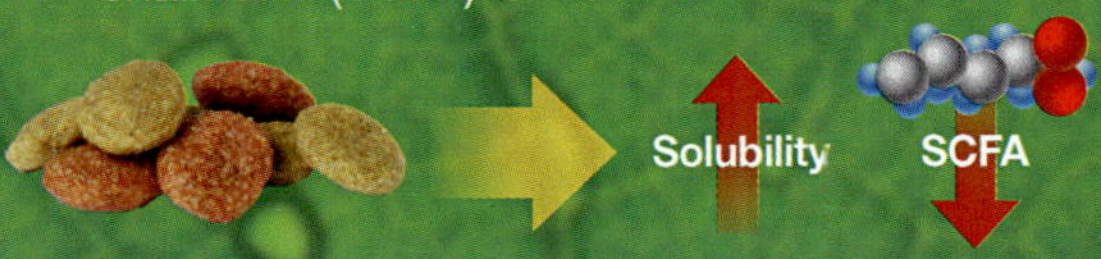

In wet foods, guar gum, from carrageenans, etc., is used in concentrations lower than 5 % of the DM as gelling agents.

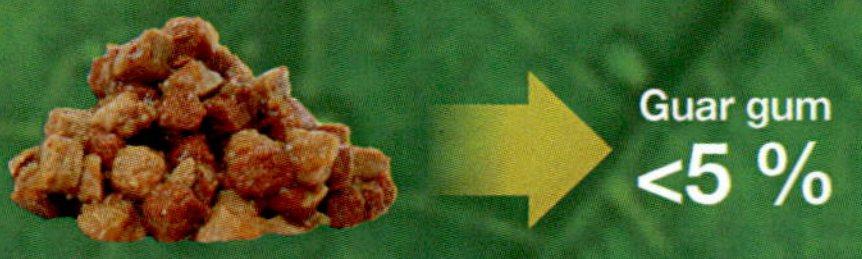

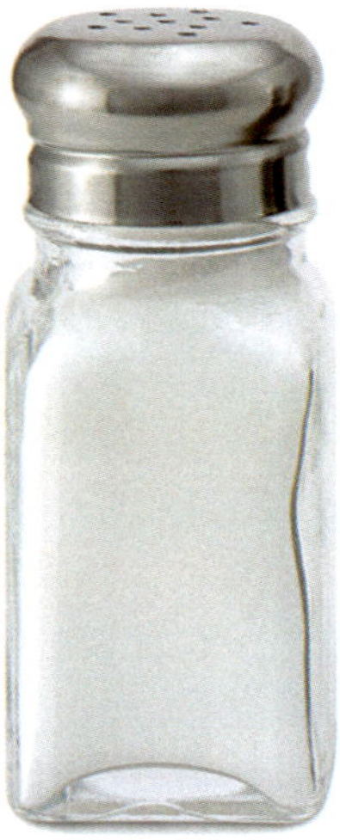

Factors that affect for vitamins

There are various concepts that explain an animal's requirements for vitamins (or other micronutrients such as minerals) based on the relationship between ingestion, their interactions, storage, their biological response, and the species (dogs or cats). It has to do with the sufficiency criteria (unlike in food-producing animals, in pets, it is not very highly developed), the dose-response curve and the pathophysiological model of response to a nutrient, the interactions and the differences between species.

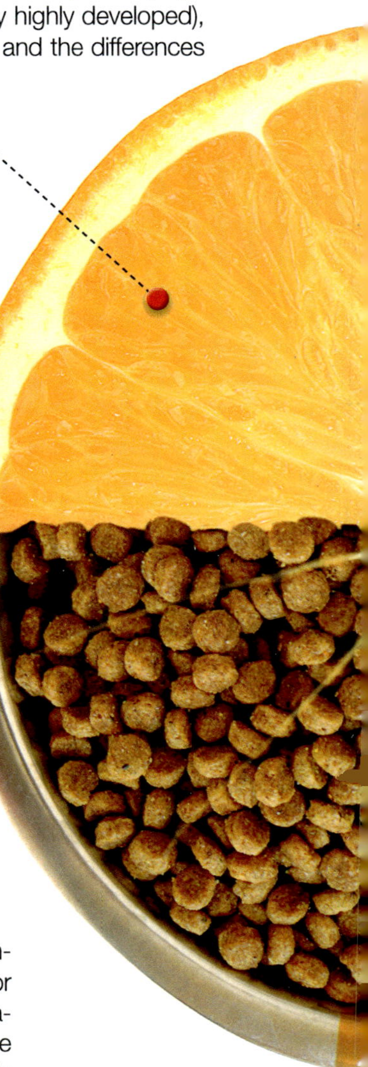

1 Differences between species

In adult cats, their requirements for certain vitamins, such as niacin, pyridoxine, and vitamin A and D are higher than in dogs due to metabolic reasons.

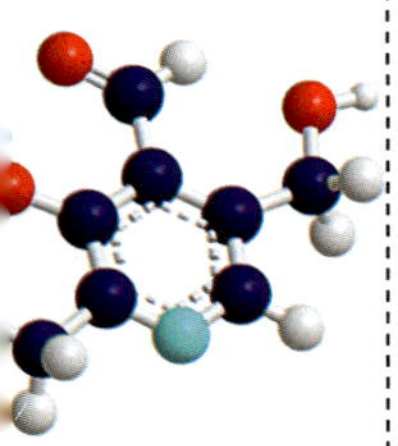

Pyridoxine

Pyridoxine is a co-enzyme of the reactions that take place in the amino acid metabolism (transamination and decarboxylation), which is higher and constantly active in cats.

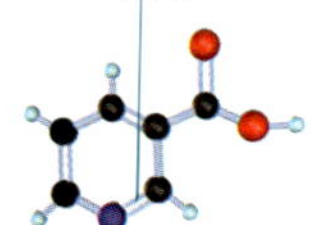

Niacin

Cats, as well as dogs, can synthesize niacin by means of tryptophan, but their requirements are much higher than their capacity to synthesize and the rate of degradation of the precursors is higher.

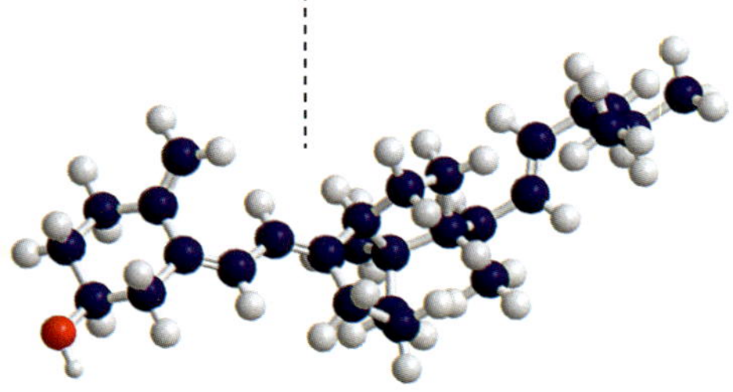

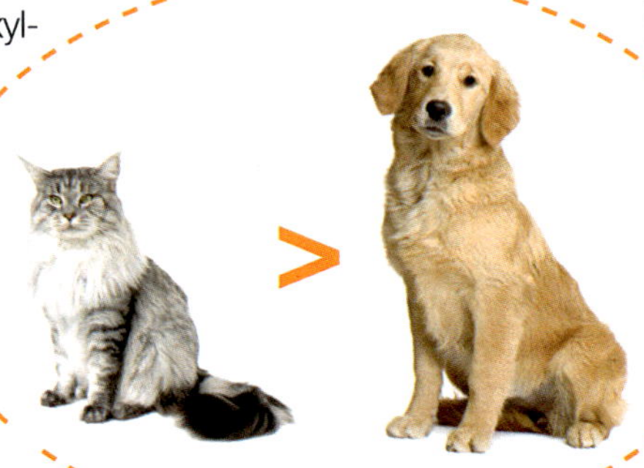

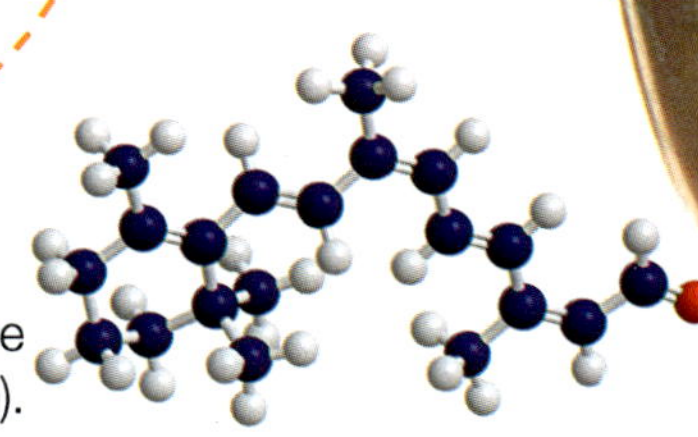

Vitamin D

The active form (D_3 or cholecalciferol) is found in animal tissues. It can be synthesized from its precursors under the influence of UV light (λ 290-315 nm). From there, it suffers two hydroxylations, in the liver and kidneys, to become the active form. Cats and dogs lack 7-dehydrocholesterol (due to the fact that there is a high level of activity of the 7-dehydrocholesterol reductase that rapidly converts its substrate into cholesterol), the precursor of cholecalciferol that is found in skin, and also, cats use the D_2 form (ergocalciferol) poorly. For this reason, both species need the active form of this vitamin. Regarding UV radiation, its light range must be taken into account in cases where the dogs ingest the precursors and live in artificially lit environments.

Vitamin A

Cats lack the monooxygenase that is responsible for the conversion of pro-vitamins (β-carotenes) into the active form of vitamin A (only present in animal tissues).

3 Dose-response curve

The dose-response curve represents the optimal dose (area between the minimum and maximum needs) and its limits. There are two areas under the curve that provide us with information on certain safety zones: the left marginal limit (of deficiency) and the upper marginal limit (of toxicity). The size of this marginal area depends on the nutrient's storage capacity. Observing the curve, we can see that there are differences between the types of vitamins according to their metabolism. Liposoluble vitamins are stored, and therefore it is rare that there are issues of deficiencies; this same characteristic favors their toxicity. In the water-soluble vitamins, the opposite is true.

Regardless of the interactions with the nutrients found in the pet's food rations, the curve moves to the left or the right depending on its chemical structure, and therefore, its bioavailability. If the latter is low, the curve will move to the right, and we will need a greater concentration to reach the same function. Not all compounds have the same activity:

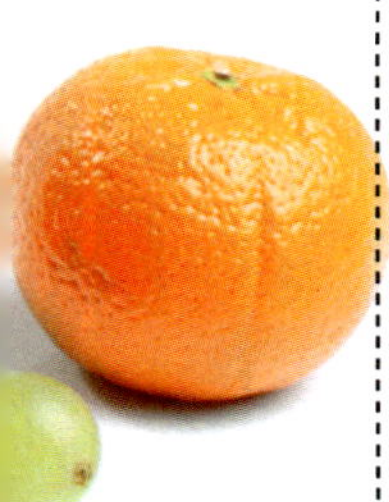

- ✓ γ, β and δ-tocopherol do not have the same biological activity as vitamin E or α-tocopherol, however they do act as an antioxidant in the foods.
- ✓ The ionic charge affects the solubility and the permeability of different transition minerals: those with a charge of 3+ are more stable than those with a charge of 2+.
- ✓ The chemical form (the organic forms are better used than the inorganic ones): Zn proteinate or propionate have better availability than Zn oxide, and Fe methionine has greater availability than Fe oxide.

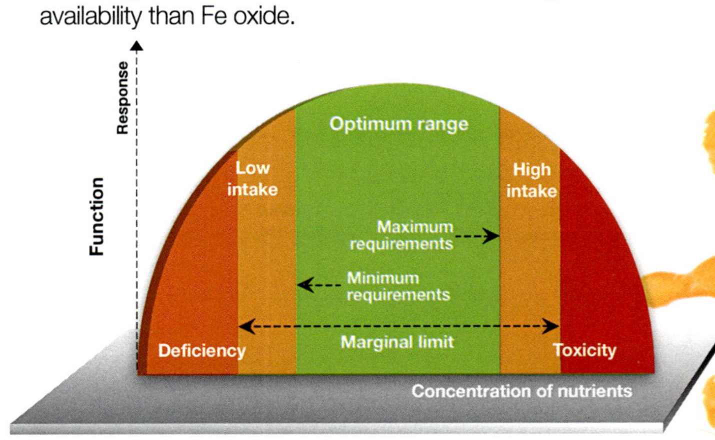

requirements and minerals

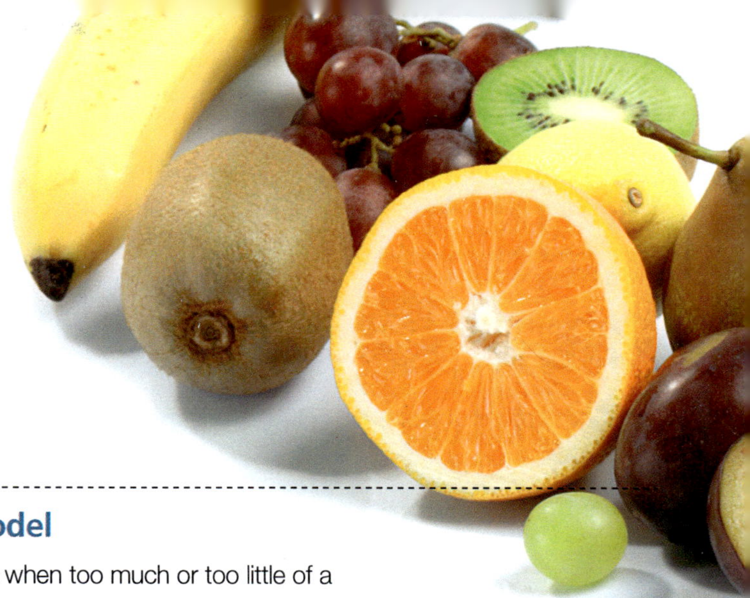

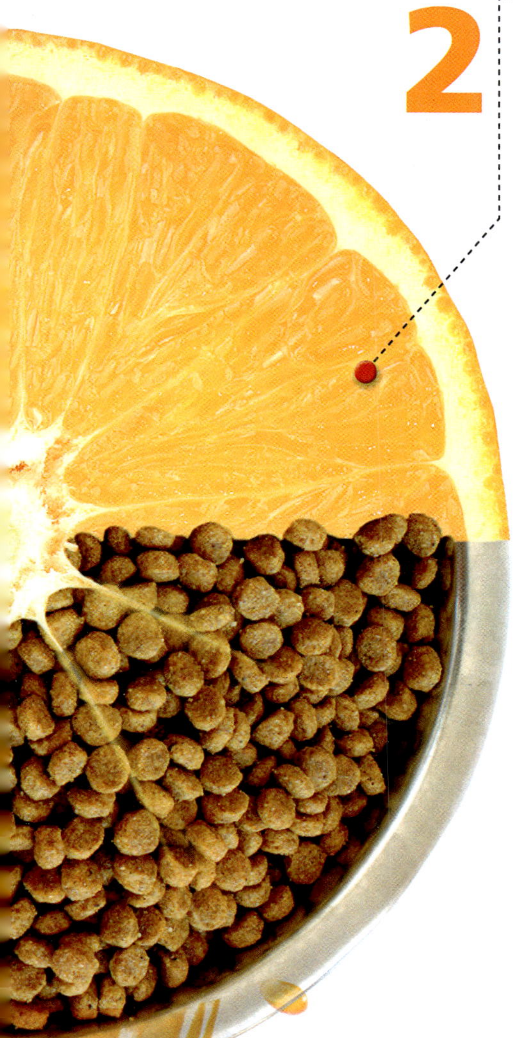

2 Pathophysiological response model

This model attempts to explain what happens when too much or too little of a nutrient is ingested.

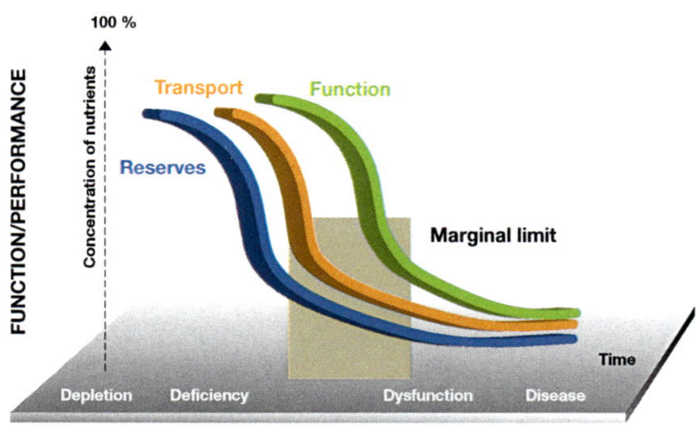

Pathophysiological response model

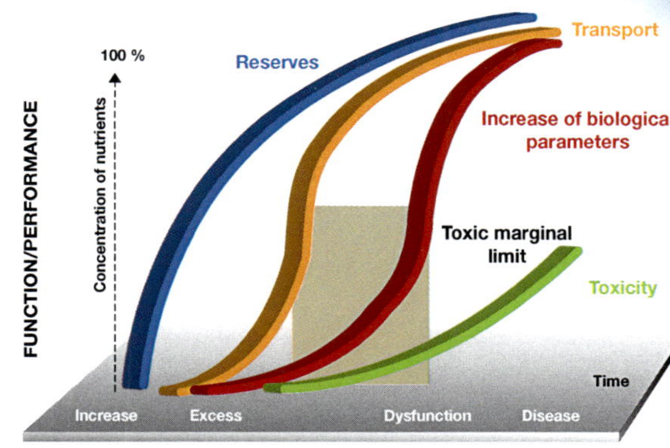

Pathophysiological response model

The area marked as the marginal limit, similar to the dose-response curve, represents the point where the functions begin to fail but without any clinical signs or symptoms. In the equilibrium and depletion phase, the use of a supplement has no effect on the animal. However, in the other phases, supplements offer possible or probable positive responses to the deficiencies. Example:

Vitamin	Cause	Depletion/ increase	Deficiency/ excess	Dysfunction	Disease/ poisoning
Vitamin D	Kidney or liver affectation. Low level of ingestion.	↓ Hepatic and renal reserves, fat.	↓ Vitamin D_3 in plasma.	Affectation of the metabolism of calcium. Osteodystrophy. Secondary hyperparathyroidism.	Fractures. Affectation of face bones.
Copper	Hereditary defect in Terriers.	↑ Hepatic reserves.	↑ ASAT, ↑ Cu in plasma.	Liver dysfunction.	Vomiting. Hemolysis. Death.

When we suspect a deficiency, from a practical point of view, we usually draw upon the use of a synthesis supplement that reverts the clinical process. Confirmation of the diagnosis will depend on laboratory analyses. We will have to send blood, plasma, urine or tissue (liver biopsy) samples to evaluate the vitamin or mineral, the intermediate substrates of its activity or the activity of certain enzymes of which they are co-enzymes.

The curve can also be affected by certain antagonists of the vitamins and minerals that interfere in its activity. Their effects are due to the following:

- ✓ Inactivation: the thiaminases degrade the thiamin. They are present in raw fish and plants of the *Pteridium* genus (ferns): important in cats.
- ✓ Competition for the same receptors: dicoumarol, found in rodenticides (responsible for episodes of vitamin K deficiency), competes with vitamin K for the enzyme responsible for the synthesis of prothrombin or coagulation factor II.
- ✓ Substitution by a similar structure: avidin, found in egg whites, competes with biotin.
- ✓ Inhibition: certain anti-fungal agents (derived from imidazole) and chemotherapy agents (anphotericin B) uptake the biological precursor of vitamin D_2.
- ✓ Inhibition and increase of the absorption of certain minerals due to the presence of vitamins: vitamin C modifies the luminal pH favoring the absorption of Fe but inhibiting that of Cu. There is a change in the solubility.
- ✓ The Na and K cations have a low affinity to form covalent bonds with carbohydrates, unlike the cations with a charge of 2+ (Ca, Mg and Fe).
- ✓ Phytates and fiber in pets' food rations form insoluble compounds with the Ca and Zn. For example, 5 % of beet pulp reduces the bioavailability of the Zn, Ca, Fe and P by between 60 and 50 %.

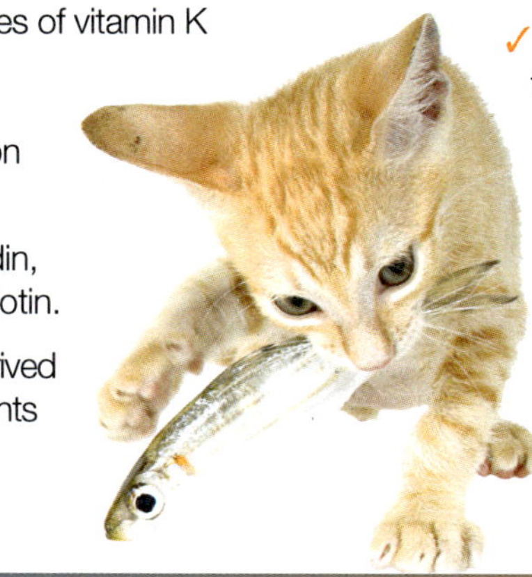

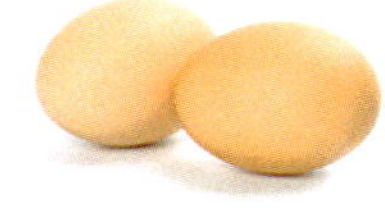

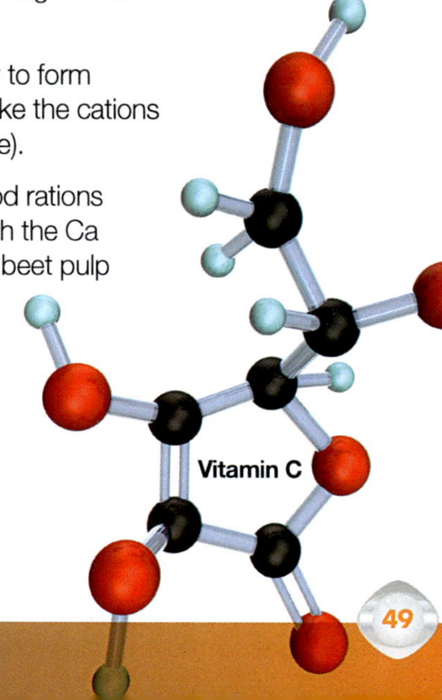

Vitamins

1 Definition and exceptions

Vitamins are a complex group of organic compounds with chemical characteristics that are different from carbohydrates, proteins and fats. They are not found in the body but are obtained through the ingestion of food, with functions that affect the metabolism (catalyzers) and are needed only in very small quantities (µg or µg per day) to ensure homeostasis.

The exception is presented by the following:

- ✓ Choline, as it is synthesized in the liver, high concentrations are needed (1 g per day) and its function is structural (it is a membrane transporter, forming part of the membranes, and it is also a neurotransmitter).
- ✓ Certain endogenously synthesized vitamins (e.g. vitamin C, K and niacin).

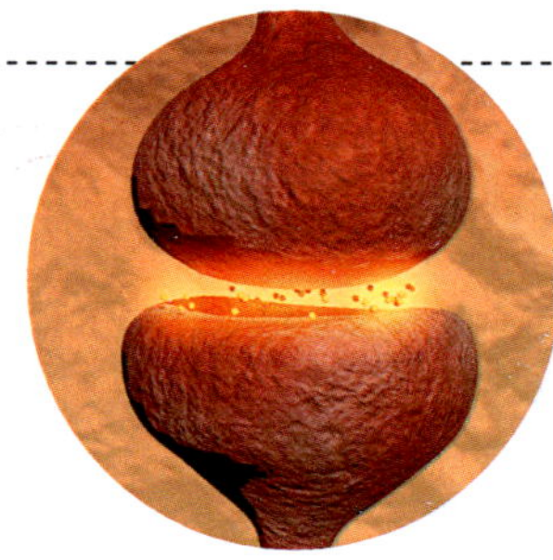

Acetylcholine

2 Classification

Traditionally, vitamins have been classified according to their solubility in water or in fat.

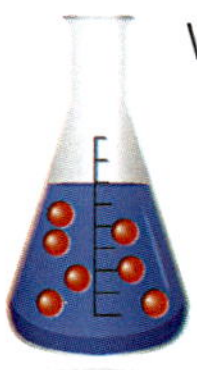

Water-soluble vitamins:

Vit. C · Choline · B group Vit. · Biotin · Folic acid

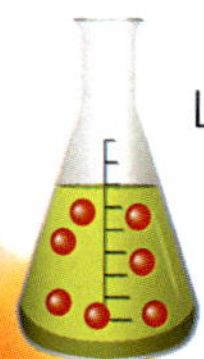

Liposoluble vitamins:

Vit. A · Vit. D · Vit. E · Vit. K

Almost all of them are considered essential with certain exceptions depending on the species:

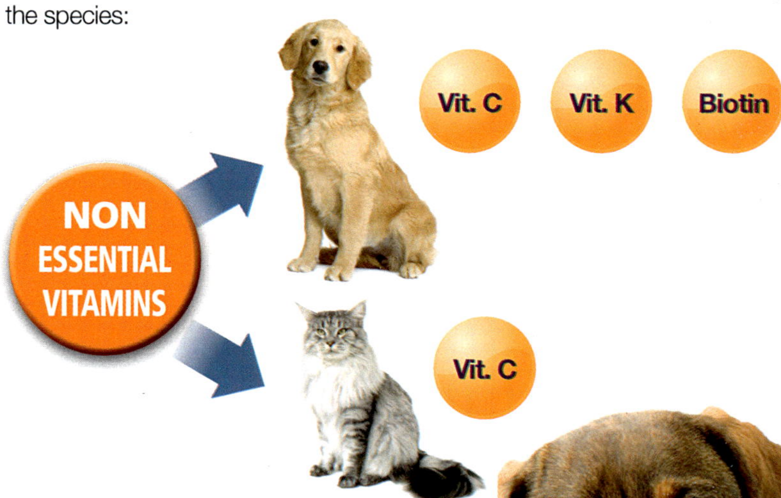

Problems caused by ingestion are very rare when the foods comply with the manufacturing guarantees.

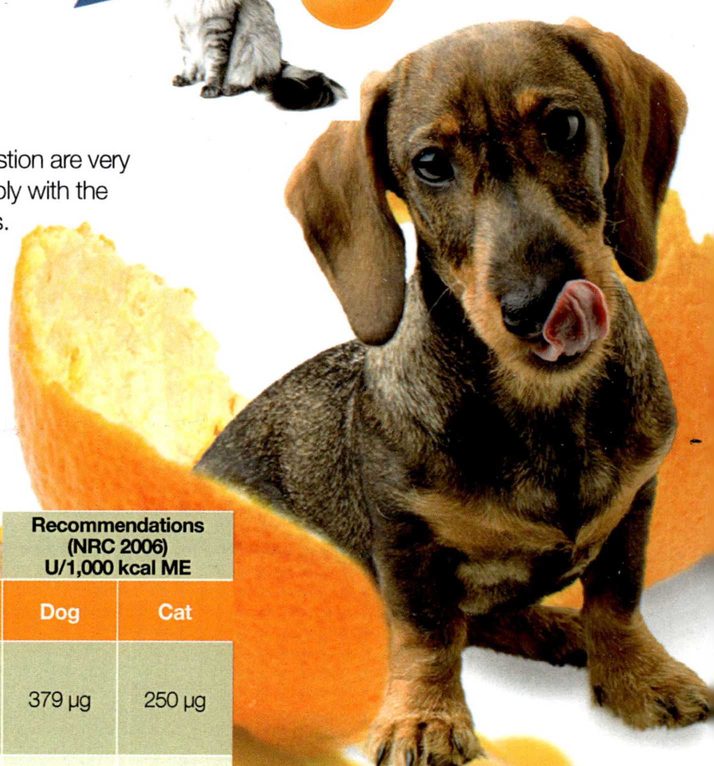

Functions, sample type for analysis and recommendations of the principal vitamins

Name and active form	Functions	Sample for diagnosis	Recommendations (NRC 2006) U/1,000 kcal ME: Dog	Cat
Trans-retinol (A)	Vision proteins. Differentiation of epithelium. Spermatogenesis. Bone resorption.	Urine: retinol	379 µg	250 µg
Dihydroxycholecalciferol, cholecalciferol, calcitriol (D_3)	Metabolism of calcium and phosphorus. Mineralization and bone resorption. Synthesis of insulin. Immune system.	Plasma: calcitriol	3.4 µg	1.75 µg
α-tocopherol (E)	In vivo antioxidant. Stabilizes biomembranes.	Tissue biopsies	7.5 mg	10 mg
Menadione (K)	Formation of fibrin: it acts on factors II, VII, IX and X. Bone mineralization (synthesis of osteocalcin).	Urine: menadione	No	0.25 mg
Thiamine (B_1)	Detoxification of CNS Krebs cycle.	Blood: transketolase	0.56 mg	1.4 mg
Riboflavin (B_2)	Component of the FAD and FMN.	Blood: glutathione-reductase Urine: riboflavin	1.3 mg	1 mg

3 Metabolism

The absorption of vitamins is intimately related with their nature:

Liposoluble vitamins: These vitamins need fat and bile salts to be digested as micelage. They are absorbed passively in the duodenum and ileum and transported by lipoproteins by means of the lymphatic system to the liver, where they are stored and distributed throughout the body, bound again to transportation lipoproteins. Some suffer modifications to their structure in other organs (e.g., the kidneys) before turning into their active form. Any excess is usually accumulated in fat and parenchymatous organs (especially in the liver).

- ✓ **Vitamin E:** This vitamin represents a special case: the concentration in all of the tissues is linear regarding its ingestion, while most vitamins present differences between different tissues and the hepatic storage. Another part can be eliminated through feces and urine.

Water-soluble vitamins: these vitamins use passive (high concentrations) or active (low concentrations) absorption and transportation systems, bound to certain transporting proteins or dependent on sodium, with the participation of ATP. Any excess is eliminated through feces and urine.

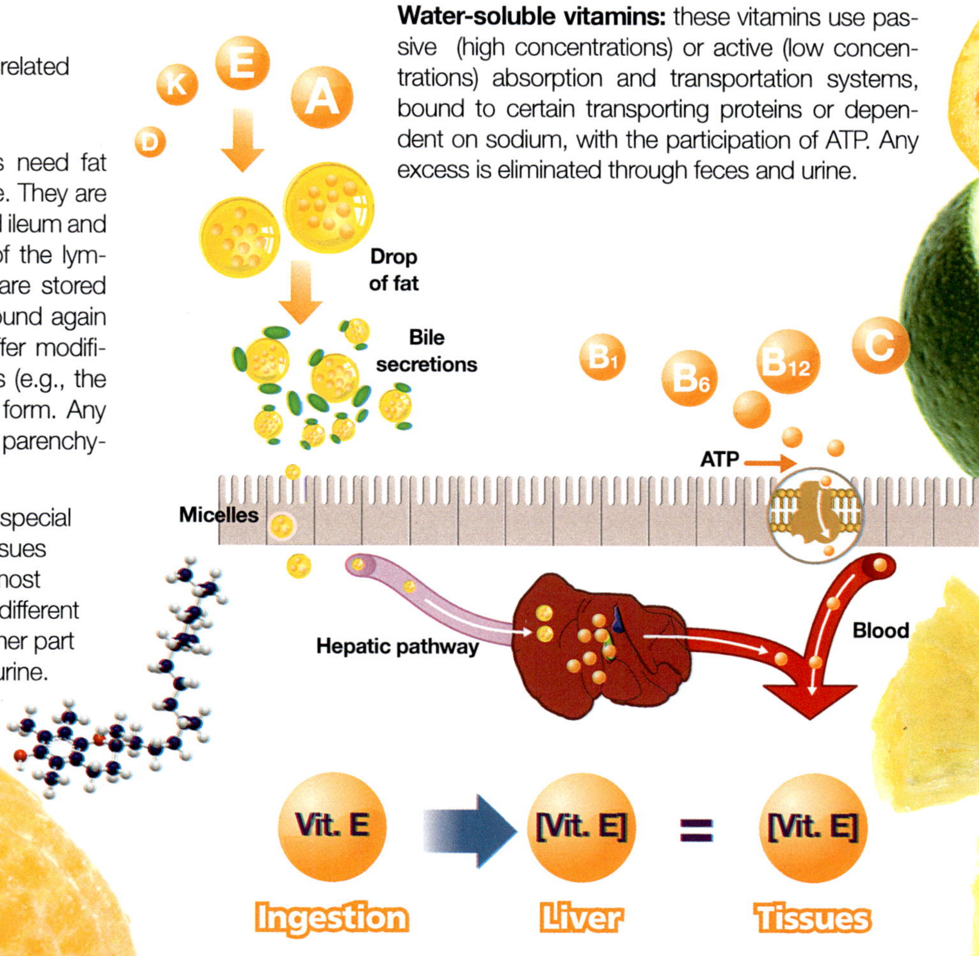

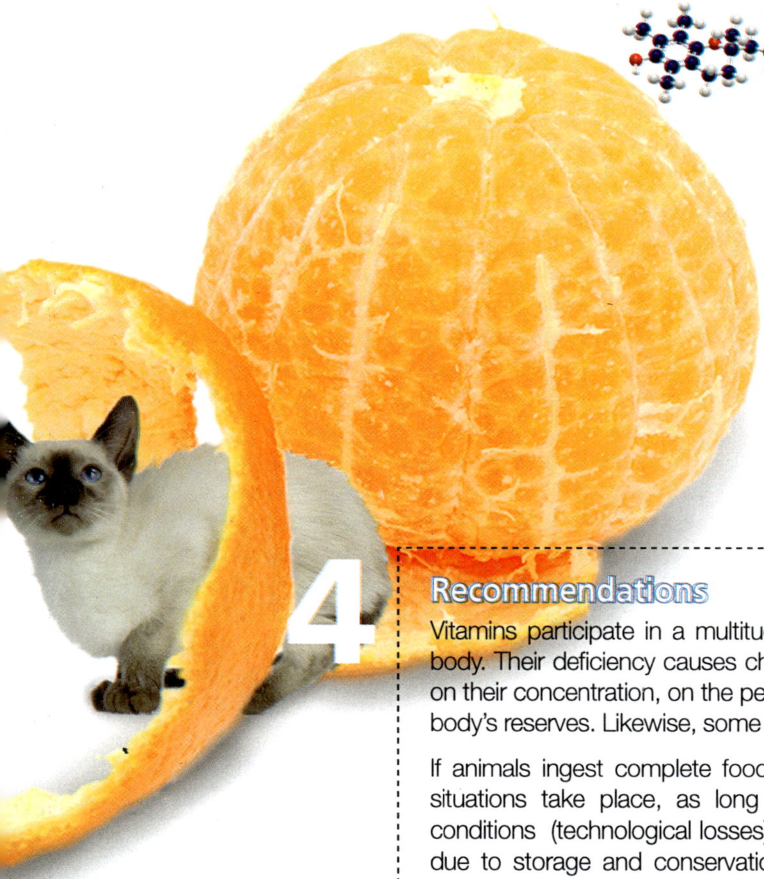

Taking into account the metabolism of the vitamins, the pathologies that affect their synthesis (the effects of antibiotics on microflora), absorption (hepatic and pancreatic affectation), metabolism (hepatic and renal affectation) and their excretion (endocrine pathologies that present with diuresis) affect the requirements of the patients.

4 Recommendations

Vitamins participate in a multitude of processes in the body. Their deficiency causes changes that will depend on their concentration, on the period of time, and on the body's reserves. Likewise, some of them may be toxic.

If animals ingest complete foods, it is rare that these situations take place, as long as the manufacturing conditions (technological losses) and those of use (loss due to storage and conservation) are respected. The foods that comply with guarantee protocols (e.g. AAFCO, CVMA and FEDIAF) are compensated, with values slightly higher than those recommended by the NRC 2006 for vitamins and minerals, and they cover the recommendations for the species and physiological condition. Supplementing the daily food rations is not therefore necessary for pets without any pathologies.

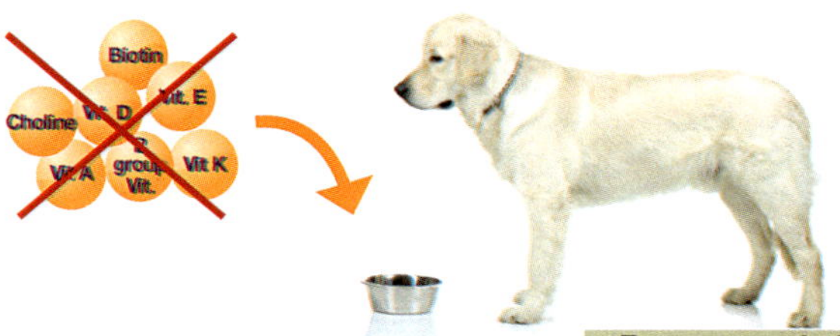

Functions, sample type for analysis and recommendations of the principal vitamins (continued)

Name and active form	Functions	Sample for diagnosis	Recommendations (NRC 2006) U/1,000 kcal ME Dog	Cat
Niacin (B_3)	Component of NAD and NADPH.	Urine: methylnicotinamide	4.25 mg	10 mg
Pantothenic acid (B_5)	Precursor of co-enzyme A. Metabolism of proteins, fats and carbohydrates.	Urine: pantothenic acid	3.75 mg	1.44 mg
Pyridoxine (B_6)	Synthesis of taurine, niacin, hemo group and L-carnitine. Co-enzyme of the transaminases and decarboxylases.	Plasma: pyridoxine Urine: pyridoxic acid	0.375 mg	0.625 mg
Cobalamine (B_{12})	Synthesis of methionine and leucine.	Blood: cobalamine	8.75 µg	5.6 µg
Folic acid	Synthesis of methionine, purines and DNA.	Plasma: folic acid	67.5 µg	188 µg
Biotin	Integrity of the epithelium.	Urine: biotin	No	18.75 µg
Choline	Forms part of the biomembranes. Neurotransmiter (acetylecholine).	Plasma: choline	425 mg	637 mg

Minerals

1 Characteristics and classification

All inorganic elements found in pet food rations are included under this name. In the immediate analysis of the foods, they represent ash, which is obtained through the complete combustion of organic material. Twenty two essential minerals have been taken into account for all mammals, but only 11 are essential in pet food rations for dogs and cats, given that the rest are present in sufficient quantities to cover their needs. Their classification will depend on their concentration in foods:

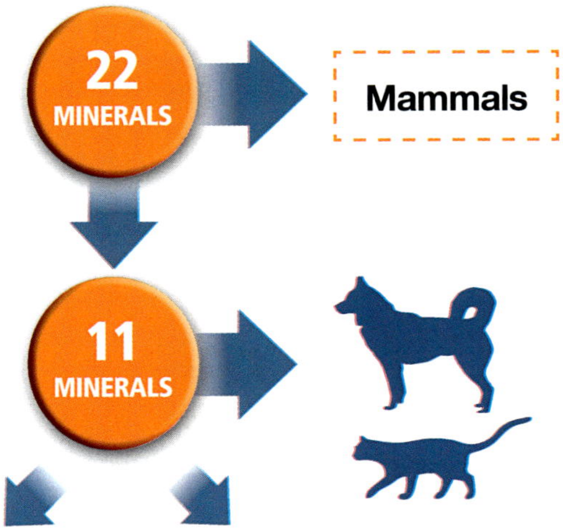

MACROMINERALS — g/1,000 kcal ME or g/kg DM

Ca, P, Mg, Na, Cl, K

MICROMINERALS — mg/1,000 kcal ME, mg/kg DM or in ppm

Fe, Zn, Cu, Mn, I, Se, Cr, B

2 Interaction between vitamins and minerals

The metabolism is very complex and the vitamins and minerals share pathways, especially those of the B group that participate in the metabolism of carbohydrates, fats, and proteins. This effect conditions the existence of a synergetic or antagonistic relationship between vitamins or minerals. A few examples:

- ✓ The absorption of vitamin B_{12} is conditioned by the levels of B_6.
- ✓ Vitamin E interferes in the absorption of vitamin K.
- ✓ Riboflavin is needed for the metabolism of B_6 and B_6 is needed for the metabolism of niacin.
- ✓ The elimination of B_6 through urine is conditioned by the levels of vitamin C.
- ✓ Vitamin C protects vitamin E from oxidation. Vitamin E protects vitamin A from the same process.
- ✓ Antagonism between the Co and the Fe or between Cu and Mo.
- ✓ Deficiencies of a mineral cause further deficiencies of other minerals: a deficiency in Ca leads to depletion of Zn in the bones.
- ✓ Cr, Mn and Fe are transported by the same protein (transferrin), for which they compete.
- ✓ The levels of ionized Ca in blood control the excretion of P and Mg at the renal level.

For these reasons, balance must be found in the ingestion of vitamins and minerals that will ensure that the pet's requirements are covered given that this way, their reserves will be optimal.

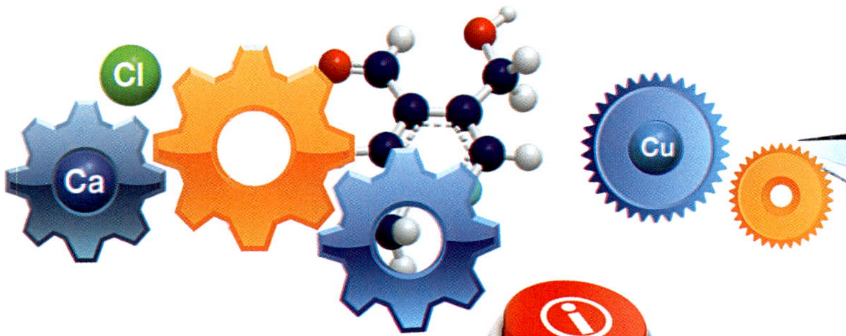

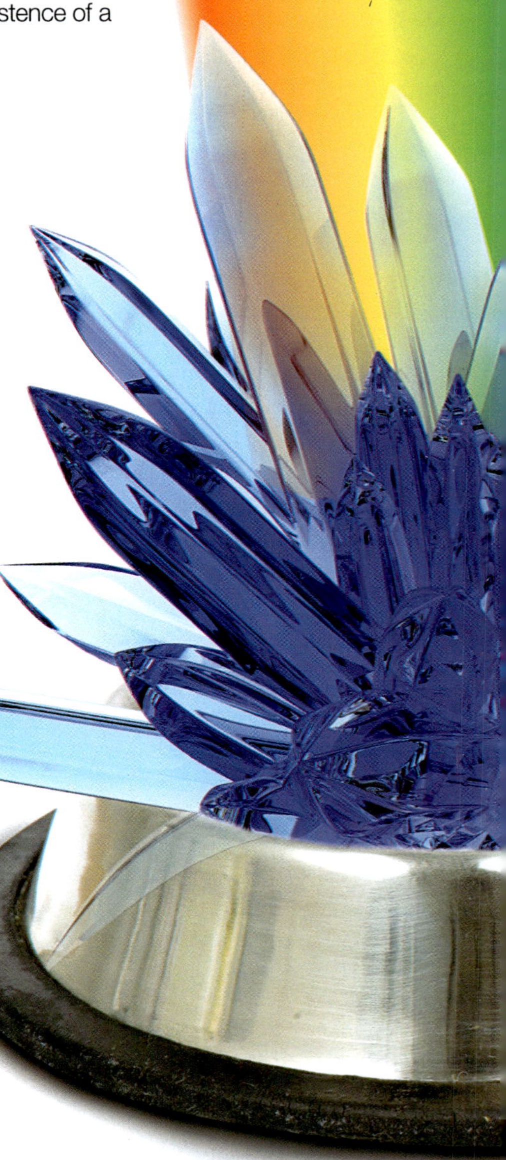

To be taken into account:

The factors that regulate the metabolism and the needs for minerals are similar to those for vitamins: sufficiency criteria, dose-response curve and the pathophysiological model of response to a nutrient, the interactions, and the differences between species. For this reason, the examples are included within the vitamins.

3

Functions

There are four principal functions of minerals in the organism:

Structural Ca P Mg

They form the skeleton, muscles and teeth of animals.

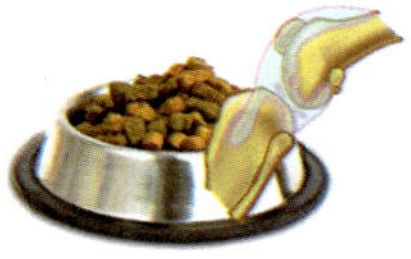

Physiological Ca Na Cl K

Electrolytes in different tissues and fluids. They are necessary for nerve impulses, acid-base balance, osmotic pressure, membrane permeability, blood and cerebrospinal fluid.

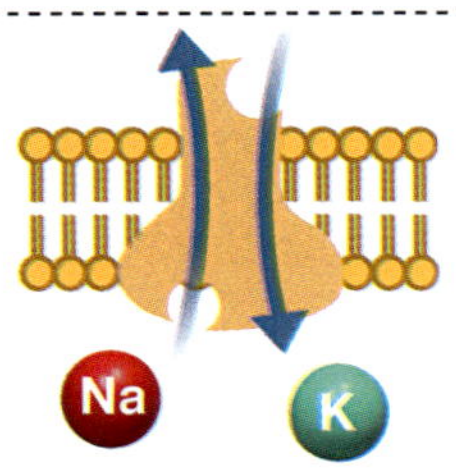

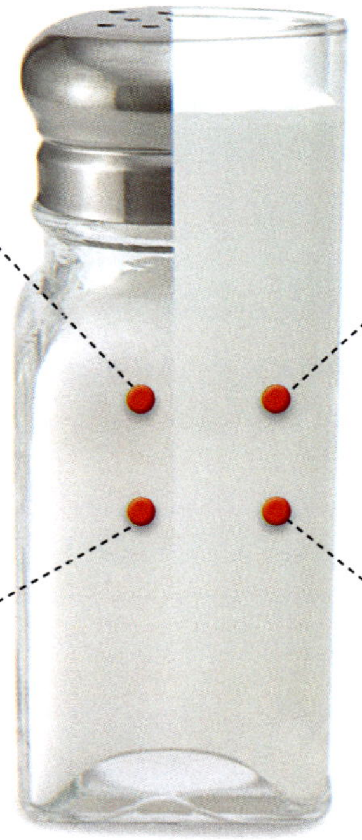

Catalytic Fe Cu Zn Mn Se

They participate as enzymatic and hormonal catalyzers, as metalloenzymes or as specific activators. A few examples: Se in the glutathione-peroxidase, Cu and Mn in the superoxide-dismutase or Zn in the alkaline phosphatase.

Regulating Ca Zn I

They intervene in cellular replication, in the metabolism of nucleic acids and in the regulation of the organism.

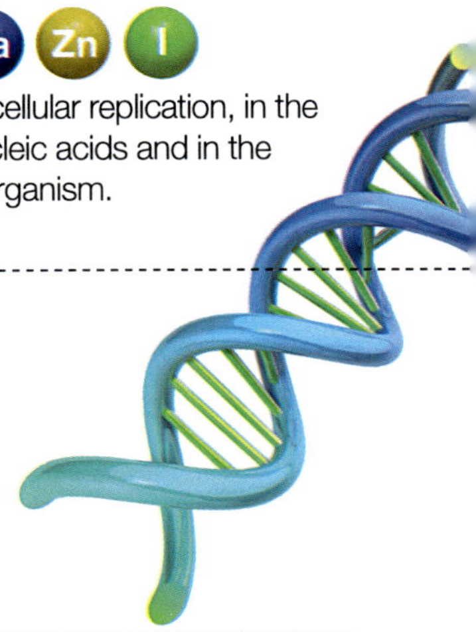

4

Functions, sample type for analysis and recommendations for minerals

Mineral	Function	Diagnosis	Recommendations (NRC 2006) U/1,000 kcal ME: Dogs	Cats
B[1]	Regulating: PTH hormone (bone mineralization: Ca, P, Mg and vitamin D). CNS activity.	–	0.5 mg	
Ca	Structural. Coagulation. Nerve impulse. Membrane permeability.	Serum	1 g	0.72 g
Ca:P	Ratio of the two minerals.	–	1:1 or 2:1	0.65:2
Cr[2]	Regulating: insulin.	–	10 kg: 13.65 µg/day 25 kg: 25.23 µg/day 40 kg: 34.56 µg/day	5 kg: 8.84 µg/day 7 kg: 11.7 µg/day
Cu	Catalytic. Structural (bone, skin and myelin). Cellular respiration.	Serum	1.5 mg	1.2 mg
Fe	Catalytic.	Serum (the hemolysis invalidates the results)	7.5 mg	20 mg
I	Regulating: triiodothyronine and thyroxine hormones.	Serum or plasma: T_3 and T_4	220 µg	350 µg
K	Muscle contraction. Nerve impulse. Acid-base balance.	Serum (avoid hemolysis)	1 g	1.3 g
Mg	Structural. Physiological. Metabolism of fats and hydrates.	Serum	150 mg	100 mg
Mn	Catalytic. Metabolism of fats and hydrates. Structural.	–	1.2 mg	1.2 mg
Na and Cl	Osmotic pressure. Acid-base balance. Nerve impulse. Metabolism of water.	Serum	200 mg (Na) 300 mg (Cl)	170 mg 240 mg
P	Structural. Metabolism of carbohydrates and proteins. Production of energy.	Serum	0.75 g	0.64 g
Se	Catalytic and regulating (synthesis of thyroxine).	Serum	87.5 µg	75 µg
Zn	Catalytic. Metabolism of proteins, hydrates and nucleic acids.	Serum or plasma	15 mg	18.5 mg

[1] There is no information for these species. Values extrapolated from human medicine and those from studies conducted on mice and chicken (< 0.3 mg/kg).
[2] There is no information for these species. Based on the daily dose for body area, values extrapolated from human medicine (0.7-3 µg/kg/day).

Acid-base balance and electrolyte balance

Physiologically, electrolytes should be considered as a whole given that the cells need to maintain a balance between cations and anions to function efficiently. All of these processes function in a very narrow pH range. The changes to the acid-base balance cause a great influence on the cellular metabolism.

Quantitatively, the acid-base balance (ABB) is expressed by the difference between its cations and anions, taking into account that the sum of all of the cations is not equal to the sum of all of the anions. Their value is from 120-200 mmol/dl.

In the digestive process, the metabolism of certain organic cations and anions from the food rations release acids and bases. respectively, that will be neutralized by their respective ions: the anions by the H+ and the cations by HCO3-. Depending on their concentration or their chemical structure, the absorption of the different minerals in the intestine represents another source of acids or bases that act on the internal balance. The process is controlled by the renal and respiratory systems.

However, not all ions act in the same manner given that some combine with others (buffer effect), considered as "weak" from the acid-base balance point of view. This would be the case of bicarbonate (HCO_3^-), hydrogen (H^+) or the hydroxyl groups (OH^-).

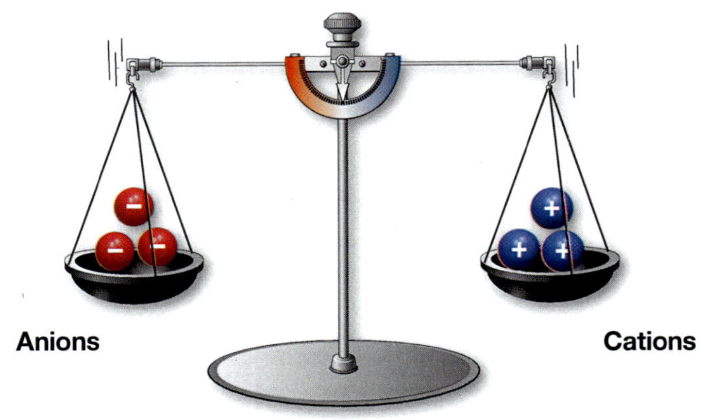

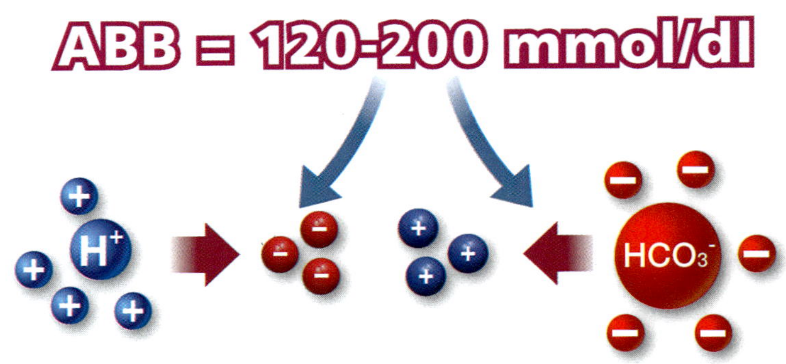

The acid-base balance of the organism is conditioned by the relationship that exists between certain ions that do not participate in the chemical reactions that take place in the plasma at its physiological pH of 7.4 (between 7.35-7.44). At this pH, these ions are completely dissociated and thus they do not perform any buffer effect. These ions, which do not participate and condition the difference between charges, are called "hard" ions and are represented by Na^+, Cl^-, Ca^{2+}, Mg^{2+}, K^+, SO_4^{2-}, PO_4^{3-} and certain organic anions (albumin, lactate, urea, hydroxybutyrate and acetoacetate). The total proteins also contribute to the maintenance of the pH: for each decrease in the concentration of albumin (g/dl), the pH increases by 0.093 in cats and 0.047 in dogs.

The modifications in the concentrations of these ions, especially Na^+, K^+, Cl^- and SO_4^{2-}, determine the metabolic acidosis or alkalosis.

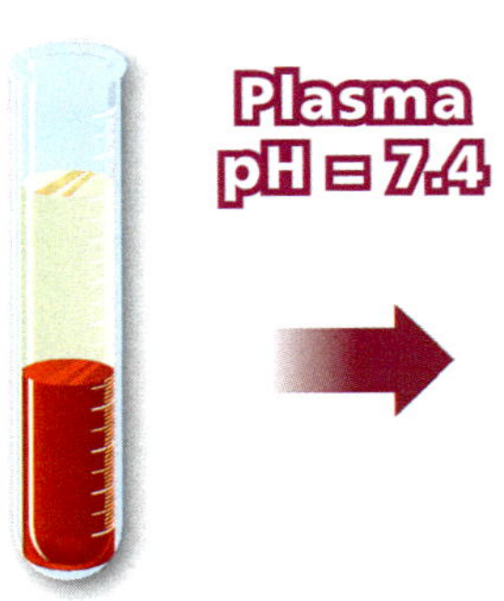

Cations $Na^+ + Ca^{2+} + Mg^{2+} + K^+$	Anions $SO_4^{2-} + PO_4^{3-} + Cl^-$ + organic anions	ABB deviation (mEq/dl)	Metabolism
Basal	Basal	Balance	Neutrality
↑	Basal	Right	Alkalosis
Basal	↓	Right	Alkalosis
↓	Basal	Left	Acidosis
Basal	↑	Left	Acidosis

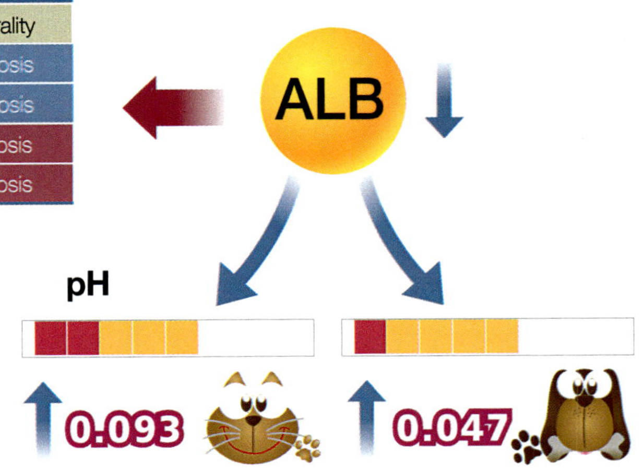

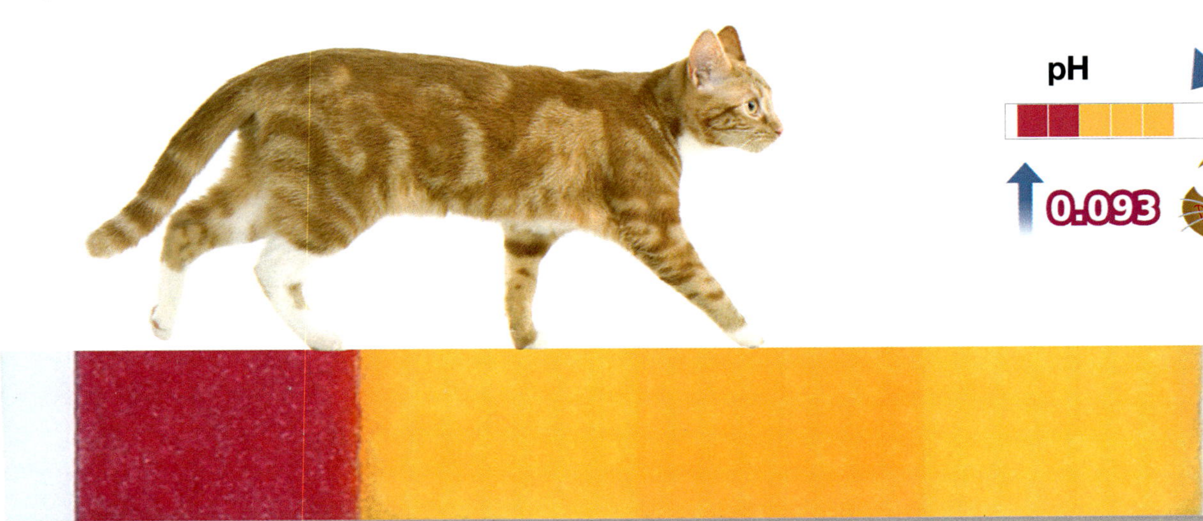

of the food ration

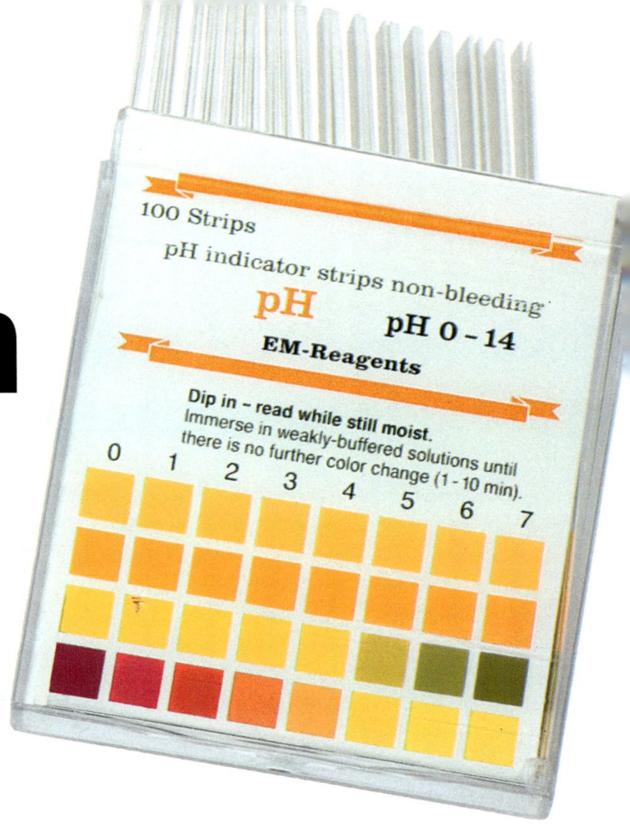

The balance is altered in a physiological manner by the amount of acids from the food rations or from bone remodeling, and they are directly related with the urinary pH. Therefore, the composition of the food ration modifies the urinary pH, which is an indicator of the endogenous production of acids.

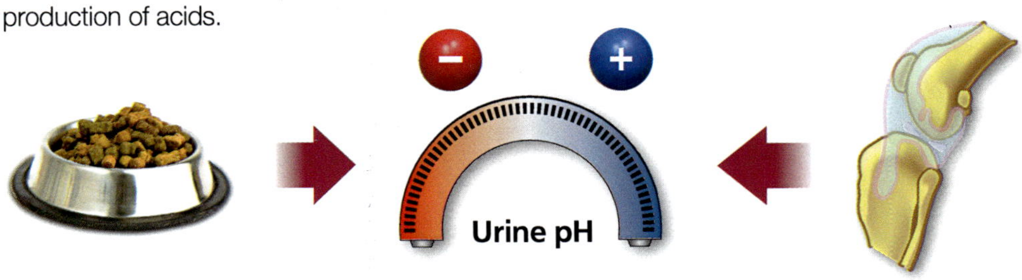

To evaluate this balance, the following is taken into account:

- ✓ The electrolyte balance of the food ration (EBR).
- ✓ The cation-anion difference (CAD).
- ✓ The excess of bases in the food ration (BE).
- ✓ The anionic interval of the food ration (AI or AG –anion gap–).

It is expressed in mmol/kg of DM. Essentially, they reflect the difference between cations and anions of the food ration.

$$EBR = [Na^+ + Ca^{2+} + Mg^{2+} + K^+] - [SO_4^{2-} + PO_4^{3-} + Cl^- + \text{organic anions}]$$

Or in a simpler manner:

$$EBR = [Na^+ + K^+] - [SO_4^{2-} + Cl^-]$$

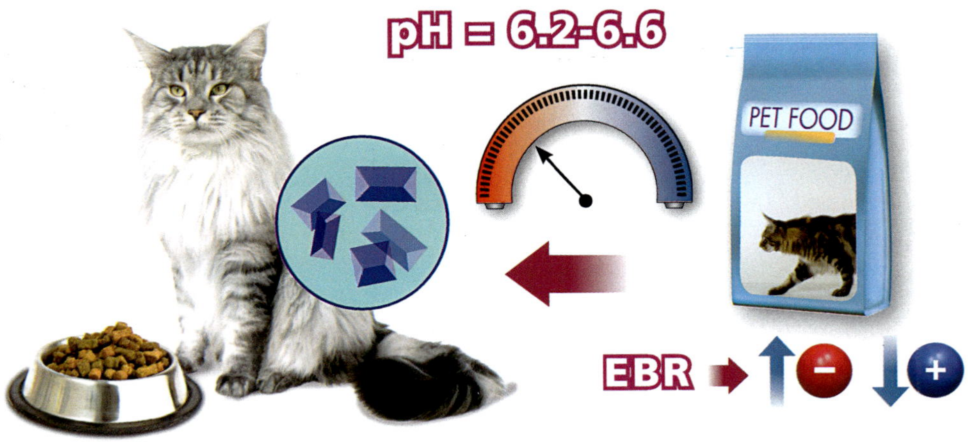

This means that we can correct the deviations of the balance by modifying the cations or anions found in the food rations depending on what we want. For example, the normal ingredients in pet food create a slightly alkaline ABB. In the case of cats, this situation is important because, together with their high capacity to concentrate their urine, they favor the presentation of episodes of urolithiasis by struvite. To prevent this pathology, the companies that manufacture foods for this species have modified the EBR, increasing the anions and decreasing the cations, creating a slight metabolic acidosis with an increase in the net excretion of acids through urine and the production of a lower urinary pH (pH = 6.2-6.6).

The pathological causes that modify the acid-base balance are varied and include primary, secondary, and yatrogenic processes. We will have to take them into consideration to correct them, as much as possible, with the animal's food. The table presents a few examples of these processes.

Ion	Alkalosis	Acidosis
Chloride	Vomit, treatment of acidosis, bicarbonate, diuretics	Diarrhea, CRI, use of KCl, parenteral nutrition, salt
Albumin	Liver disease, entero/ nephropathies with loss of protein	–
Organic anions	Dry commercial foods	Diabetes, CRF, protein
Phosphates	–	CRF, ARF, diarrhea
Calcium	Dry commercial foods	Vitamin D and A, supplements

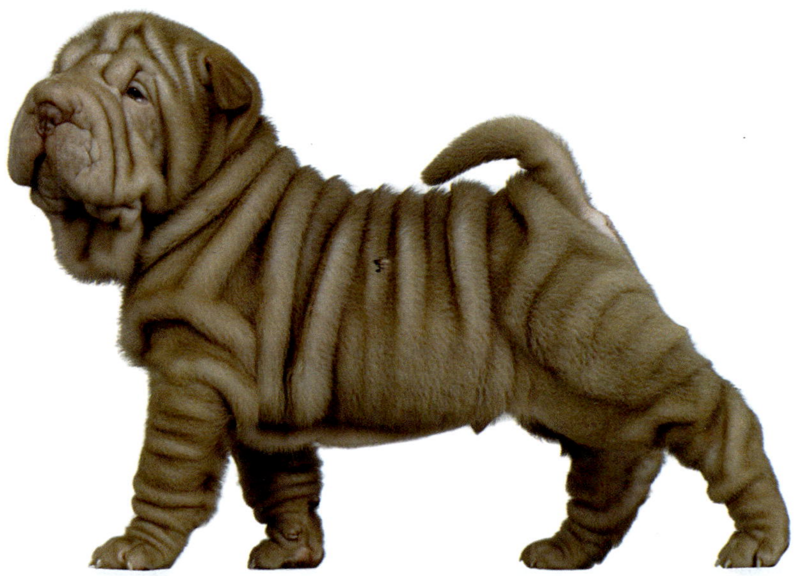

How do we express the of pets?

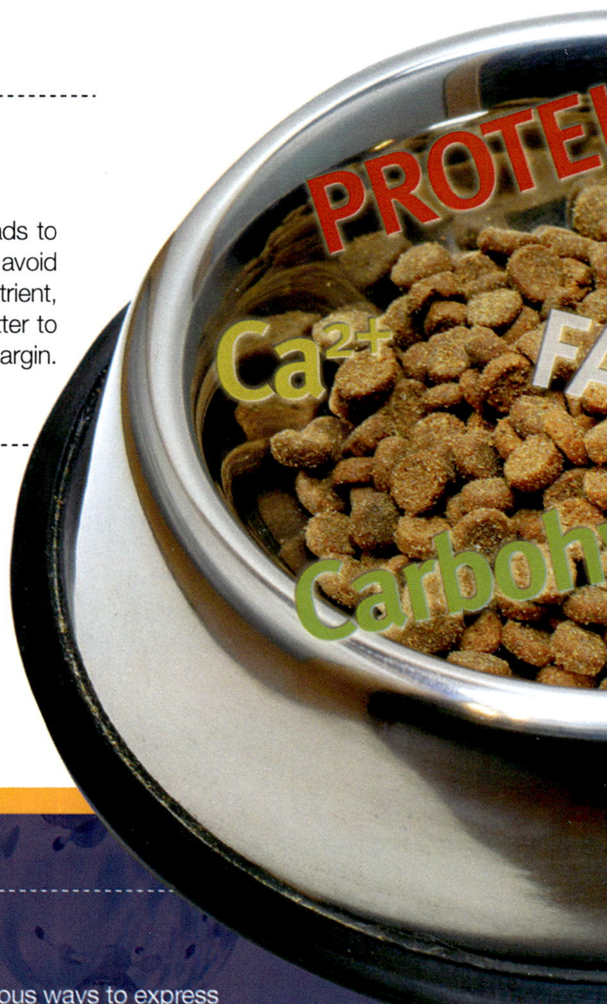

1

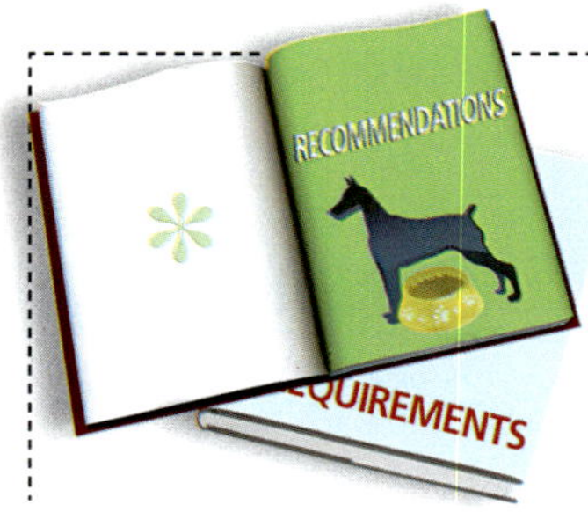

Recommendations are better than requirements

The concept of "requirements" is very restrictive and leads to certain errors derived from different existing research. To avoid the variability of the population, the bioavailability of the nutrient, as well as the specificity of the experiment itself, it is better to talk about "recommendations", which includes a safety margin.

2

NRC The National Research Council

NRC requirements table

The information on the requirements of animals appears in the Requirements tables, such as the those published by the National Research Council (NRC). For dogs and cats, there are NRC publications dating back to 1974, revised in 1985 (dogs) and 1986 (cats). The last edition is from the year 2006: *Nutrient requirements of dogs and cats.*

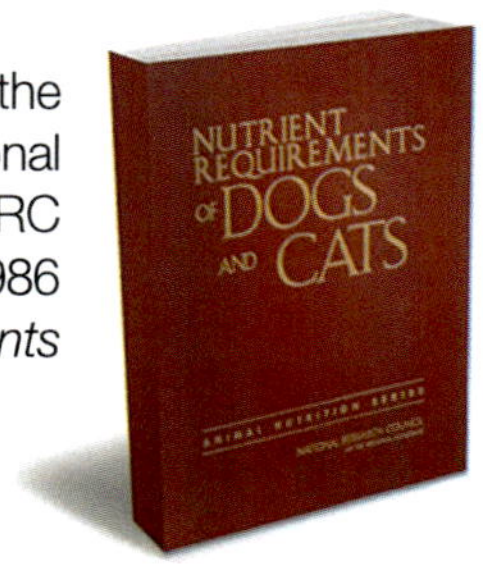

4

Which methods should we select?

When creating a balanced food ration from the tables, we can see that there are various ways to express the different nutrients, making it difficult to choose. The three expression methods are as follows:

1. Nutrient unit (%, g or mg) for every 1,000 kcal of metabolizable energy (ME)

2. Nutrient unit per kg of dry material (DM)

Generally for a food ration with an average density of 4,000 kcal of ME. In this case, it must be taken into account that modifications of the concentration of the nutrient in the food ration are produced when its energy concentration varies. Also, these variations may affect the provision of nutrients, given that the recommendations depend on the pet's metabolic weight. This effect is hardly noticeable in cats, but highly evident in dogs.

Examples

What happens with calcium? Ca^{2+}

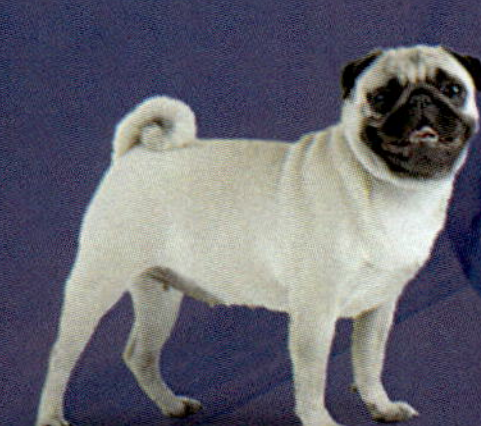

Adult dogs in maintenance → The tables recommend 4 g of calcium per kg DM (in a food of 4,000 kcal/kg DM).

Case 1 **What would happen if the energy concentration was modified?**

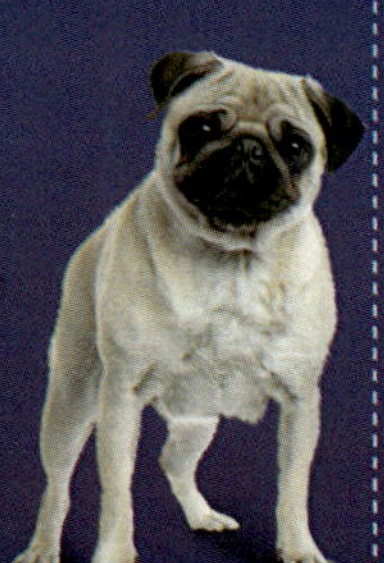

Dog of 7 kg with a MER of 568 kcal ME/day and daily calcium recommendations of 0.56 g

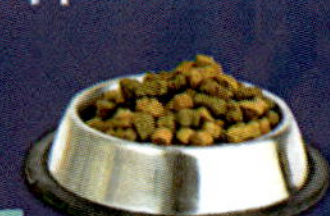

Density: **4,500 kcal/kg DM**
Daily food ration for the dog: **0.126 kg.**
With the recommended proportion of calcium, we provide **0.50 g/day.**

In this case, the calcium requirements would not be met. To meet them, a content of **4.43 g of calcium per kg of DM** would have to be provided.

The calcium requirements would not be met.

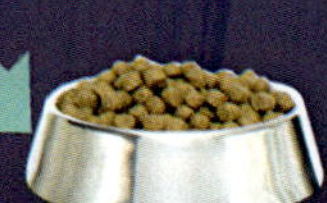

Density: **3,000 kcal/kg DM**
Daily food ration: **0.189 kg**
With the recommended proportion of calcium, we provide **0.75 g/day.**

We are increasing by nearly 34 % the calcium recommendations for our patient. To cover the animal's requirements of calcium, we must **reduce 1.05 g of calcium per kg of DM.**

Increase of nearly 34 % of calcium

nutrient requirements

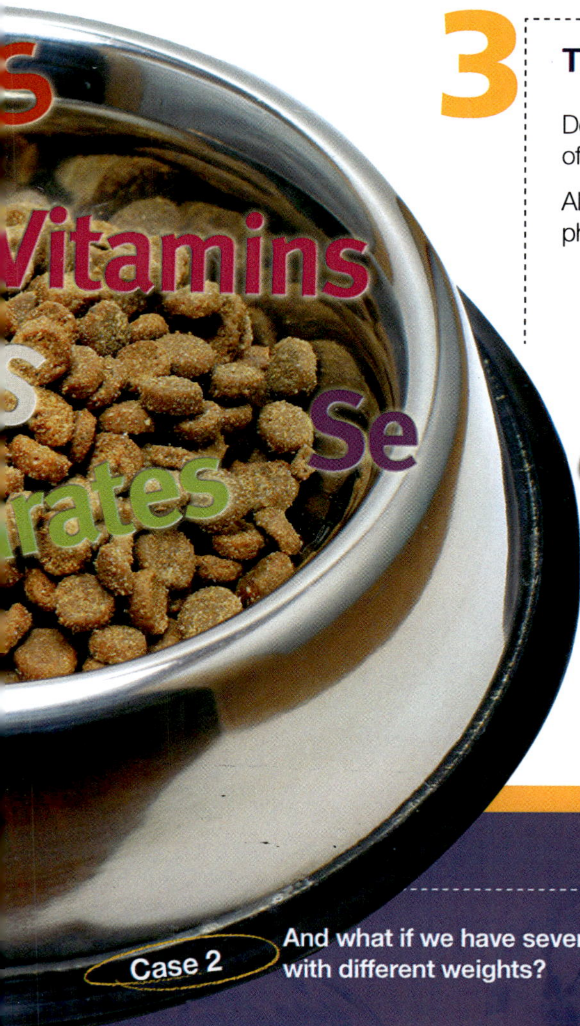

3 This is formulated according to the energy provided by the nutrients

Dogs and cats ingest food until they satisfy their energetic requirements. For this reason, in the formulation of the food rations, the content in nutrients is done according to the energy content.

Also, we must keep in mind that the proportions of the different nutrients, just like with energy, vary with the physiological or pathological state of the animals,

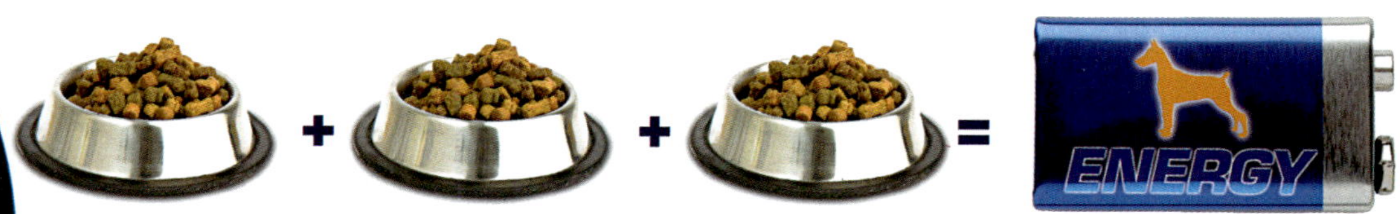

Energy needs covered

Case 2 And what if we have several dogs with different weights?

Density of the food ration: 4,500 kcal/kg DM

	Dog weight	MER (kcal ME/day)	Calcium (g/day)	Ration (g/day)	Calcium (ration g)
	5 kg	441.4	0.4	98	0.39
	10 kg	742.3	0.7	165	0.66
	15 kg	1,006.1	1	223.5	0.89
	20 kg	1,248.4	1.2	277.4	1.10
	25 kg	1,475.8	1.5	327.9	1.31

As you can see, the amounts provided are lower than the requirements as we increase the weight of the animal.

Balanced kilocalorie: all the nutrients are adjusted to a content in ME

Although both expressions (1 and 2) are valid to create generic food rations, the use of the nutrient unit expression/1,000 kcal ME is preferable to avoid the variations that are produced with the modifications in the energetic density of the food ration. This way, we avoid under or overfeeding when we increase or decrease the energetic density, respectively.

Continuing with the same previous example, the tables recommend 1 g of calcium for every 1,000 kcal of ME.

A

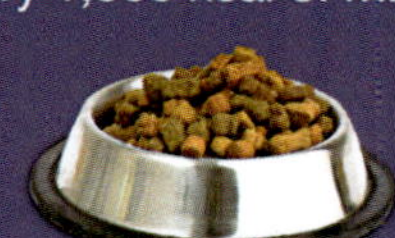

If the food ration has a density of 4,500 kcal/kg DM, there will be 4.5 g of calcium. Our patient will ingest the needed 0.56 g of calcium.

B

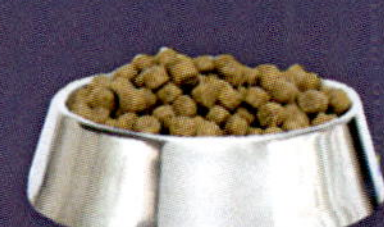

If the food ration has a density of 3,000 kcal/kg DM, there will be 3 g of calcium. Similar to the previous case, the animal will ingest the needed 0.56 g of calcium.

3. Nutrient unit per kg of metabolic weight

Dogs: Nutrient unit/kg body weight$^{0.75}$

Cats: Nutrient unit/kg body weight$^{0.67}$

Its use is restricted for the individual formulation of food rations. In this case, we elaborate a food ration according to the specific needs of the animal. The different nutrients would be adjusted according to the energy they provide.

In our example, the dry material ingested would have to provide 568 kcal of ME, of which 8.7 % would be in the form of protein (14.11 g), 11.5 % in the form of crude fat (7.68 g) and 79.8 % as carbohydrates (129.5 g), to cover the energy, protein and fat requirements of our dog. Regarding calcium, we would have to determine what amount would be provided by the ingestion of the dry material and make up for the difference until reaching the 0.56 g needed with a mineral supplement.

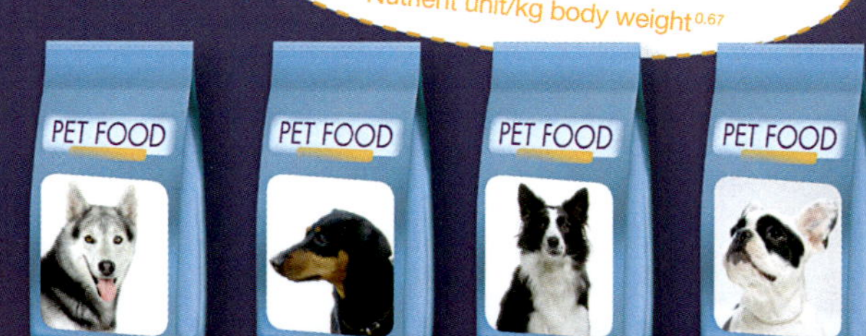

The label of the package (I)

The publicity and sales

The publicity and sales techniques offer us with different manners to offer products to consumers.

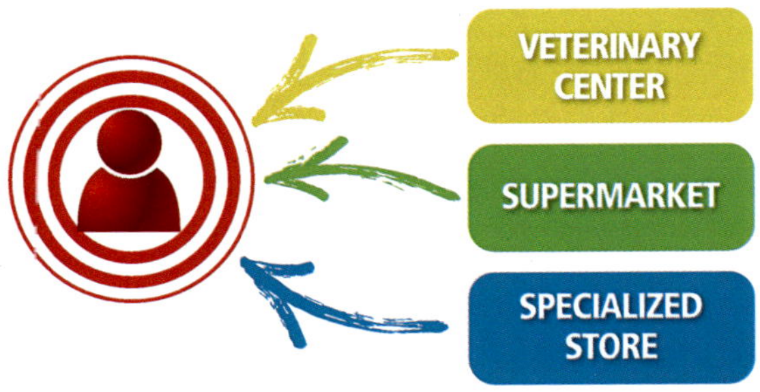

Primary panel

The primary panel is the greatest publicity claim and it describes the identity of the product.

Name of product (1)

Manufacturer (2)

Net weight (average net weight, in EU) (3)

Brand name (4)

Species identifier (5)

Declaration as a prescription dietary food

Best before date (6)

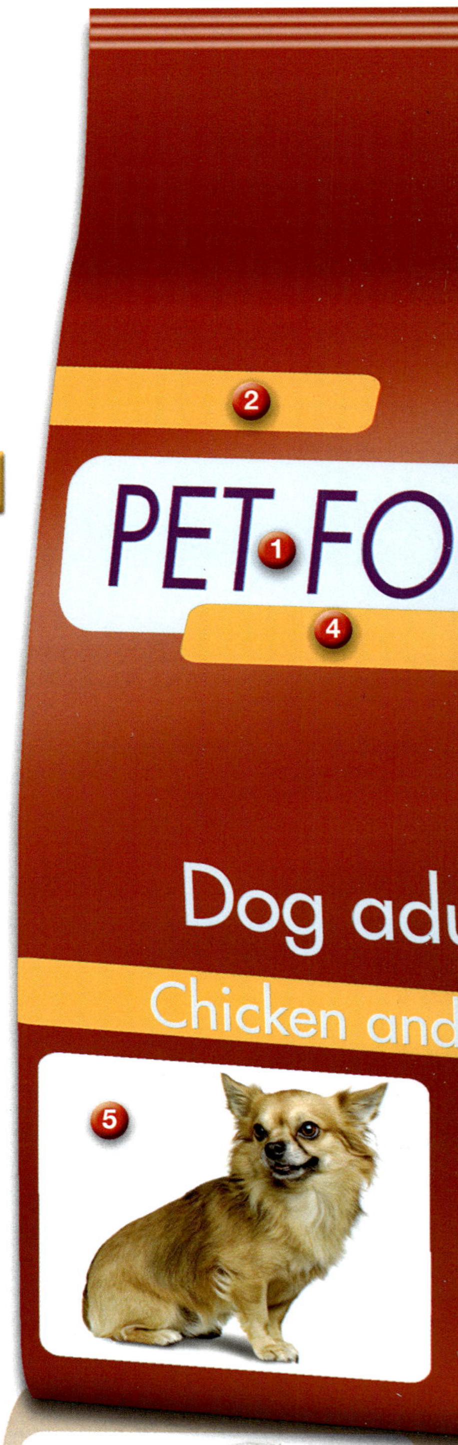

1

Name of product

Describes the food. It is related with the list of ingredients and its proportion in the food. It represents, together with the sales price, one of the principal selection criteria for owners. We can have various options according to the name. For example, with "meat", we find different proportions depending on how its indicated:

Meat | Rich in meat | Meat-based food | With meat | With meat flavor

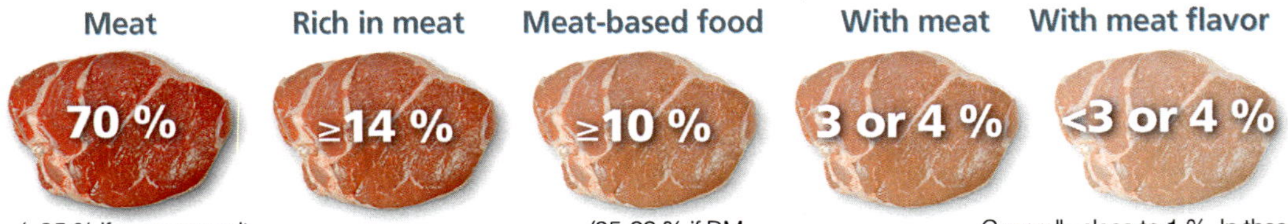

(>95 % if we express it as dry material –DM–). In Europe, only sauce or gelatin are allowed.

(25-29 % if DM is considered).

Generally close to 1 %. In these cases, the only objective is that the animal recognize the characteristic flavor and smell.

2

Species identifier

Whether it is directed at dogs or cats and for a specific physiological state. Also, certain nutrition details are typically included such as the concepts of "complete" or "complementary" and "food with natural ingredients":

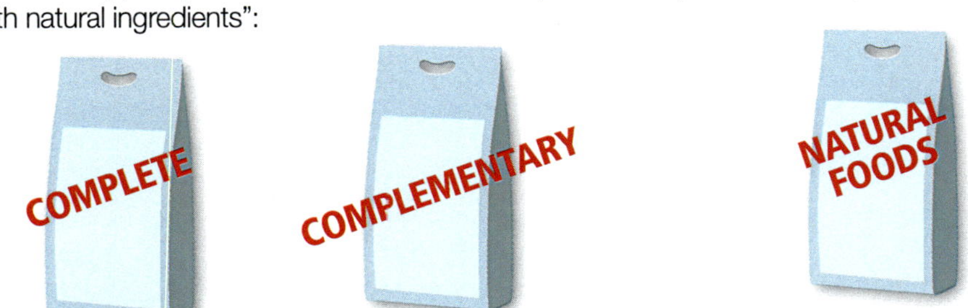

Its composition claims to cover all daily nutrition needs of the target species. Specifying for which physiological state the food is for is sometimes necessary.

It does not cover daily nutrition needs although it includes high proportions of certain ingredients. It can cover the daily food ration in combination with other foods.

Ingredients of animal or plant origin. They allow for treatments such as extraction, hydrolysis and fermentation. It cannot contain synthetic ingredients, food coloring, or flavor-enhancers. Synthetic nutrients (taurine) can be included as long as they are listed. A differentiation must be made from the "organic food" denomination. In this case, the ingredients included would be included within the concept of "ecological", that is, free of hormones, fertilizers, antibiotics, genetic modifications...

3

Prohibited

Certain terms for normal foods (not prescription) cannot be used when there is another food of similar characteristics on the market. For example: if foods A and B have similar compositions and are for adult dogs, we cannot say that A is healthier because it prevents ageing.

The information panel

The information panel provides qualitative and quantitative information about the different ingredients and nutrients.

It appears on the back or lateral sides of the food packaging.

Also, it offers information about the following:

- ✓ **The nutrition sufficiency.**
- ✓ **Food recommendations or recommended daily quantities.**
- ✓ **Additives.**
- ✓ **Information from the manufacturer, importer and distributor of the food.**
- ✓ **Certifications from competent bodies.**
- ✓ **International product codes.**
- ✓ **Barcodes.**
- ✓ **Manufacturing date.**

1 The recommended daily quantities

The recommended daily quantities represent the table that indicates the grams of food per day that should be offered to the pet, depending on their body condition, age and breed.

DOGS		CATS	
Weight	**Daily food ration**	**Weight**	**Daily food ration**
3-5 kg	50-70 g	4 kg	55 g
20-25 kg	180-210 g	5 kg	70 g
45-50 kg	310-355 g	6 kg	80 g
75-80 kg	440-460 g	7 kg	95 g

2 Dietary foods

Dietary foods are designed for the prevention and treatment of certain pathologies, based on research, and their administration can only be done under veterinary supervision. The legislation is similar to that for the rest of foods, but also includes the following:

- ✓ Its prescription or indication (weight loss, elimination of uroliths…).
- ✓ Under veterinary prescription.
- ✓ Specific nutrition characteristics (e.g. low in sodium).
- ✓ Target species.
- ✓ Time that this diet will be used (e.g. up to 12 months).

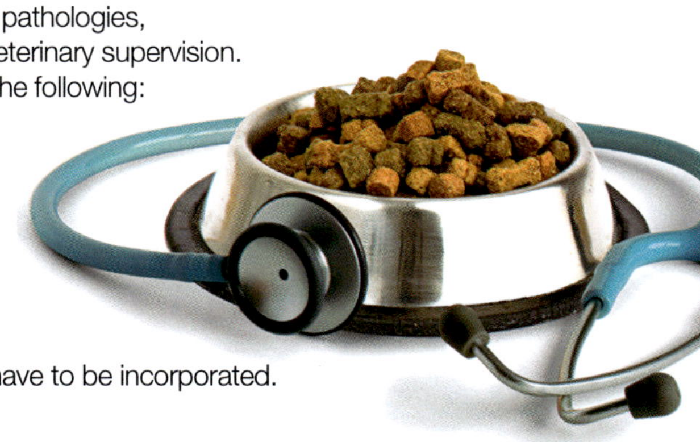

The table of the recommended daily quantities (food guide) does not have to be incorporated.

3 The nutrients are divided into 6 categories

The nutrients are grouped according to the approximate analysis of the foods.

Six categories have been established:

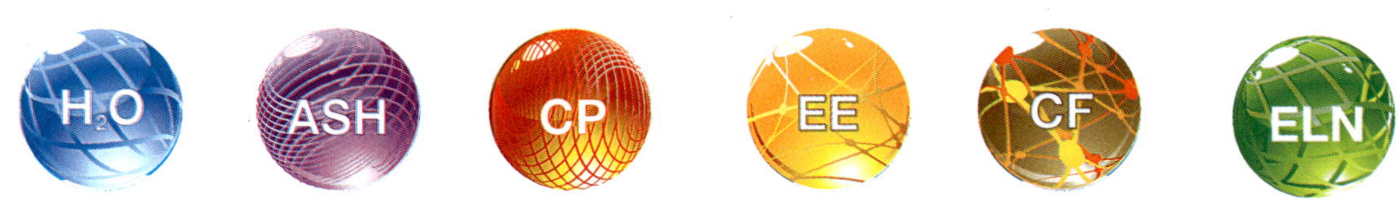

Moisture | Ash content | Crude protein | Crude fat or ether extract | Crude fiber (in some cases as cellulose) | Nitrogen free extracts

The list of ingredients

The list of ingredients reflects the raw materials or ingredients that have been used. Its expression includes basic ingredients, that is, with their water content.

It is mandatory that they appear in decreasing order according to their proportion or weight in the food.

The declaration of the list of ingredients is done as follows:

By groups (EU and Canada):

- ✓ *Grains and by-products.*
- ✓ *Plant protein extracts.*
- ✓ *Plants and by-products.*
- ✓ *Meat and by-products: it is permitted to be derived from slaughter animals. When it is from another species (turkey, deer, or rabbit), this should be reflected in the list of ingredients. Its quality is highly variable depending on the anatomical base; muscle is the most ideal, while bone flour and connective tissue present the worst quality.*
- ✓ *Milk and by-products.*
- ✓ *Eggs and by-products.*
- ✓ *Fish and by-products.*
- ✓ *Fats and oils: from animal or plant origin.*
- ✓ *Sugars.*
- ✓ *Yeasts.*
- ✓ *Minerals.*

Individually (USA, EU and Canada as certified product): corn, poultry meat, soy flour, oats, poultry by-products, animal fat, calcium carbonate…

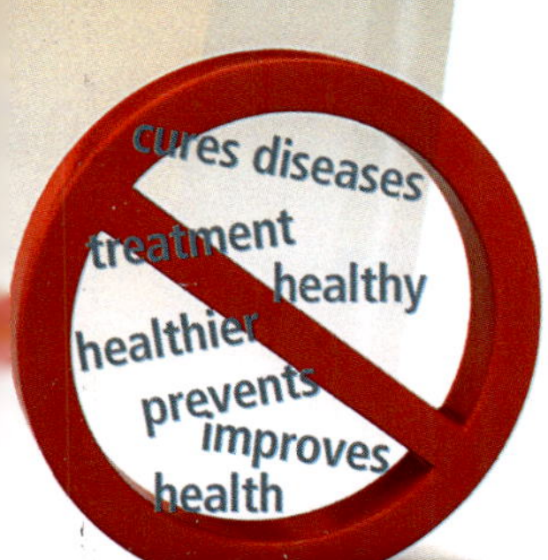

The label of the package (II)

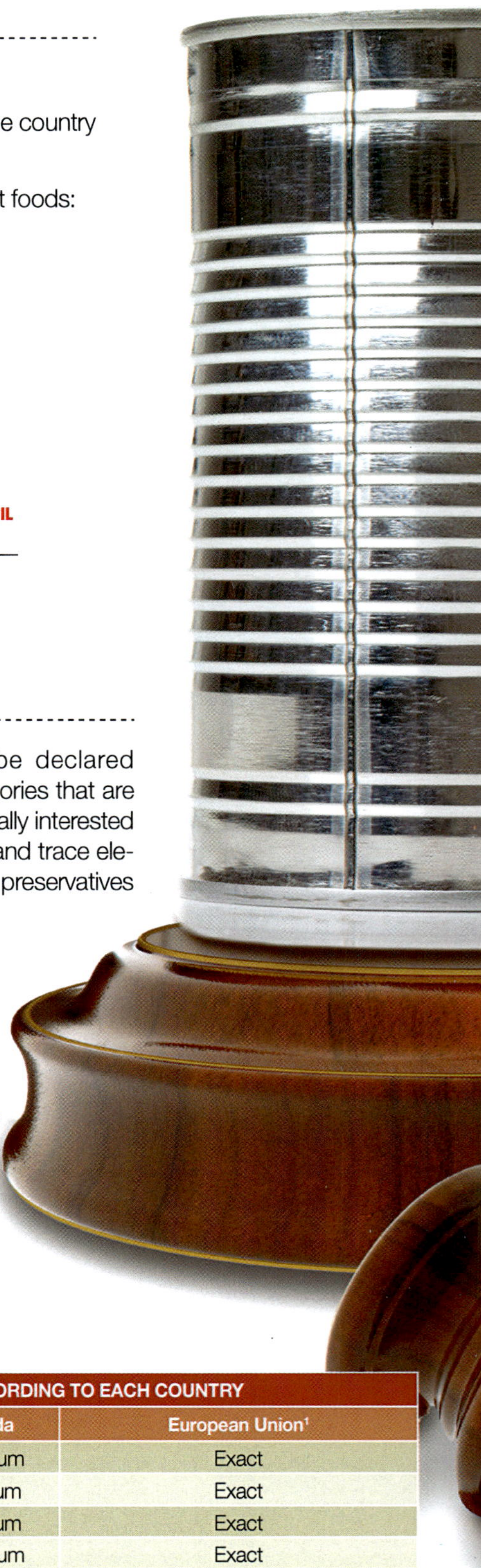

1 The edition of the label

The edition of the label is regulated by the law and is a legal document. The legislation depends on the country and varies if it is for foreign trade, importation or for local sale.

These are some of the different organisms, both official or independent, that monitor the safety of pet foods:

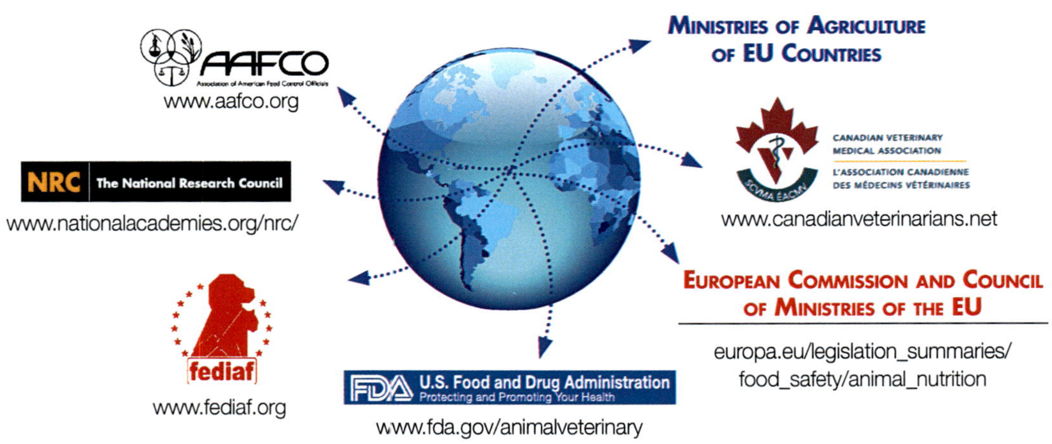
AAFCO
Association of American Feed Control Officials
www.aafco.org
NRC The National Research Council
www.nationalacademies.org/nrc/
fediaf
www.fediaf.org
FDA U.S. Food and Drug Administration
Protecting and Promoting Your Health
www.fda.gov/animalveterinary
Ministries of Agriculture of EU Countries
CANADIAN VETERINARY MEDICAL ASSOCIATION
L'ASSOCIATION CANADIENNE DES MÉDECINS VÉTÉRINAIRES
www.canadianveterinarians.net
European Commission and Council of Ministries of the EU
europa.eu/legislation_summaries/food_safety/animal_nutrition

2 The information according to countries

Depending on the country, there is an obligation to report about certain nutrients (e.g., protein, fat, moisture, ash, additives, vitamins and minerals), as well as of the minimum or maximum guaranteed content or of the exact content of a nutrient, that is obtained from the average from various laboratory determinations.

Expressions such as range of values are not permitted, for example:
Nutrient X: from 18 to 22 %.

The expression of the additives in the labels varies with the size of the package:

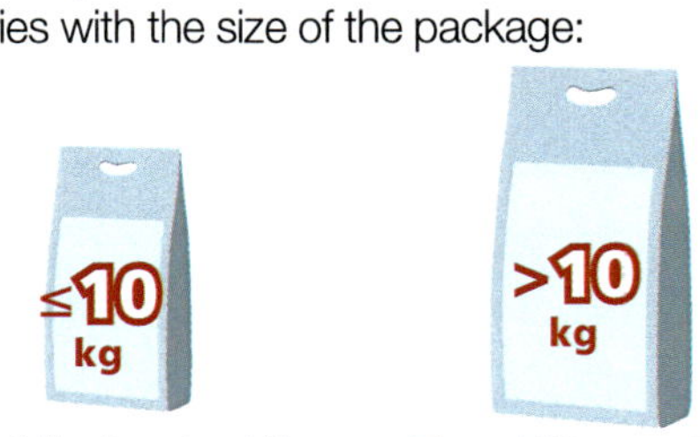

The following should be specified:"contains X additives authorized by the EU"

The additive must be specified: "contains food coloring X"

Nonetheless, some food manufacturers follow the norms established by the independent organisms (FEDIAF) where the minimum and maximum levels are recommended for the different ingredients.

On the other hand, any other nutrient that is added to the list of nutrients or is part of the commercial name must be highlighted as a "non-essential nutrient" and be included on the list.

In the EU, it is mandatory that additives be declared (1831/2002/EC). They are classified in four categories that are then divided into functional groups. We are especially interested in the categories of nutritional additives (vitamins and trace elements) and technological additives (food coloring, preservatives and antioxidants).

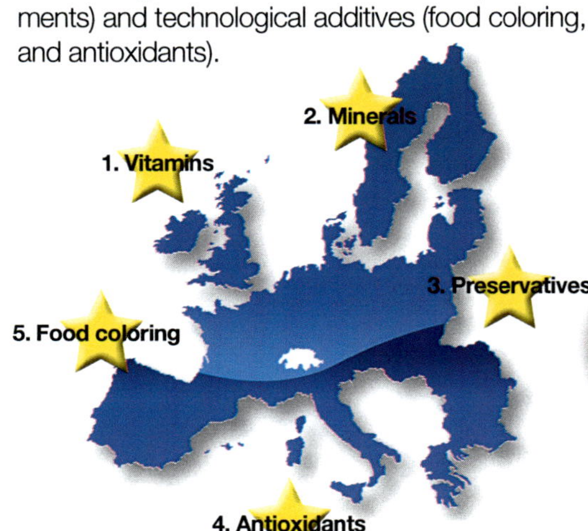

INFORMATION REQUIREMENTS ACCORDING TO EACH COUNTRY			
Nutrient (%)	USA	Canada	European Union[1]
Moisture	Maximum	Maximum	Exact
Crude protein	Minimum	Minimum	Exact
Crude fat	Minimum	Minimum	Exact
Crude fiber	Maximum	Maximum	Exact
Ash content	–	Maximum	Exact
Additives	–	–	Mandatory
Vitamin A (IU or mg/kg)	–	–	Exact
Vitamin E (IU or mg/kg)	Minimum	–	Exact
Vitamin D_3 (IU or mg/kg)	–	–	Exact
Copper (mg/kg)	–	–	Exact
Antioxidants	–	–	Authorized
Food coloring	–	–	Authorized
Caloric content (kcal ME/kg)	Mandatory in light or low calorie foods	Not needed	Mandatory in certain dietary foods (weight loss, obesity and convalescence)

[1] The legislation is similar for livestock animals and for pets.

3

Of interest for clinicians

From a practical point of view, the list of ingredients, the guaranteed or typical analysis and the statement of nutrition adequacy are of interest to clinicians.

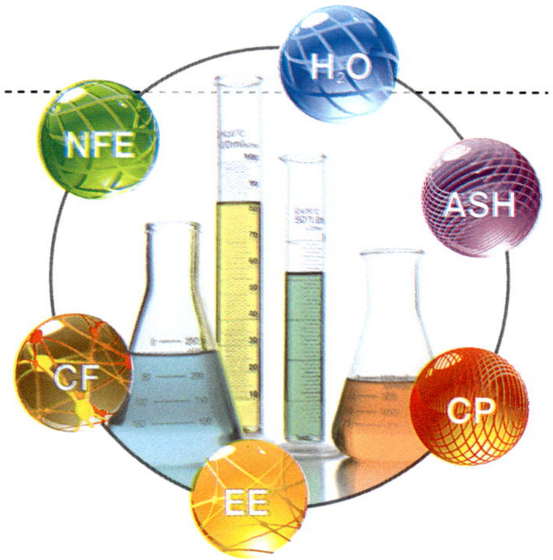

- ✓ The **guaranteed analysis, typical analysis, analytical constituents, average analysis or average composition**, provide information about the nutritional characteristics of the food (6 categories of nutrients).

- ✓ The **statement of nutritional adequacy** ensures that the food meets the **AAFCO regulations** (Association of American Feed Control Officials) and those of the **FEDIAF** (The Europe Pet Food Industry). This means that its efficiency as a basic food ration has been proven scientifically with the required protocols for the different categories established: adults (maintenance), gestation/lactation (reproduction) and growth. If a food covers the needs for reproduction and growth, it is valid for all physiological states. Text that indicates that

The foods have passed the AAFCO tests, are complete and balanced and that they are manufactured specifically for X (physiological state) should appear on the label.

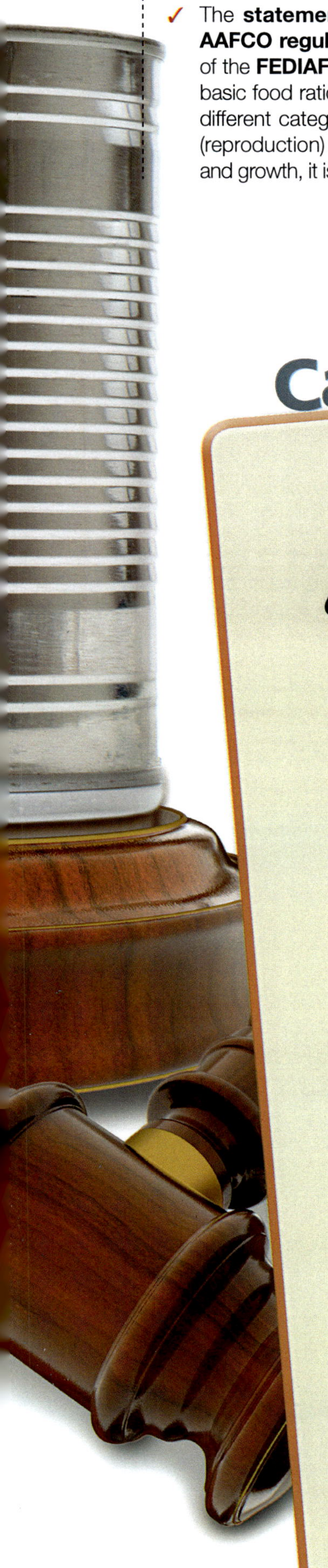

Caution!

I

Ingredients

- ✓ We can see different presentations of an ingredient or different ingredients from the same category listed separately or in intermediate or final positions, but the sum of all of them is greater than some of the first majority ingredients. Example:

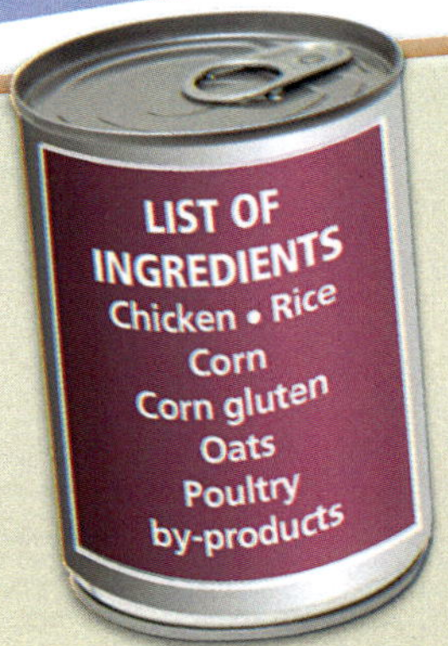

LIST OF INGREDIENTS
Chicken • Rice
Corn
Corn gluten
Oats
Poultry
by-products

If we read the list, we can see that the sum of the grains has a greater proportion than that of chicken. In this case, the quality and quantity of the protein is not primarily from animal sources.

BI

Base ingredients

- ✓ As the list is created according to the base ingredients, that is, with its content in water, some ingredients with a low moisture content occupy intermediate positions in the list, when they are actually majority ingredients if we evaluate them based on the dry material. Example:

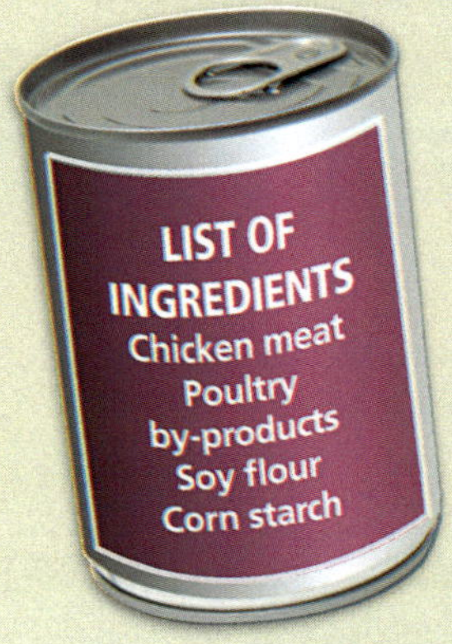

LIST OF INGREDIENTS
Chicken meat
Poultry
by-products
Soy flour
Corn starch

Meat and its by-products have elevated moisture proportions (≈70 %) and low protein concentration as a base food (15-20 %), and they are the first to appear on the list. Soy flour, which has a low moisture (12 %) and high concentration in protein (44 %), will appear in later positions, however, if we compare it as dry material, the quantity of soy flour is much greater than that of meat. In this case, the same would occur as in the previous case regarding the protein.

CP:ASH

Protein:ash ratio

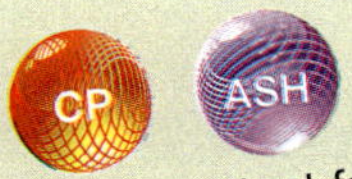

- ✓ The protein:ash ratio is an important factor in the formulation of dry foods, especially in the case of cats. The choice of an ingredient low in protein and rich in ash (e.g., meat flour, meat and bone flour, lamb meat, fish flour) could present us with difficulties to cover the protein needs of a strict carnivore like cats, aside from the undesirable effects of the high proportion of magnesium and phosphorus.

Dry foods

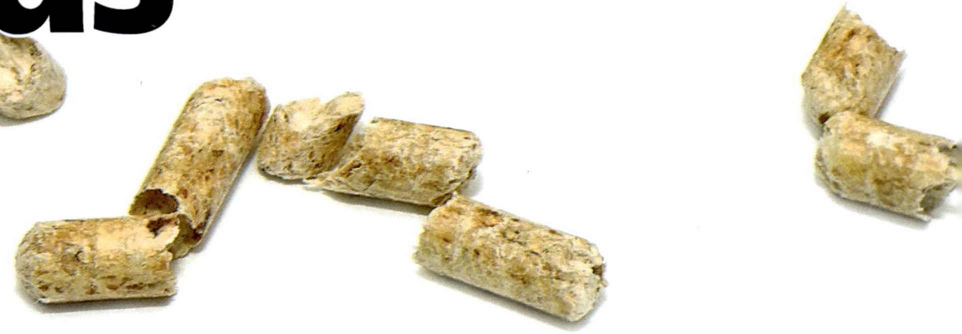

Data sheet

Moisture: 3-12 %

Energy density:
2.7-7 kcal/g.

Raw materials:
plant and animal origin, vitamins and minerals.

Commercial category:
complete foods.

Price (cost/calorie)

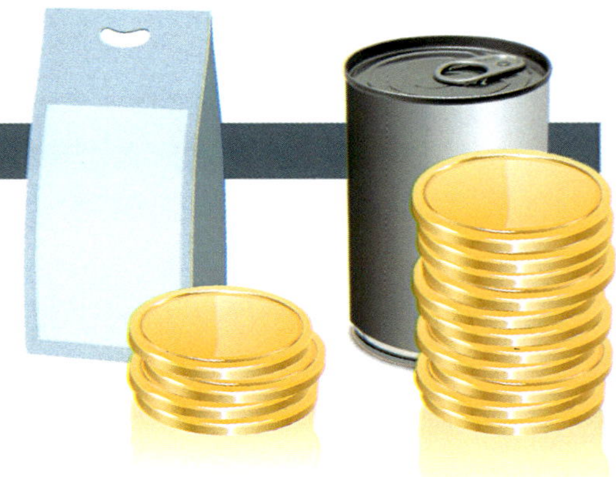

- ✔ Lower water content.
- ✔ Cheaper packaging materials.
- ✔ More economical distribution costs.

1/3 more economical than wet foods!!

Example:

	A	B
Moisture	12 %	75 %
Energy	3.40 kcal ME/g	0.96 kcal ME/g
Price	35 €/kg	35 €/kg
Cost/g	0.035 €/g	0.035 €/g
Cost per calorie as a complete food	0.035/3.40 → **0.010 €/kcal**	0.035/0.96 → **0.036 €/kcal**

General characteristics of dry, wet and semi-moist foods

The general characteristics of the three principal types of food found in the market are summarized in this table: dry, wet and semi-moist.

	Dry (extruded)	Semi-moist	Wet
Moisture (%)	>12 %	15-35 %	>60 %
Protein (% DM)	Low	Average	High
Fat (% DM)	Low	High	High
Carbohydrates (% DM)	High	High	Low
Minerals (% DM)	Low	Low	High
Energy (DM)	Low/medium/high	Medium	High
Food energy	Low/medium/high	Medium	Very low
Majority ingredient	Grains/meat	Grains/meat	Meat
Palatability	Low	High	High
Texture	Kibble, star, etc.	Meat portions	Portions, paté, sauces, vegetables, semi-liquid, etc.
Complete food ration	Yes	No	Occasionally
Exogenous supply of water	Needed	Conditioned	Conditioned
Cost (€/calorie)	Low	Medium	High
Appearance in the market	Dry food	Sausage, hamburger, treats	Cans, tubs, packets, sausage
Food type	Complete	Complementary	Complete
Moisturizing substances	No	Yes	Yes
Technology	Extrusion	Extrusion	Cooking (25-85 °C)
Time: cooking temperature	High	High	Medium

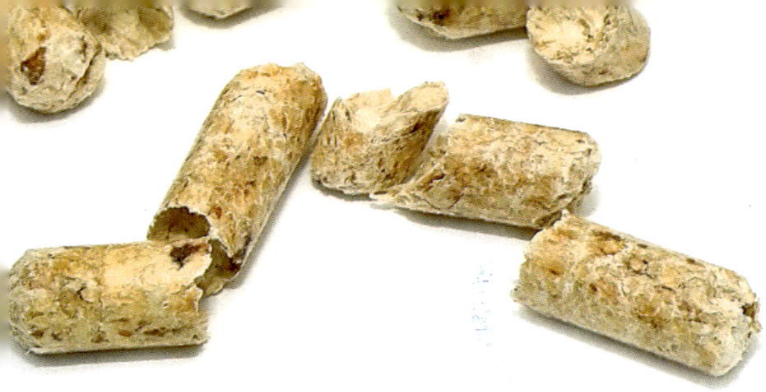

Extruded The most common in the market

Granulated Lower cost than extruded

Kibbles Called "menu" or "mix"

Crushed and cooked Currently not used

Manufacturing technology

1 Extruded

During the manufacturing, processes are included that incorporate the following:

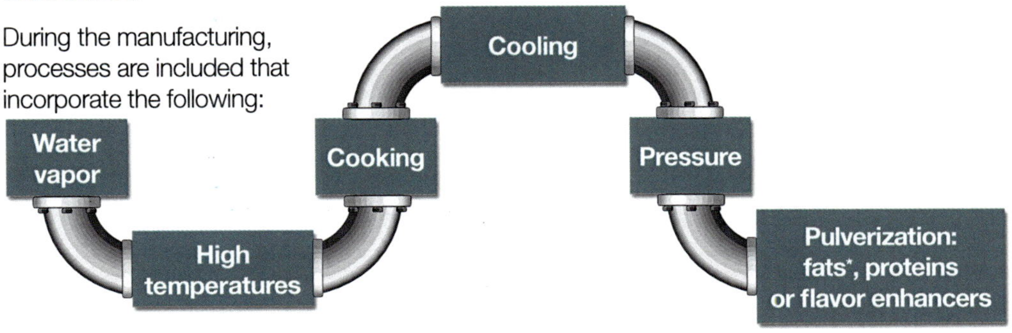

* Levels of incorporation of 5 to 15 %.

With these effects, the following is achieved:

- ✔ **Gelatinization of carbohydrates**: this ensures better hydrolysis of the starch and, therefore, better digestion.
- ✔ **Reduction of contaminating microorganisms**.
- ✔ **Greater half life of the product**.

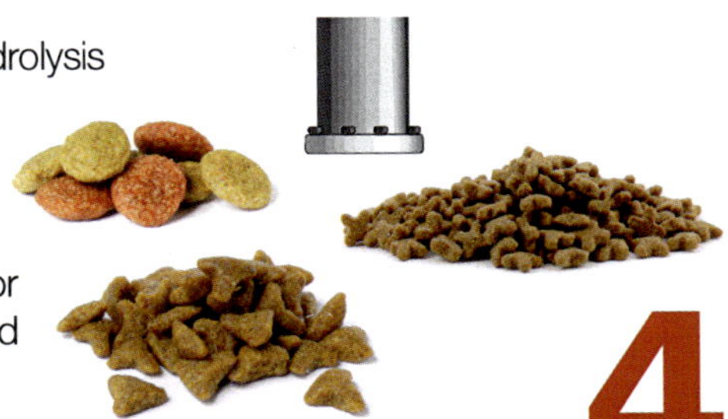

This type of manufacturing allows for modifications of the color and the final form of the food according to the market demand criteria of the owners (anthropomorphism).

2 Granulated

Conventional manufacturing technology.
In this case, the cooking time and temperature is less:

- ✔ **The starch is not completely hydrolyzed,** which causes digestive problems in some cases.
- ✔ **A correct mixture of the fat is not produced in the liquid phase**.
- ✔ **Microorganisms may develop**.

They are frequently used in the elaboration of foods for ruminants, horses and rabbits.

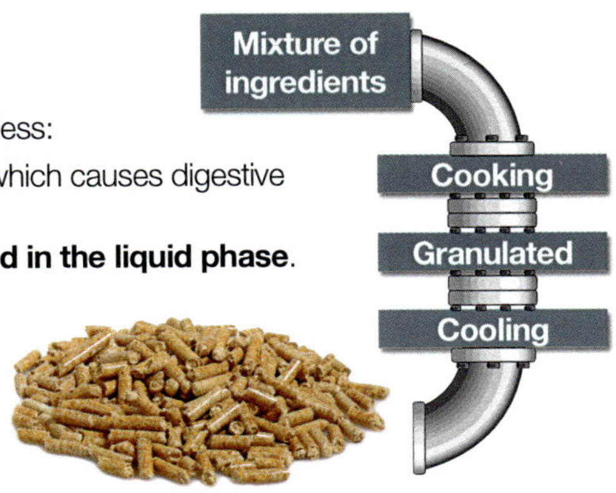

3 Flakes

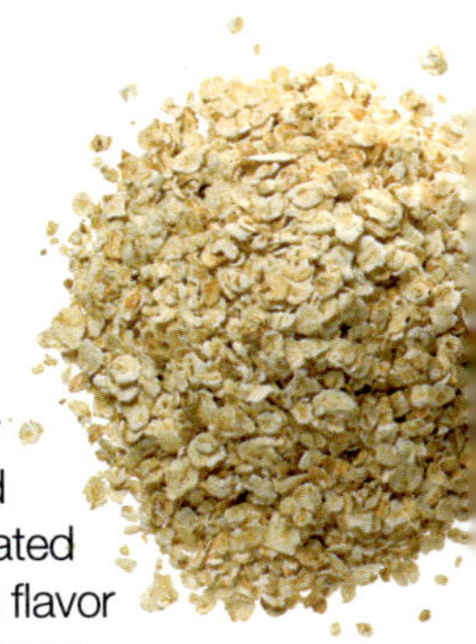

The flakes are the result of the dry mixture of the different ingredients, primarily thermally treated grains and sources of granulated proteins, to which flavor enhancing substances or fatty substances are added.

4 Crushed and cooked

They are processed in a traditional manner, incorporating high levels of grain-based flours (>50 %) and a limited proportion of meat and fat derivatives. They were the first foods created specifically for pets at the beginning of the last century.

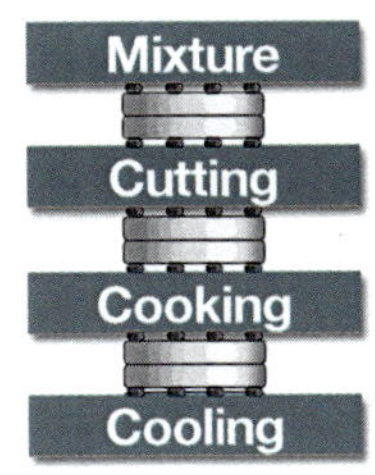

	Dry (extruded)	Semi-moist	Wet
Sterilization	Extruder <200 °C <5 minutes 35 atmospheres	Extruder <200 °C <5 minutes 35 atmospheres	Retort (autoclave) 121 °C 3 minutes
Advantages of extrusion	Hydrolysis of carbohydrates Emulsion of fats	Hydrolysis of carbohydrates Emulsion of fats	Not produced
Preferential species	All	Dogs	Cats, dogs of small breeds
Type of packaging (approx.)	0.4 kg up to 25 kg	0.5 kg up to 1 kg	0.25 kg up to 1 kg
Storage at home	Simple	Requires space	Requires space
Storage (open)	Dry environment	Refrigerated	Refrigerated
Storage (closed)	Room temperature (RT)	RT, sensitive to freezing	RT, sensitive to freezing
Half life (closed)	12 to 18 months	9 to 12 months	<36 months
Half life (open)	Long	4 to 24 hours	<48 hours
Loss of vitamins	Storage	Storage	Processing
Acceptance by owner	Medium	High	High
Volume of the food ration	Small	Excessive	Excessive
Therapeutic use	Yes	No	Yes

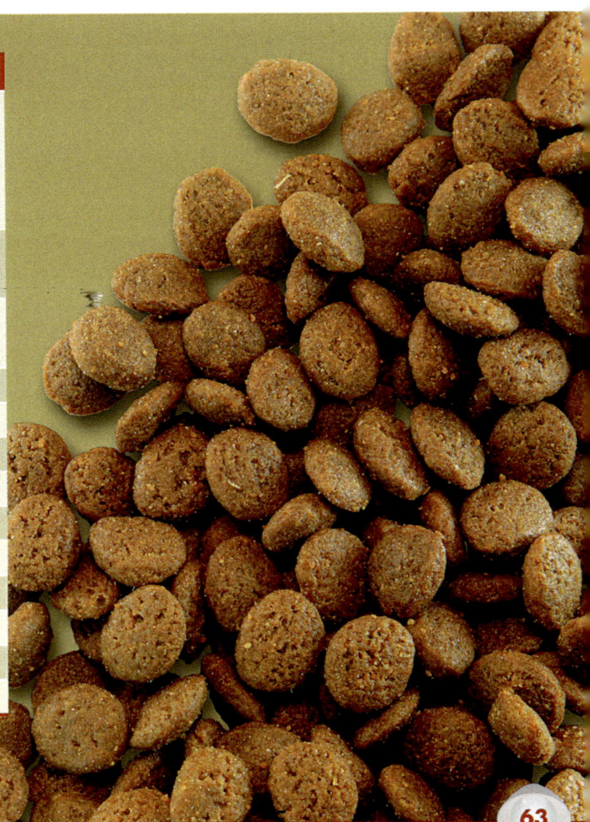

Data sheet

Moisture: 15 - 35 %

Energy density:
Intermediate between dry and wet foods, from 2.7 to 3.8 kcal/g.

Raw materials:
Highers quantities of protein or fatty ingredients (30-50 % of the total) that ensure a greater proportion of crude protein (>30 %) and fat (15 %) per unit of DM.

Additives:
Moisturizing substances to uptake the free water.

Commercial category:
Complete and complementary foods.

SEMI-MOIST

Semi-moist

15 - 35 %

1 Moisturizing substances

The elevated moisture decreases the half life of these products. For this reason, moisturizing substances are added to control the activity of the water (a_w):

- Sugars
- Sodium chloride
- Potassium sorbate
- Glycerin
- Organic acids
- Low molecular weight alcohols

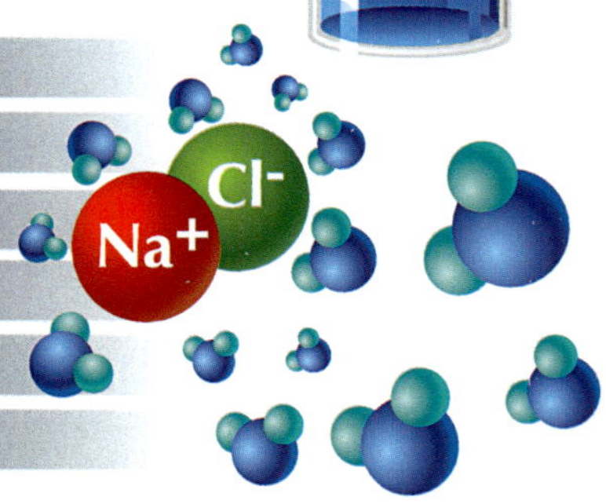

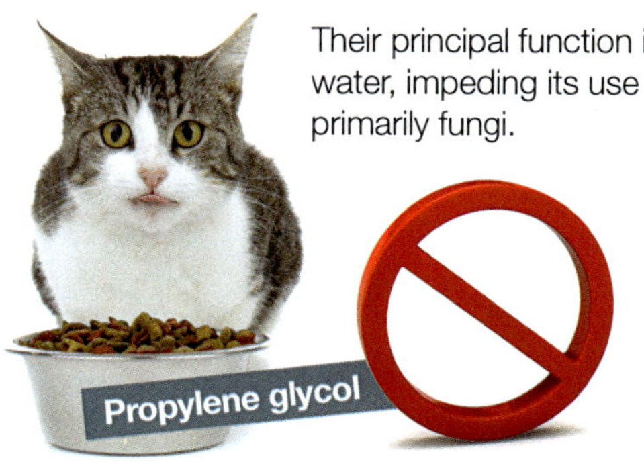

Their principal function is to uptake the free water, impeding its use by contaminating flora, primarily fungi.

It is a good idea to review current legislation regarding this issue given that there are restrictions in some cases (e.g. propylene glycol is prohibited in cats).

WET

Moisture: >60 %

Energy density and nutrients concentration per unit of DM:
Higher than in dry foods.

Raw materials:
Most of the ingredients (50-75 %) are of animal origin. Sometimes concentrated plant protein with meat-like texture are used. This allows lower costs.

Additives:
Moisturizing substances to uptake the free water.

Commercial category:
Complete foods.

Price (cost/calorie): high

- ✔ Low energy density as a food.
- ✔ Costs of manufacturing process and packaging.
- ✔ Greater distribution costs.

1 Be careful with excesses

- ✔ Their poor use can lead to overfeeding and obesity.
- ✔ Although they are complete and balanced foods, they are generally used as a protein complement with certain foods rich in carbohydrates: this situation may cause nutritional imbalances.
- ✔ They are also used to increase the palatability of dry foods in animals with reduced or difficult appetites (as its texture is variable depending on the principal ingredient and its content in "sauces").
- ✔ In some cases, especially with sausages, they may be complementary foods rich in protein and minerals, with a very short half life.

Complete and balanced food

High palatability

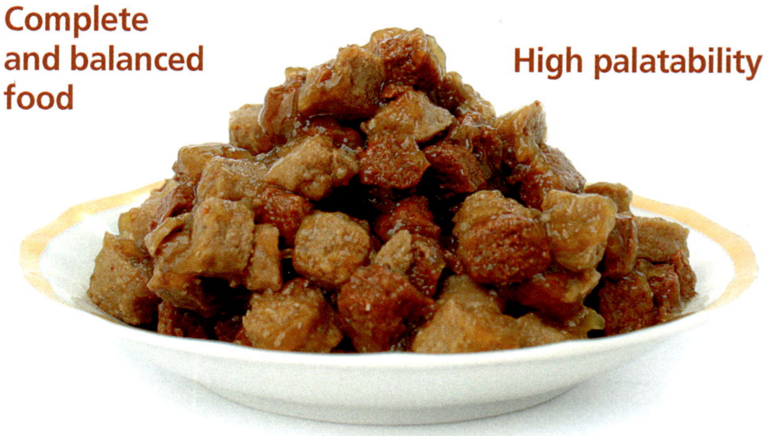

and wet foods

2 Manufacturing technology

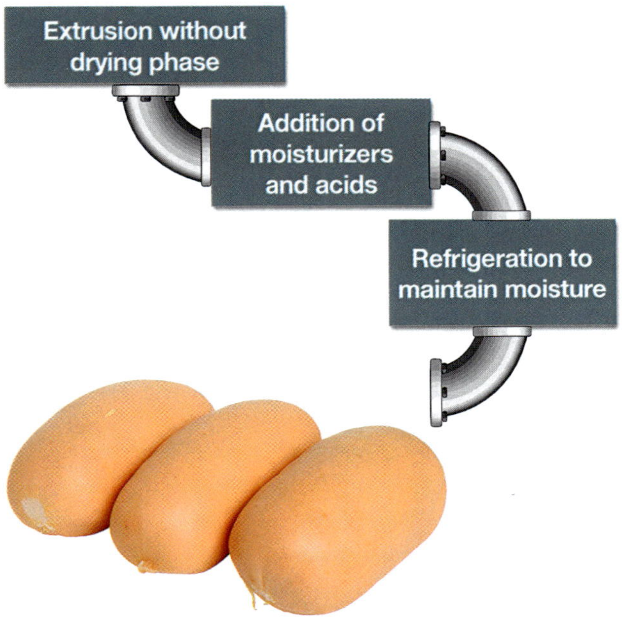

Their manufacturing technology is also by extrusion, but in this case, after the extruder, there is no drying phase. From this moment, the moisturizers and acids are added, to later be refrigerated, and thus maintain the moisture.

3 Product evolution

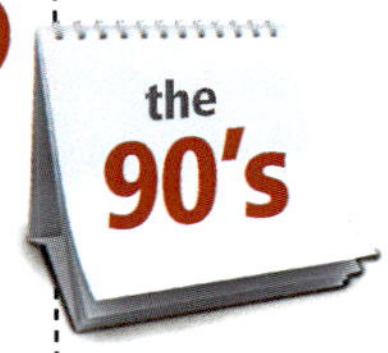

- ✔ Since the 1990's, their presence at stores has noticeably fallen.
- ✔ Currently, they are included in treats or prizes for pets, due to the high level of flavor enhancers used in their formulas.
- ✔ Their presentation has an appearance similar to meat.
- ✔ They have a high palatability for pets.
- ✔ At stores, we find them in vacuum-sealed packages with a physical form that is greatly accepted by owners (sausage, hamburger) and their size ensures a complete meal.

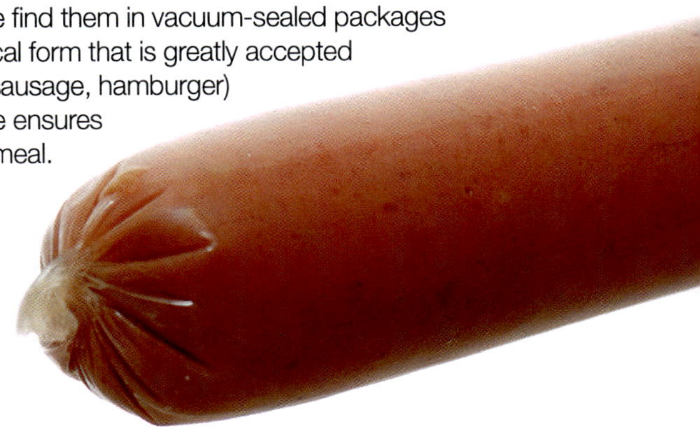

2 Manufacturing technology

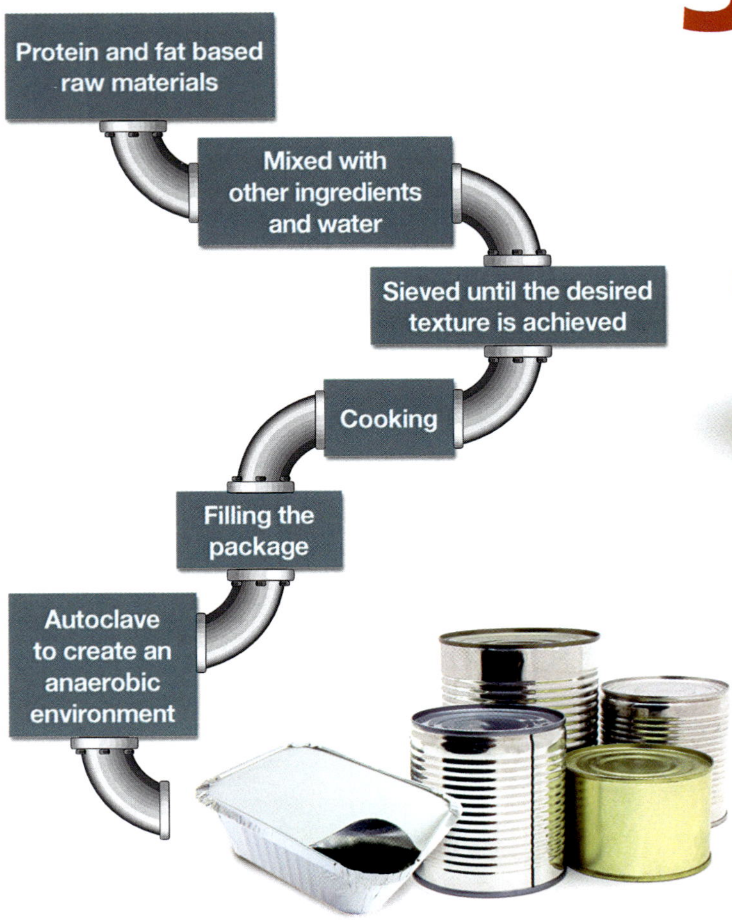

3 "Gourmet" products

Wet foods have become very important to owners as special high quality "gourmet" products for their pets, especially in miniature breed dogs and cats, and therefore, their physical form (tubs, packets, cans, tubes) and their texture (paté, kibbles, portions, stews, sausages, cooked natural foods, cooked vegetables) are varied.

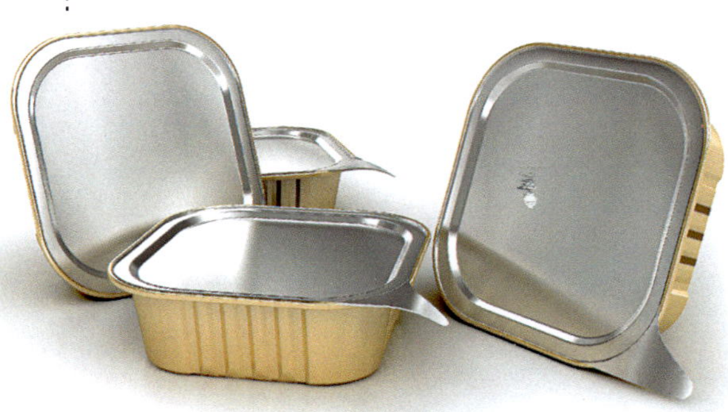

To be taken into account

The high content in raw materials from animal sources makes us doubt about dietary safety.
To ensure the absence of microbial contamination, manufacturing must be done according to current legislation for semi-acid canned products.

Criteria for selection

1 Selection factors

Evaluating and selecting pet foods depends on certain important factors:

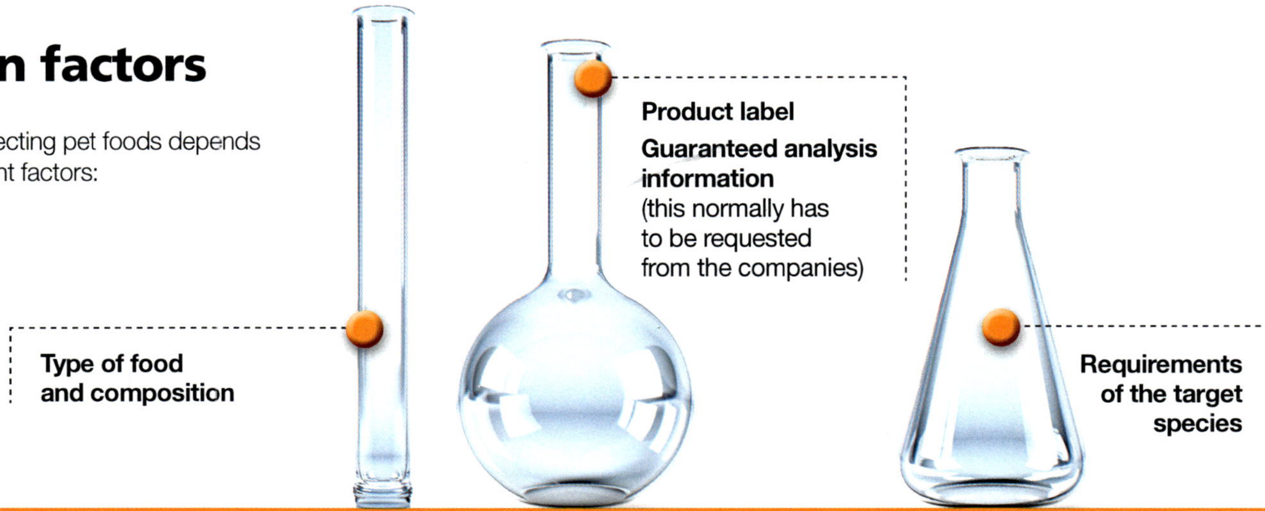

3 Information on the nutrient content

The information on the nutrient content is found on the product label and it is adjusted to current legislation and even to certain criteria established by independent organizations (e.g. AAFCO –Association of American Feed Control Officials– and FEDIAF –The European Pet Food Industry Federation–). This information is obtained from the results of laboratory analyses following a standardized reference method.

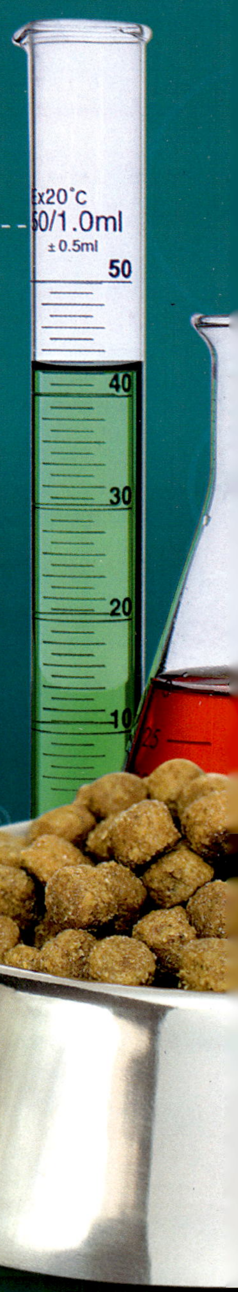

The most common method is proximate analysis

This method, developed by Henneberg and Stohman in the Weende Experiment Station (Germany) in 1864, is a simple, fast and cheap method that provides us with information on the composition in nutrients, however, it does not analyze nutrients but rather groups together substances with common chemical characteristics.

It establishes six components:

- **Water** (H_2O)
- **Ash content** (ASH)
- **Crude protein** (CP)
- **Crude fiber** (CF)
- **Crude fat** (or ether extract) (EE)
- **NFE** (nitrogen free extracts) (NFE)

If we observe food packaging, we can see that it corresponds exactly with the description of "analytical constituents", "average analysis" or "average composition", etc. It is not a perfect method as it possesses certain errors, but it can give us a fast idea of the composition.

For a deeper understanding of the methodology for its determination, we refer readers to the AOAC manual –Association of Official Analytical Chemists– (www.aoac.org).

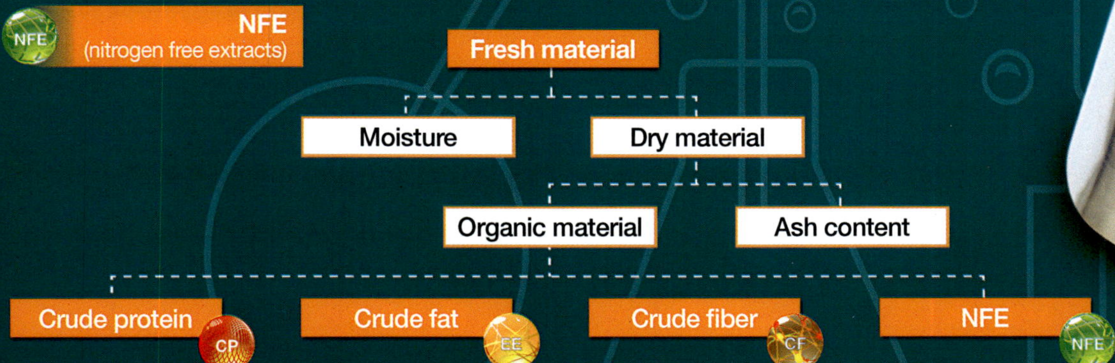

and comparison of foods

2 Systems to express the value of the foods

There are three systems to express the value of the foods and to compare them.

An evaluation of the cost of the food must be carried out on any of the three bases.

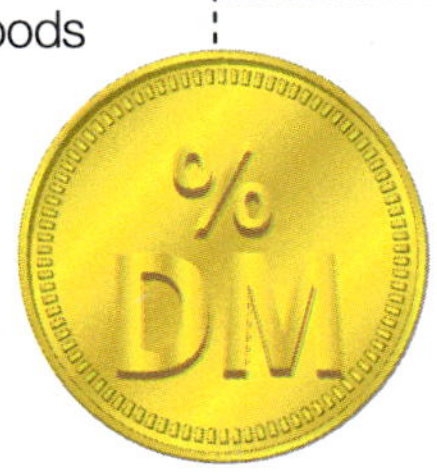

Depending on the dry material
(% DM)

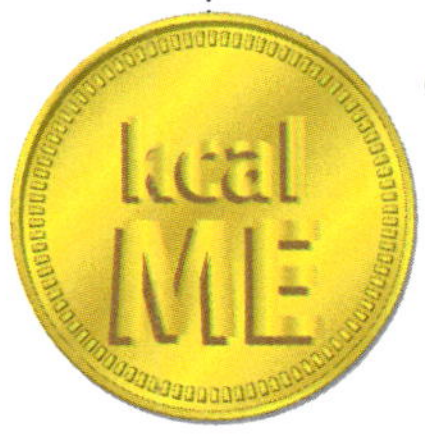

Depending on the energy
(% energy provided by the nutrients regarding the kcal of ME of the food)

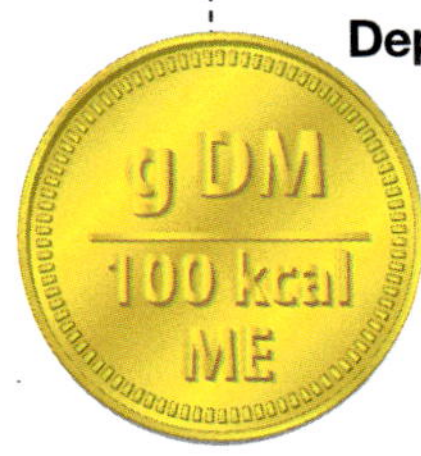

Depending on the dry material for a defined energy density
(g nutrient as DM/100 kcal of ME of the food as DM)

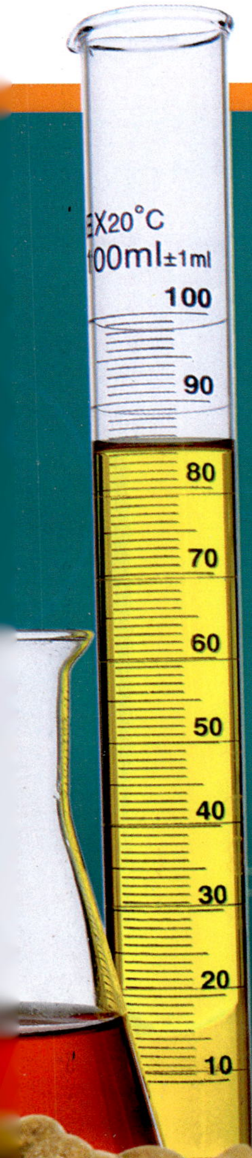

Nitrogen free extracts

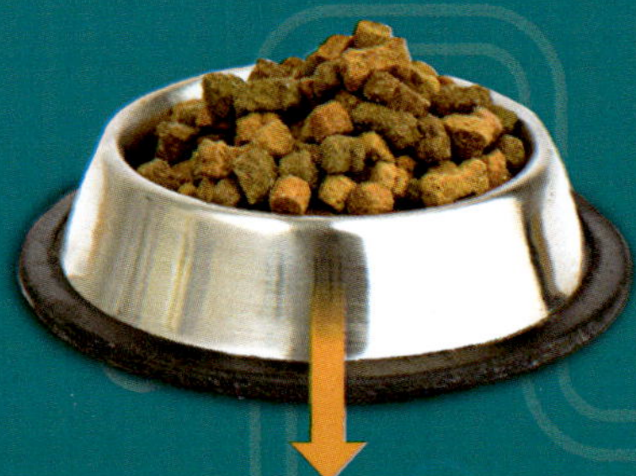

We start with a fresh sample (a food) that represents 100 % of the total. The rest are percentages of this food. Five of the six categories are determined in the laboratory: moisture, protein, fat, fiber, and ash. The NFE are obtained by the difference of the aforementioned. In our example, for food A:

100 – 12 – 22 – 15 – 8 – 5 = 38

NFE + CF = Carbohydrates

Limitations of the method

This method is not very precise nor does it provide information on the quality of certain nutrients, however it does provide information on a food's content and, as we previously mentioned, it is shown on all labels. Let's look at some examples of its limitations:

CP The technique to determine protein actually measures the nitrogen in the sample and extrapolates to crude protein by multiplying by the factor 6.25 (100 g of protein contains 16 % of nitrogen), that is, no difference is made between true protein (bound by peptide bonds) from non-true protein (free amino acids, nitrites, nitrates, urea, ammoniac...), or about the quality (biological value) of the true protein.

EE The complete extraction of the fat with ether is not sufficient. This does not provide us with any information about its profile (saturated or unsaturated) or about its rancidification.

ASH The ashes group together all of the minerals present, but there is no information about their composition or quality.

CF The crude fiber could be a reflection of the digestibility and of the content in net energy of the food ration, but only in cases where we have a special interest. The fermentation of fiber in pets is reduced compared with other animals. In this sense, a greater fiber content leads to lesser digestibility and less content in net energy. This point may be especially interesting when feeding patients with digestive problems, overweight or diabetics. However, there is no differentiation between soluble-fermentable fiber and non-soluble-non-fermentable fiber.

NFE The NFE include the starch and non-starch carbohydrates. They are determined by the difference of the previously mentioned: the calculation errors that we may have committed are accumulated at this point.

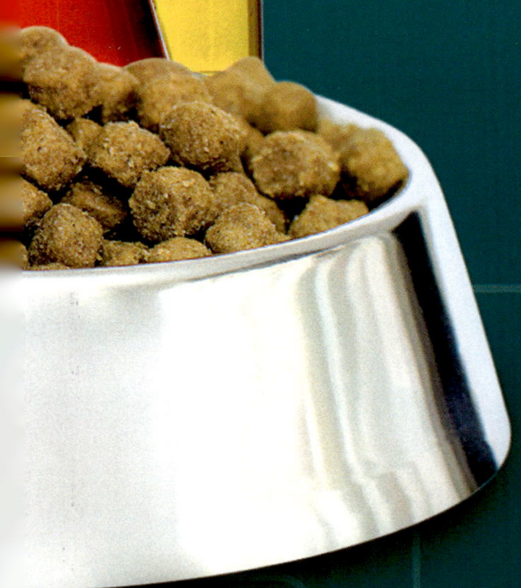

Comparison of foods with

1 The nutrients must be expressed as dry material

Handling the different concepts fluently is of great interest given that to compare foods with different moisture contents, it is necessary and indispensable to express it as dry material. The grams of a nutrient may be the same, but not its proportions. An explanation using a diagram makes it very simple to understand:

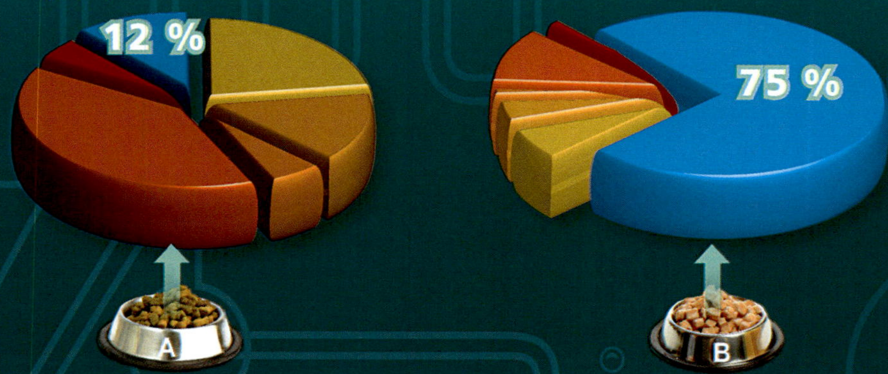

In these two foods, the percentages of nutrients regarding the DM are the same, although their amounts vary noticeably.

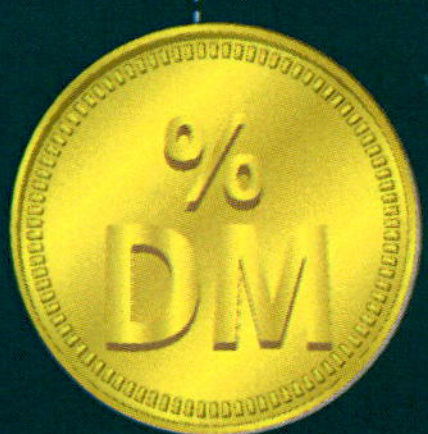

%
DM

3 Example of food comparison regarding dry material

	FOOD (FM)		FOOD (DM)	
NUTRIENT	A (%)	B (%)	A (%)	B (%)
Moisture	12	75	0	0
Dry material	88	25	100	100
Protein	22	6.25	25.00	25.00
Fat	15	4.26	17.05	17.04
Fiber	6.2	1.75	7.05	7.00
Carbohydrates	39.8	11.32	45.23	45.28
Ash	5	1.42	5.68	5.68

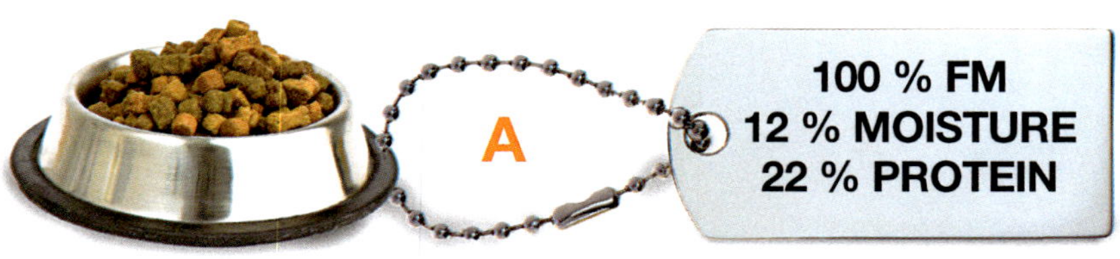

A
100 % FM
12 % MOISTURE
22 % PROTEIN

100 – 12 = 88 % of DM

Protein → $\frac{22\ \%}{88\ \%\ DM}$ = **25 % of protein (DM)**

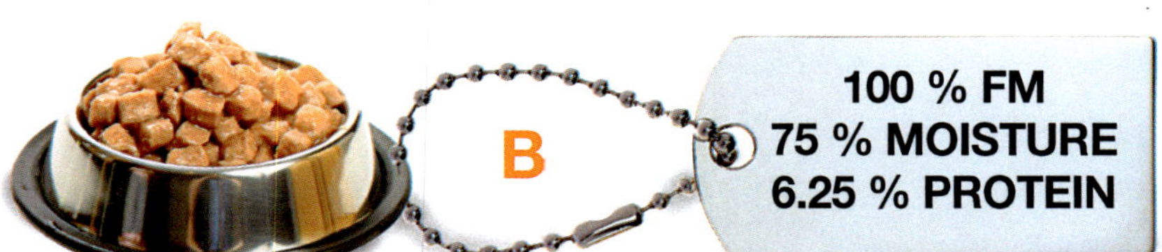

B
100 % FM
75 % MOISTURE
6.25 % PROTEIN

100 – 75 = 25 % of DM

Protein → $\frac{6.25\ \%}{25\ \%\ DM}$ = **25 % of protein (DM)**

and so on with the rest of the nutrients.

In this example, we can see that the use of the dry presentation (A), with a 12 % of moisture, has the same content in nutrients expressed as dry material as a canned food (B), with a moisture of 75 %. Apart from the other considerations, either one of the two foods has a very similar nutrient composition. One is not better than the other.

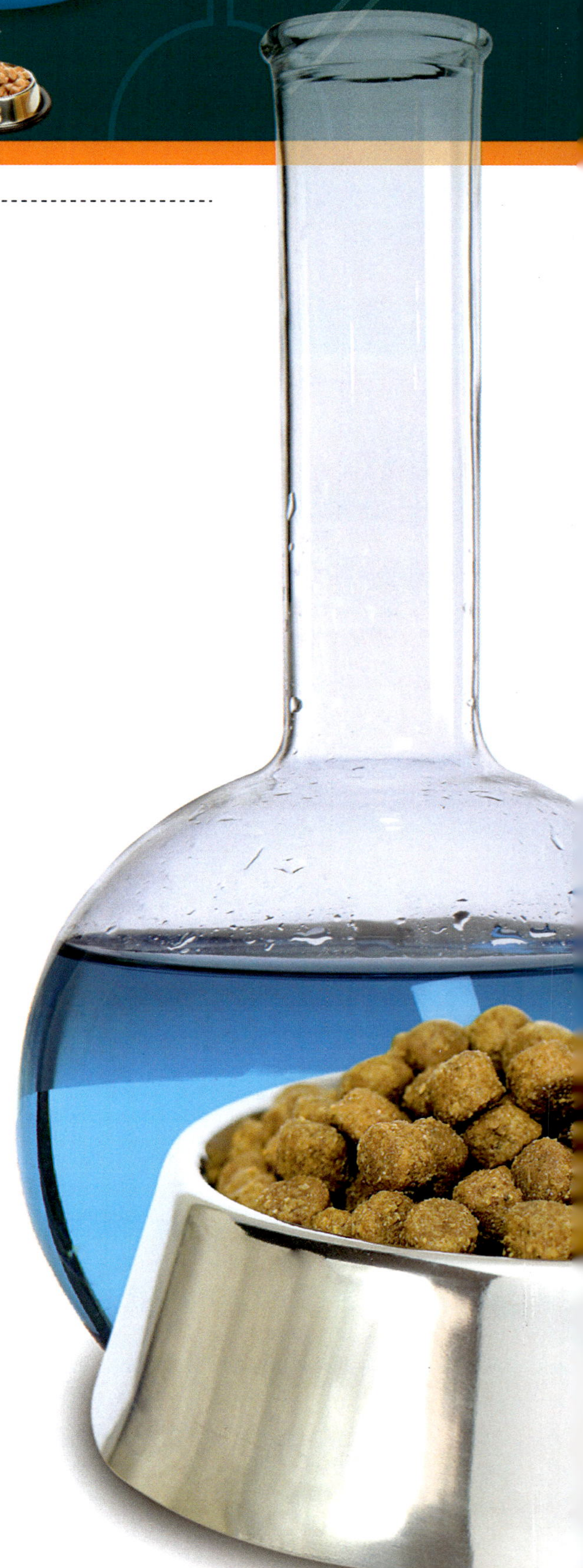

different levels of moisture

2

Determination of the dry material (DM) of the foods

We perform the conversion of the value of the different nutrients expressed depending on its water-free content.

A. The first step consists of knowing the percentage of dry material of the food:

100 % FM – % moisture = % DM

B. Below we express the value of the fresh nutrient as if 100 % of the sample were dry material:

% nutrient (FM)/% DM = % nutrient (DM)

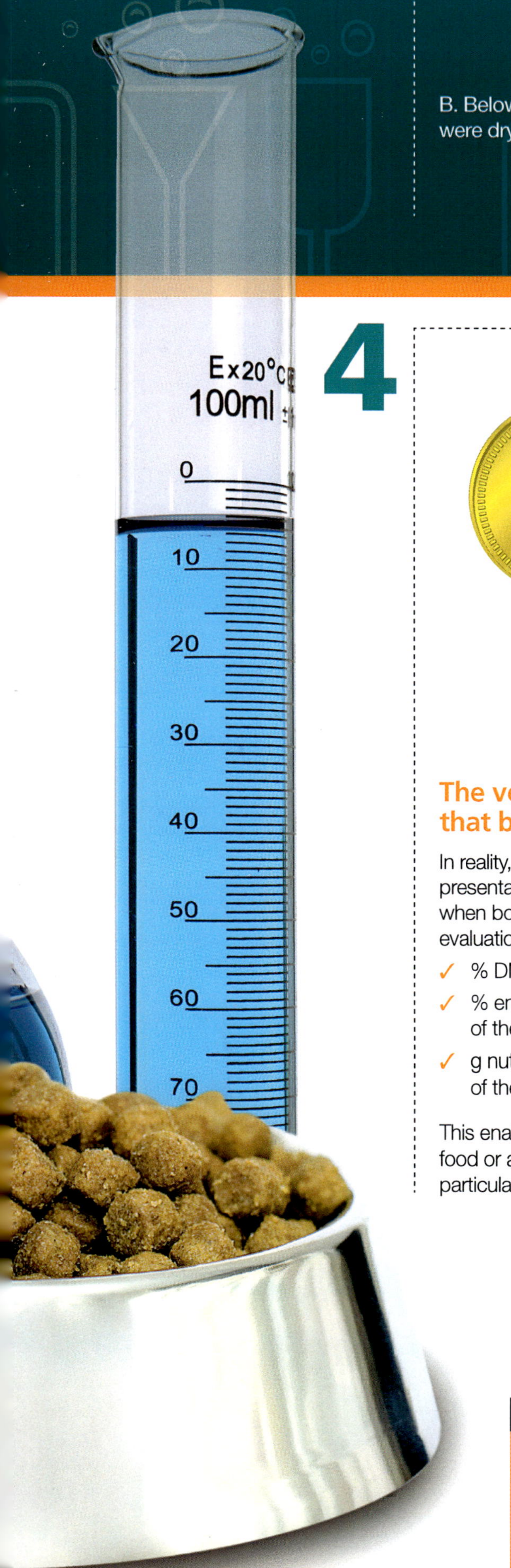

4

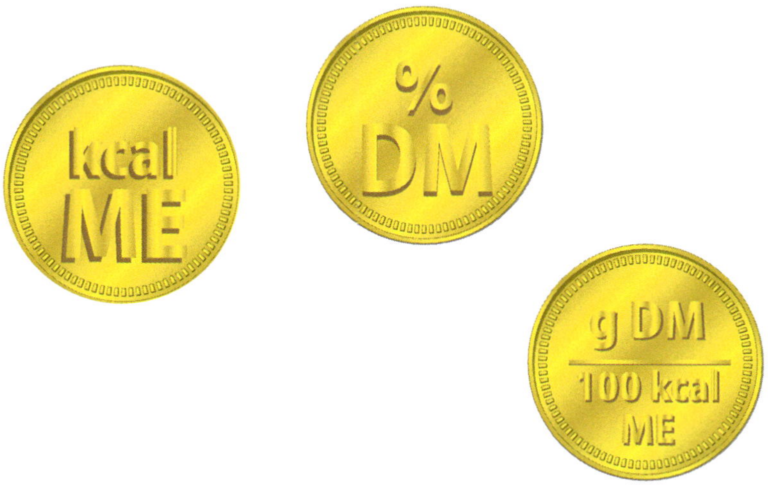

The veterinarian can select the method that best adapts to the patient

In reality, the same food from the same brand with its two presentations, dry and canned, is not exactly the same when both presentations are compared with any of the three evaluation methods:

- ✓ % DM.
- ✓ % energy of the nutrients regarding the kcal of ME of the food.
- ✓ g nutrient (DM)/100 kcal of ME of the food (DM).

This enables the veterinarian to choose one food or another depending on the nutritional particularities of each patient.

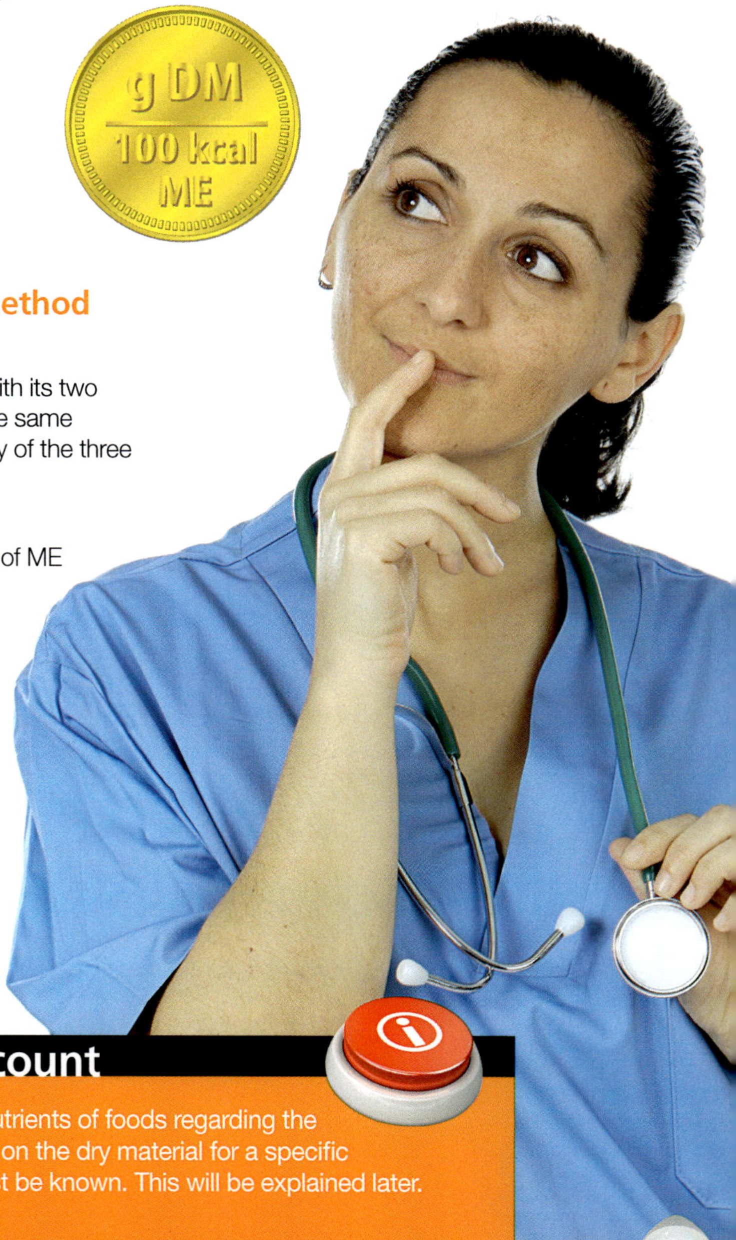

To be taken into account

In order to express the content in nutrients of foods regarding the metabolizable energy or depending on the dry material for a specific energy level, its energy content must be known. This will be explained later.

Other methods

Energy and nutrient per unit of energy

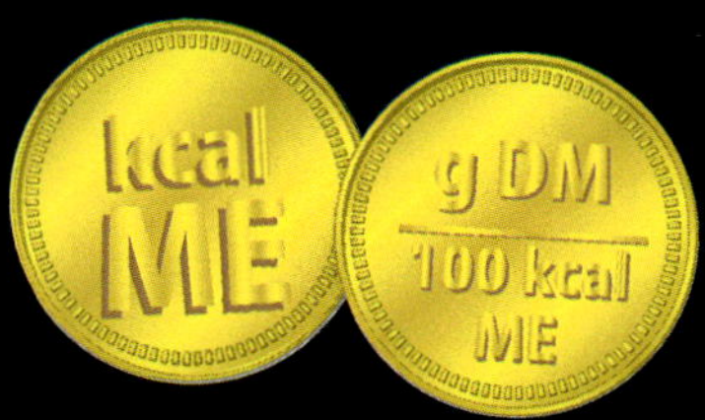

Sometimes we find that the composition of a food is expressed as **energy (%)** or as **nutrient per unit of energy (g/100 kcal)**. Depending on the situation, this assessment can be interesting given that it determines the choice of one food over another regarding the balance of nutrients and the energy it provides.

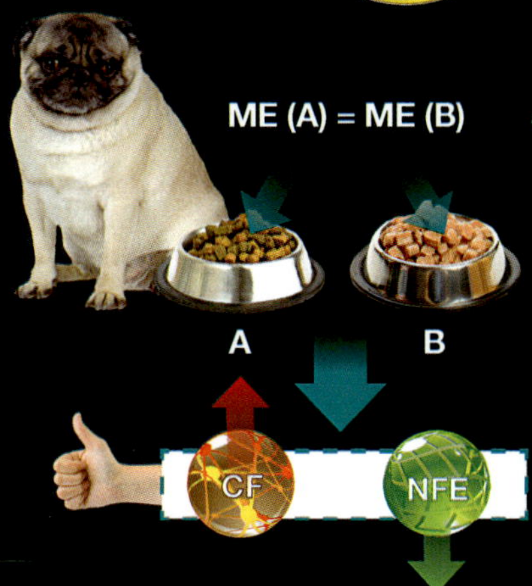

Example:

In a diabetic animal, when given the possibility of two different presentations, dry food and canned food, with a similar ME (DM) level, we are faced with the question of which would be best.
We would be interested in high and similar fiber levels, but lower NFE levels to avoid decompensating glycemia levels.

We previously saw how the ME of a food is calculated. Here we will see how the nutrients are expressed in the two following ways:

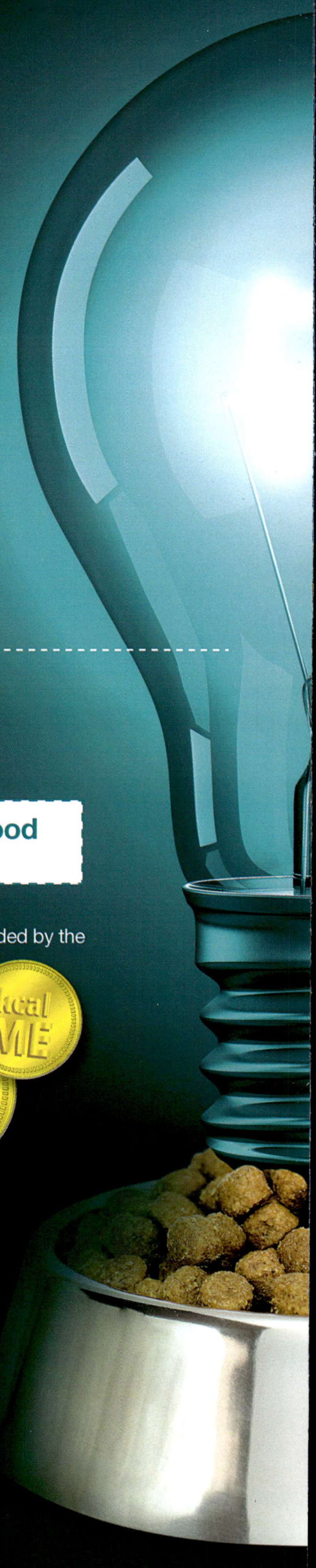

1 As a percentage of the energy of the food

The calculation is simple and based on determining the energetic value of the nutrient and comparing it with the energy that the food provides. To do so, first we have to know the ME that the nutrient provides:

$$\% \text{ nutrient} \times \text{Atwater factor}_{\text{modified}} \text{ (kcal/g of nutrient)} = \text{kcal ME of the nutrient/g of food}$$

Once obtained, it is divided by the total ME of the food, which is obtained by the sum of the energies provided by the three nutrients, and this is how we obtain the relative proportion that the nutrient provides.

$$\frac{\text{kcal/g of food}}{\text{ME g of food}} = \% \text{ kcal from the nutrient}$$

Example:

If we take into account the values from the following table:

Nutrient	FS (%)	Modified Atwater	ME (kcal/g)	Energy (%)	g/ 100 kcal
CP	21	3.5	0.735	23.08	6.59
EE	10	8.5	0.85	26.69	3.14
NFE	45.7	3.5	1.56	50.23	14.35
Total ME			3.18		

FS: fresh sample

For the case of protein, it would be:

$$\frac{21}{100} \times 3.5 = 0.735 \text{ kcal/g of protein}$$

$$\frac{0.735 \text{ kcal/g of protein}}{3.18 \text{ kcal/g of food}}$$

Protein provides 23.08 % of the energy of the food

to evaluate the energy in foods

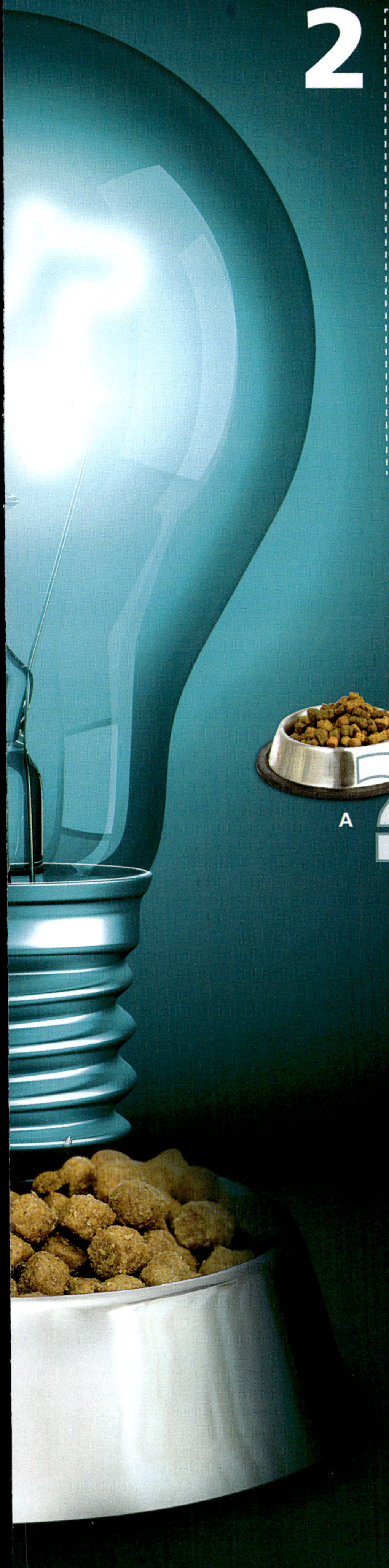

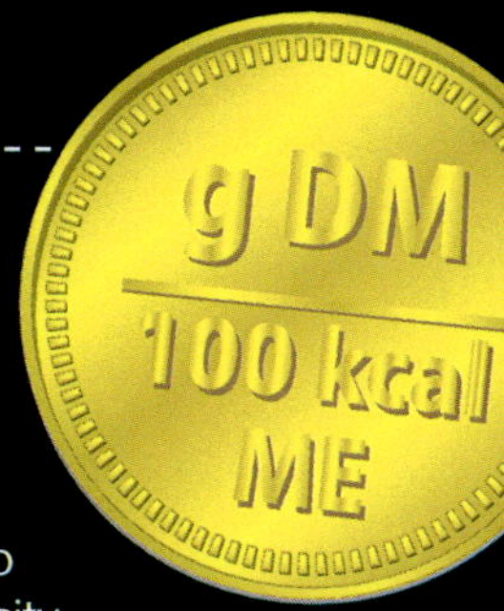

2 As unit of nutrient per unit of energy of the food

This system of expression sometimes appears in the "average analysis" provided by manufacturers, just as the requirements in dogs and cats are expressed in the NRC. Like the previous case, it is a relative method and is generally expressed as g of nutrient per 100 kcal of food.

For calculation, you simply have to determine how many grams of a nutrient are needed, with the proportion that they represent over the total of the energy of the food, to obtain a food with an energetic density of 100 kcal:

$$\frac{\%\ \text{nutrient energy}}{\text{Atwater factor}_{\text{modified}}} = \text{g of nutrient/100 kcal of food}$$

Following with our example:

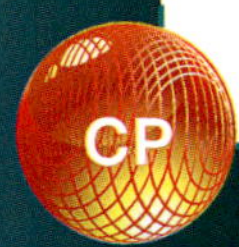

$$\frac{23.08\ \%}{3.5} = 6.59\ \text{g of protein/100 kcal of food}$$

Additional factors in the selection of foods

Aside from the nutritional point of view, there are other factors that help us to decide which is the best option for the pet and the owner:

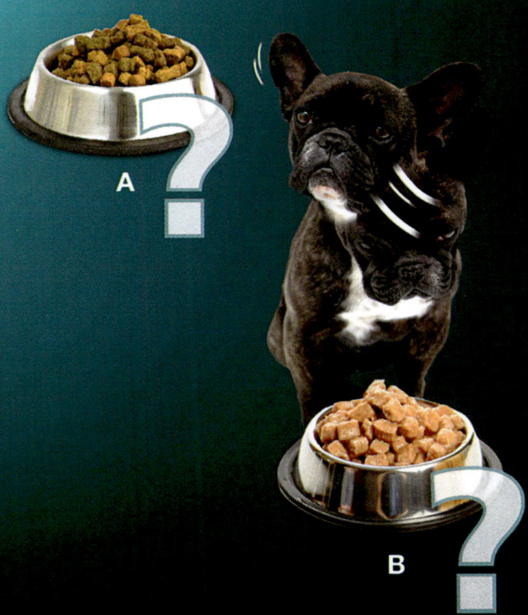

Preference and acceptance tests

Brands make decisions based on these tests on which foods they will commercialize. We can do the same using a few references that we believe are appropriate, allowing the animal to choose which option is most palatable (smell, taste, and texture). This is very interesting in animals with a picky appetite (when it has not been altered by the owner, for example, with homemade food...) and in patients with consumptive chronic diseases.

This consists of presenting the different references A and B in two plates for 2 or 3 days and measuring the ingestion of each one of the foods. Also, we can quantify the results using the following ratio: **rate of ingestion = A/(A+B)**. In practice, simple observation on behalf of the owner is sufficient.

The pet's preferences usually are related with the content in nutrients, with the manufacturing technology and with the presence of palatability enhancing substances.

Storage conditions and cost of feeding

These are defined by the water and fat content of a food as well as the energy content per unit of base food, respectively. These aspects have previously been explained in the section on pet foods.

Quality of the feces

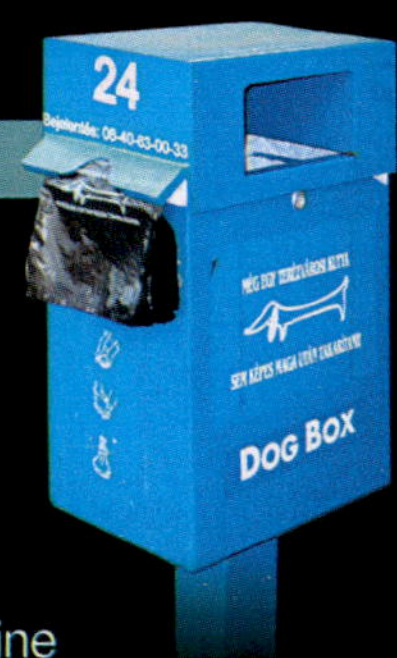

Social manners and legislation force us to eliminate our pet's excrements from public areas. Likewise, the ease of cleaning dog runs or kitty litter boxes is an important aspect for owners, breeders and people that run canine and feline residencies. The quality of feces (frequency, form, size and consistency), determine the selection of a food. It all depends on the content in moisture and in the quantity and quality of the fiber found in the food.

How do we calculate the daily food ration?

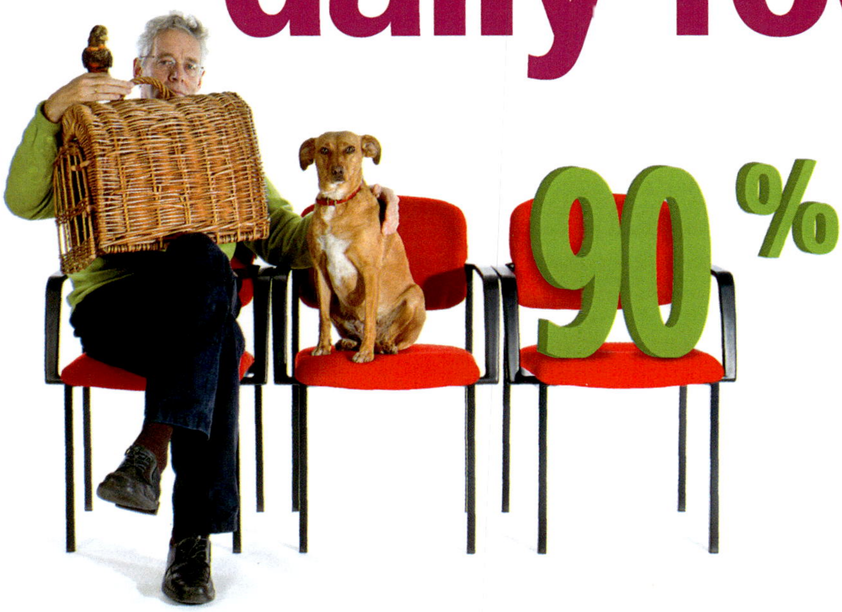

Ninety percent of owners would prefer that their veterinarian provide them with advice regarding this issue

One of the primary factors of the loss of trust in a veterinarian as a consultant in nutrition for dogs and cats is because owners' questions have been answered by reading the label on the pet food packaging or by the information presented in the "product leaflet" by the manufacturing company. This is curious given that an estimated 90 % of owners would like their veterinarians to provide guidance on this topic, although only 54 % have actually sought this service out.

To add value to the nutrition and feeding consultations, more has to be done. The steps to follow are simple; here we see how it is done with an example:

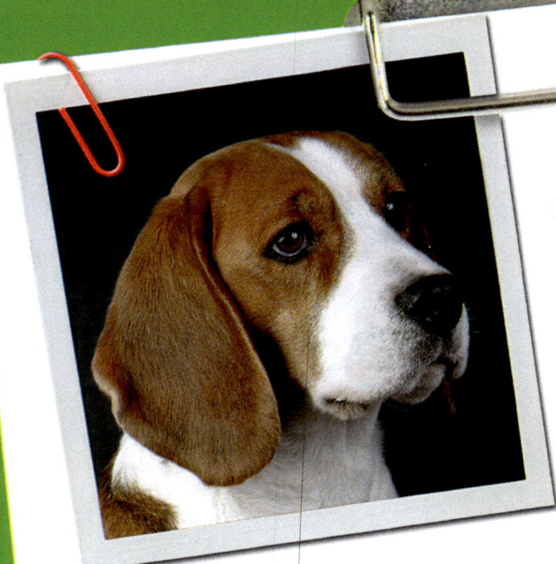

Patient: *Tobby*, Beagle breed.

History: Sterilized, insulin-dependent diabetic, with a body weight of **18.4 kg**.
The dog's body condition is **5/9**.
It has an **abdominal circumference of 45 cm** and a **paw length of 12.5 cm**.
Tobby lives in a yard in the southern part of Spain where the average maximum temperature is **35 °C**.

Which of these two complete foods for adult dogs would we recommend, A or B?

What would the daily food ration of the selected food be?

	Moisture (%)	Protein (%)	Fat (%)	Ash (%)	Fiber (%)
A. Dry	8	21	10	6.2	9.1
B. Wet	78	5.21	3.03	2.51	3.27

1 Determine the weight and body condition

After weighing the animal, we classify it with the body score system: level 5/9. He is at his optimal weight.

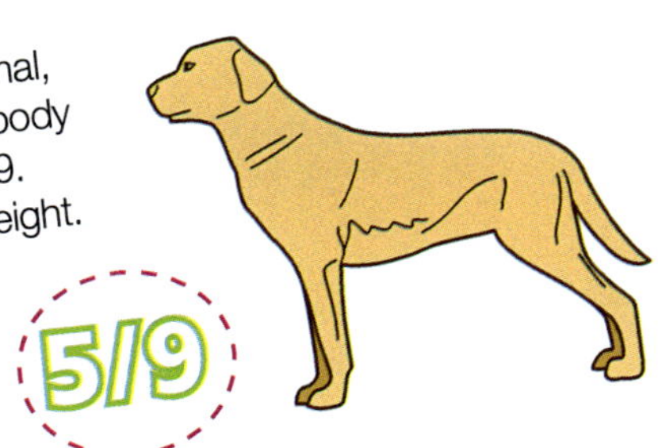

With this information and the morphometric measurements, the dog's body fat has a value close to 20.

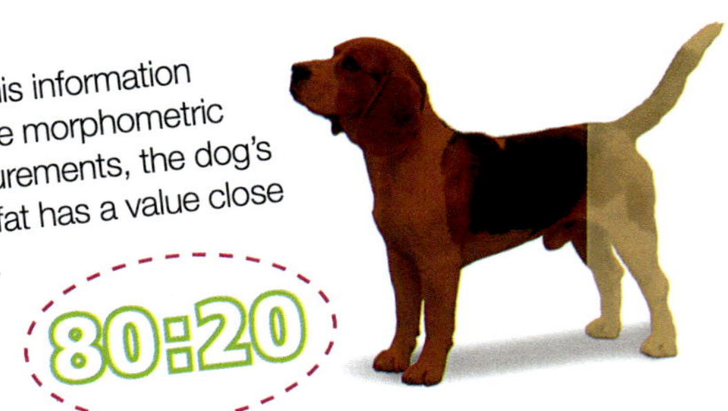

2 Calculate the nutrition requirements for maintenance

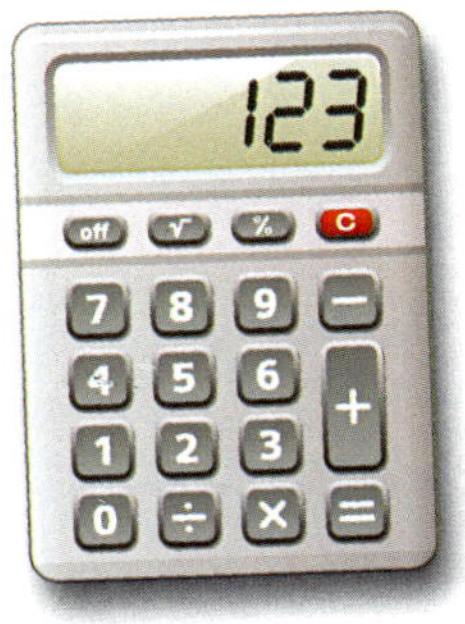

$$MER\ (kcal\ ME/day) = 132\ (kcal) \times body\ weight\ (kg)^{0.75}$$

$$MER = 132 \times 18.4^{0,75} = 1{,}172.7\ kcal\ ME/day$$

However, the **daily requirements** that should be taken into account are the following:

- Sterilized animal **0.8**
- The dog lives outdoors **1.06**
- High temperatures **1.1 to 1.3**

$$DER = MER \times 0.8 \times 1.06 \times 1.2$$

$$DER = 1{,}172.7 \times 0.8 \times 1.06 \times 1.2 = 1{,}192.7\ kcal\ ME/day$$

Ingestion of water to maintain body temperature

	ml water: ME	% body weight	50-60 ml × body weight
18.4 kg	1.2 liters	1.2 liters	1.01 liters

However, we must correct the value as the temperatures are high (35 °C) and the dog lives in an outdoor yard.

$$Water\ (Temp. > 30\ °C) = 6\ ml/kg\ body\ weight^{0.75}/day/°C$$

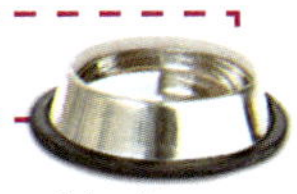

$$Water = 6 \times 18.4^{0.75} \times 5 = 266.5\ ml$$

The following amount of daily water should be provided:

1.2 liters + 0.266 liters = 1.46 liters/day

3 Compare the foods, estimate the energy value and take into consideration the nutritional profile that best adapts to the patient

A. Dry

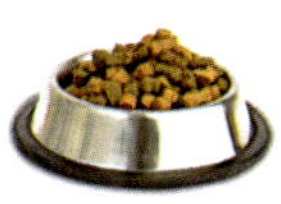

B. Wet

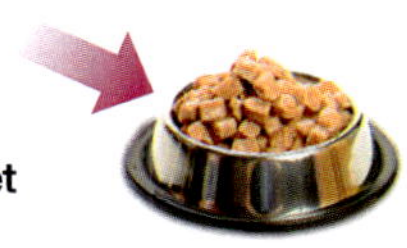

	A. Dry Label	A. Dry DM	A. Dry % Energy	A. Dry g/100 kcal	B. Wet Label	B. Wet DM	B. Wet % Energy	B. Wet g/100 kcal
Moisture	8	0			78	0		
CP	21	22.83	23.08	6.59	5.21	23.68	25.35	7.24
EE	10	10.87	26.69	3.14	3.03	13.77	35.81	4.21
ASH	6.2	6.74			2.51	11.41		
CF	9.1	9.89			3.27	14.86		
NFE	45.7	49.67	50.23	14.35	7.98	36.27	38.83	11.10
*ME kcal/g	3.18	3.46			0.72	3.26		

*Estimate by modified Atwater ME kcal/g = 3.5 x (CP + NFE) + 8.5 x EE.

Without performing an in-depth analysis of the nutritional profile of a diabetic, in our case, we prefer food B for the following reasons:

- ✔ **The energy concentration per unit of DM is scarcely variable (5 %).**
- ✔ **Provide a similar amount of protein.**
- ✔ **A lower content in NFE.**
- ✔ **A greater content in CF.**

4 Determine the daily food ration

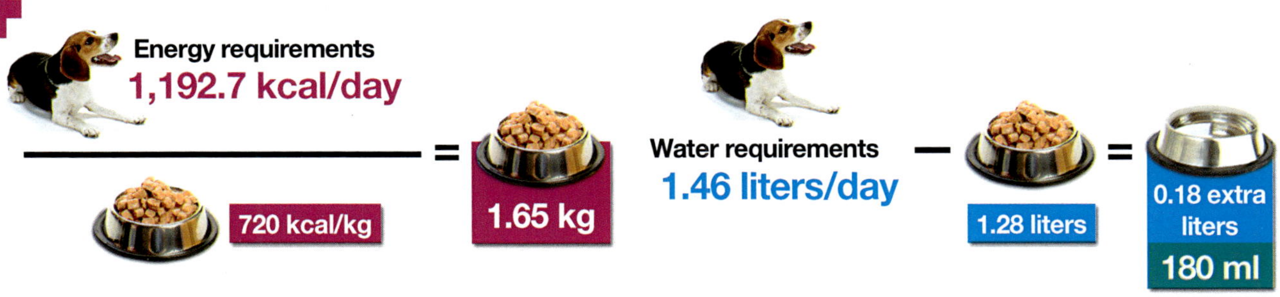

Energy requirements
1,192.7 kcal/day
───────────── = **1.65 kg**
720 kcal/kg

Water requirements 1.46 liters/day − **1.28 liters** = **0.18 extra liters 180 ml**

Administration

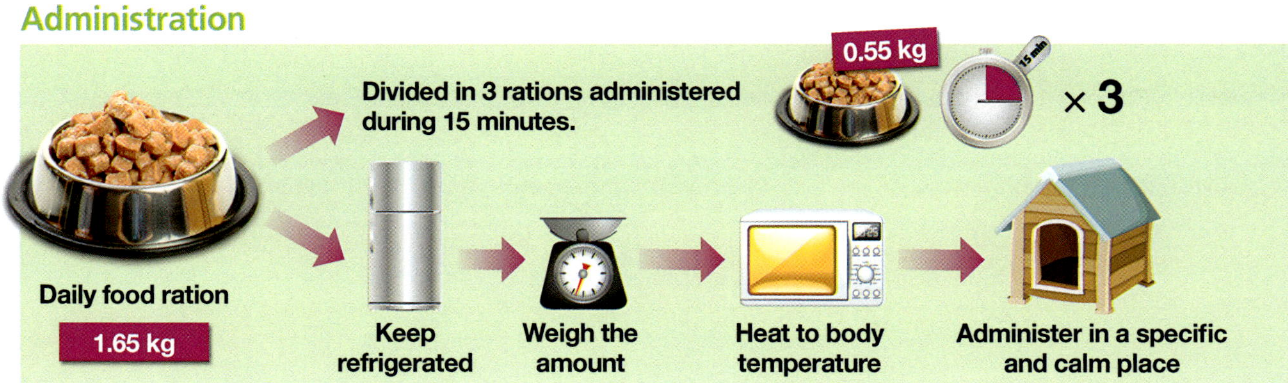

Food "extra"

1

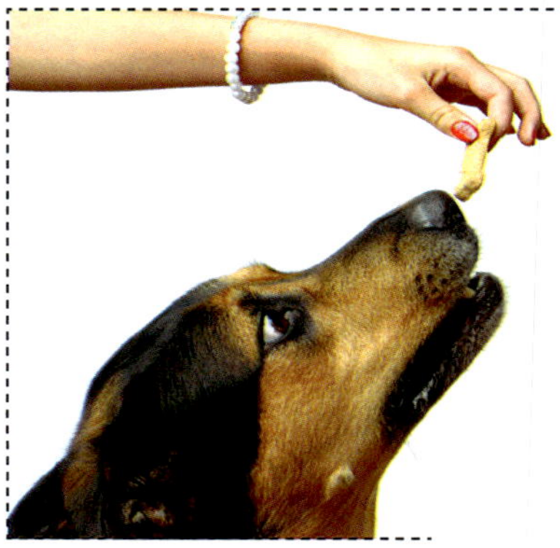

60-90 %

Between 60-90 % of pets receive treats throughout their lives.

The presentation of these products is highly varied: specific (treats, snacks), wet foods, table scraps, etc. The primary justification is emotional.

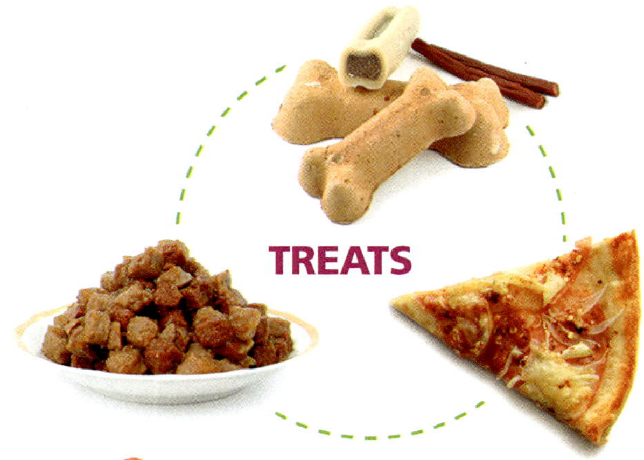

2

Food as a gift

Food plays an important role in human relationships. We share our food as a sign of friendship within the organization of social groups. It has been demonstrated that sharing a meal represents social equality. Likewise, there is a tendency toward man-animal interaction through food, as the first form of contact or as a sign of caring. It is also true that food is sometimes used as a reward for a job well done: it is a tool –a positive reinforcement– during the learning process. However, many owners consider food to be a gift, undervaluing the calories provided and the consequences in pets' energy balances.

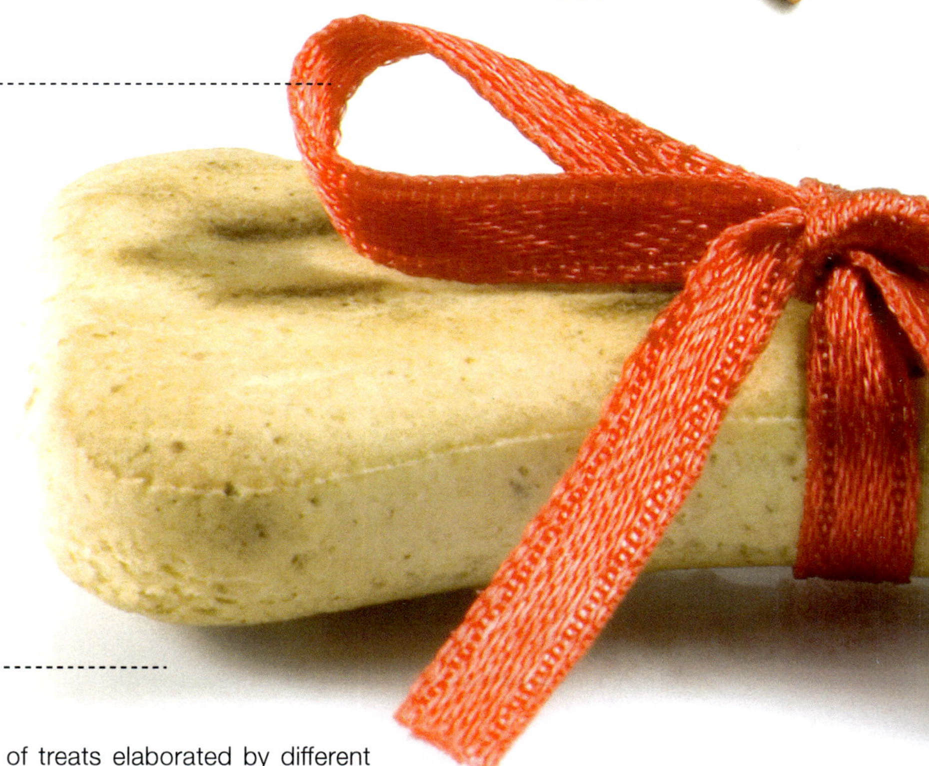

3

Energy content of treats

The composition, and therefore the energy content, of treats elaborated by different commercial brands is highly varied. The use of 10 g of a treat of this type is equal to 5 or 10 % of the dogs' or cats' requirements, respectively.

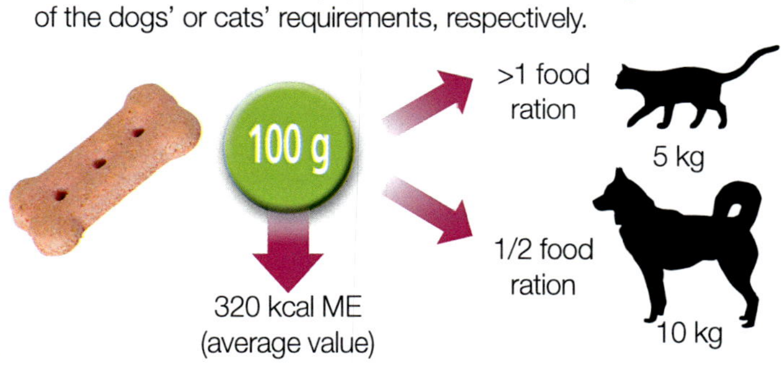

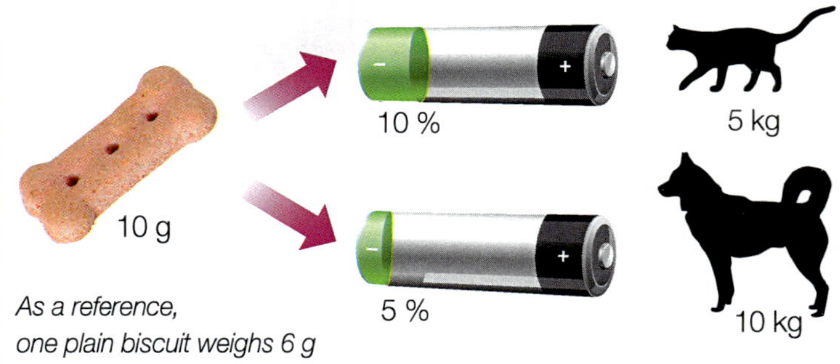

4

Exceptions

Some treats sold to the public that are rich in protein of little biological value (tendons, cartilage) could be used for their low digestibility and calories. One inconvenience that this type of treats presents is the fermentation of non-digested protein in the posterior sections of the digestive apparatus, with the elimination of gases (derivatives of sulfur, indole and skatole, methane) that have an unpleasant effect on those nearby.

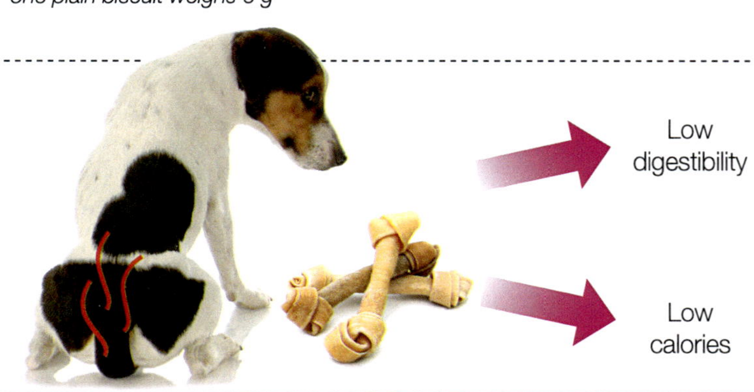

5 Careful with the excess of energy

One of the problems that we see in our clinical practice today is the lack of coherence between the food requirements of pets and how their owners feed them. The perception on what implications a food may have and its true nutritional value is very different. Most of them do not know or undervalue the caloric value of the food offered and its implications in the animal's energy balance. All of these "treats" provide energy, even those labeled as light.

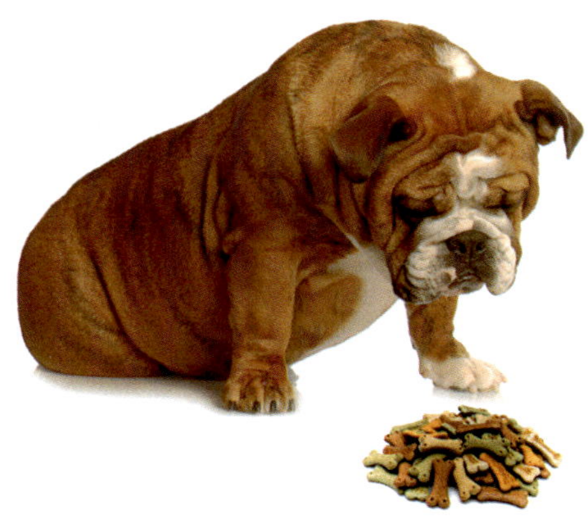

6 Be careful with table scraps

The situation is even more complicated when we use table scraps of homemade food or human foods. Here we see some comparisons of the energy value provided and the proportion that they represent regarding the maintenance requirements (M) of dogs and cats:

					"Hamburger equivalent" (210 g unit)	
Food	**Amount**	**kcal ME[1]**	**% M dog[2]**	**% M cat[2]**	**Dog (10 kg)**	**Cat (5 kg)**
Small piece of cheese	20 g	70	9.4	23.8	1/2	1
Milk	1/2 of a glass	58	7.8	19.7	1/3	1
Bread	1/2 of a baguette	270	36.4	91.8	1.5	Not routinely
Toast	Unit	145	19.5	49.3	1	2
Apple	1/4	20	2.7	6.8	-	Not routinely
Cookies	3 units (× 6 g)	87	3.9	9.9	1/2	1.2
Cookies with chocolate	Unit (24 g)	114	15.4	38.8	2/3	1.5
Baked ham lunch meat	Slice (20 g)	43	5.8	14.6	1/4	3/4
Sausage	Unit	189	25.5	64.3	1	3
Paté	Can (80 g)	260	35	88.4	1.5	3.5
Potato chips	1 handful (15 g)	77	10.4	26.2	1/4	Not routinely
Popcorn	1 handful (10 g)	50	6.7	17.0	1/2	Not routinely
Tuna/sardines	Can (80 g)	180	24.2	61.2	1	2.5
Beef	1/2 fillet steak (85 g)	225	30.3	76.5	1.2	3
Lunch meat	Slice (10 g)	37	5.0	12.6	1/4	1/2
Meat-filled pasta	Ration (125 g)	125	16.8	42.5	1	1.5

[1] Calculated using the modified Atwater equation (NRC 1985).
[2] NRC 2006.

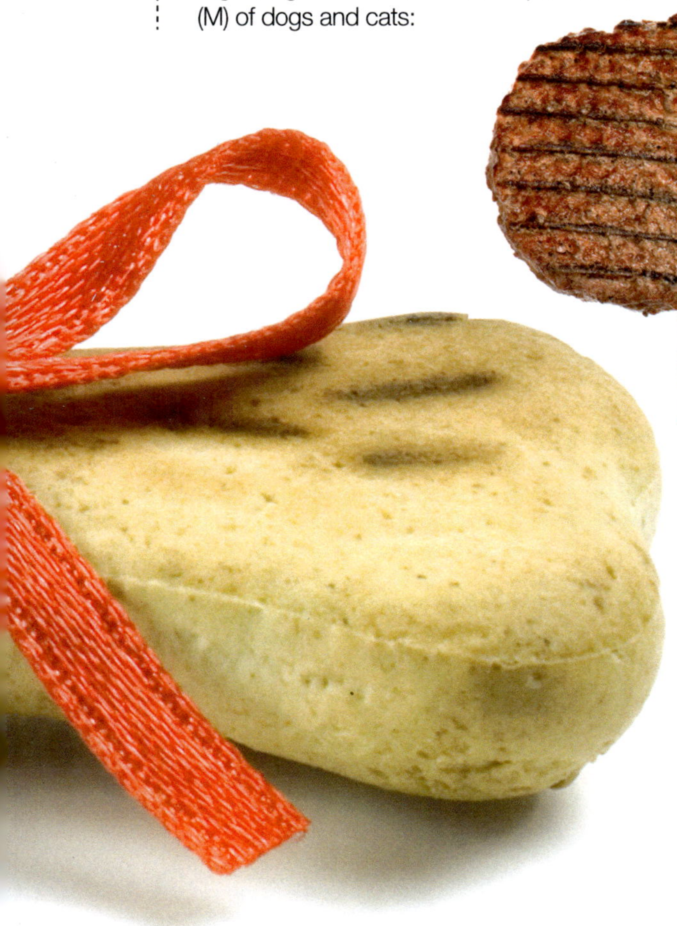

7 Use not recommended

Generally, the use of "extra" foods is not advised when animals are eating a complete and balanced diet. In these cases, they could be used substituting up to a maximum of 10 % of the animal's energy requirements. That said, we do not recommend their use as they modify the normal palatability of foods and create bad habits (asking for food or begging).

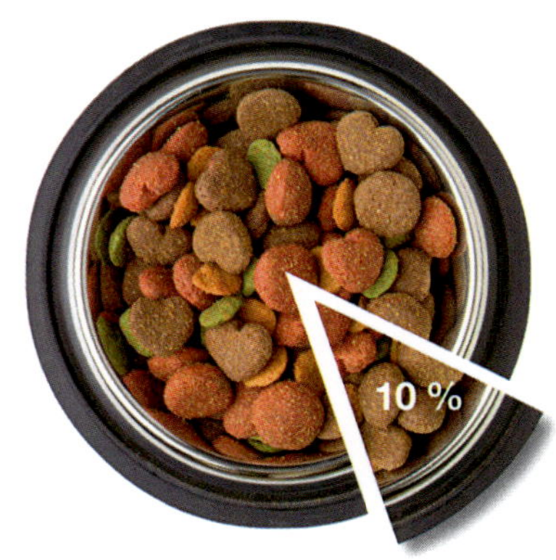

8 The "hamburger equivalent"

The use of an intelligible unit and its equivalence in humans, such as a 210 g hamburger (the normal size at establishments that serve this type of food) may help owners understand what the treats that they give to their pet truly represent. According to the table, a Frankfurt-type sausage offered to a cat daily is the same as if a pet owner ate three hamburgers every single day, or a piece of breakfast toast, with butter and jam, for a 10 kg dog, represents the daily ingestion of one hamburger for us humans.

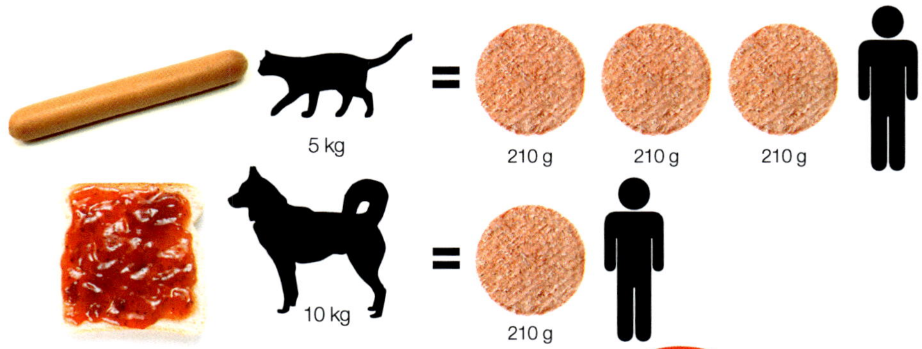

To be taken into account

The use of treats as a tool during the training period of a dog or cat does have a clear purpose.
What would be its ideal use? There are two possibilities:

- Subtract its energy value from the animal's daily ingestion.
- Use part of the animal's daily food ration as treats.

Diet changes

1 Reasons to make changes

Throughout the life of pets, their feeding may need to be changed as a consequence of an imbalance in their initial food ration, because their requirements have changed (different physiological stages or presence of pathological processes) or because of a personal decision on behalf of the owner independent of our recommendations.

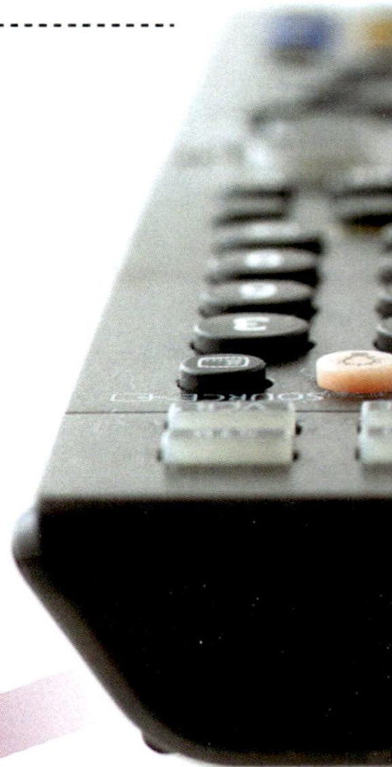

2 Substitution may lead to dysbiosis

In most healthy animals, these changes can be implemented from one day to the next without causing any digestive problems. However, sometimes digestive symptoms with a sudden presentation may be produced. Initially taking into consideration only healthy animals, the cause of this process is a dysbiosis due to the substitution, incorporation or modification in the proportions of the ingredients and nutrients.

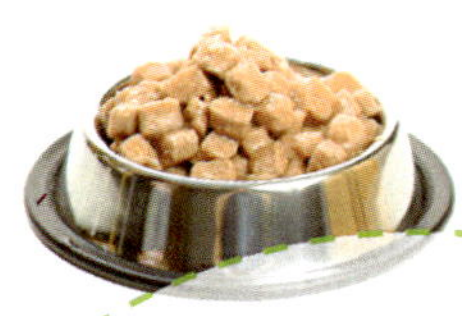

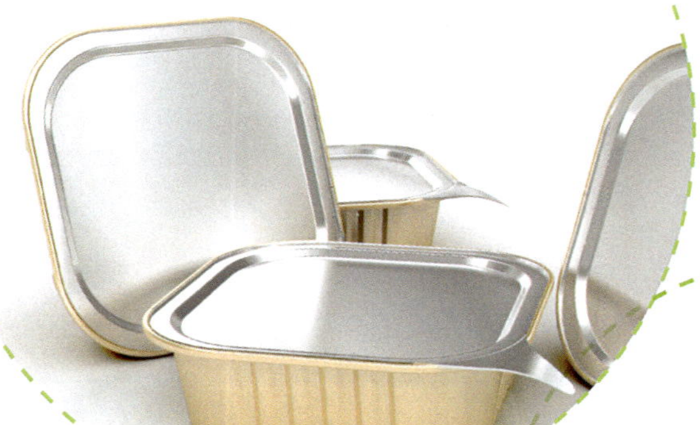

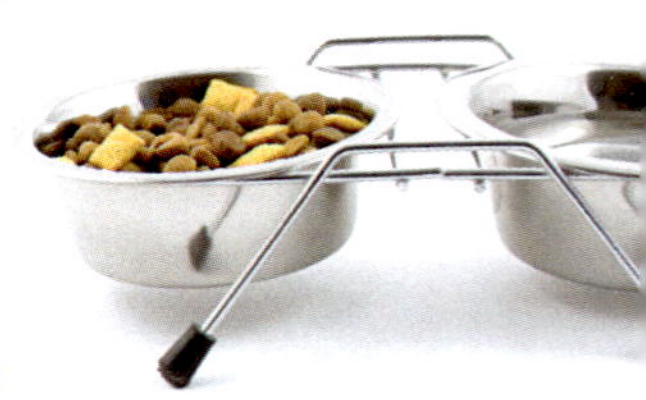

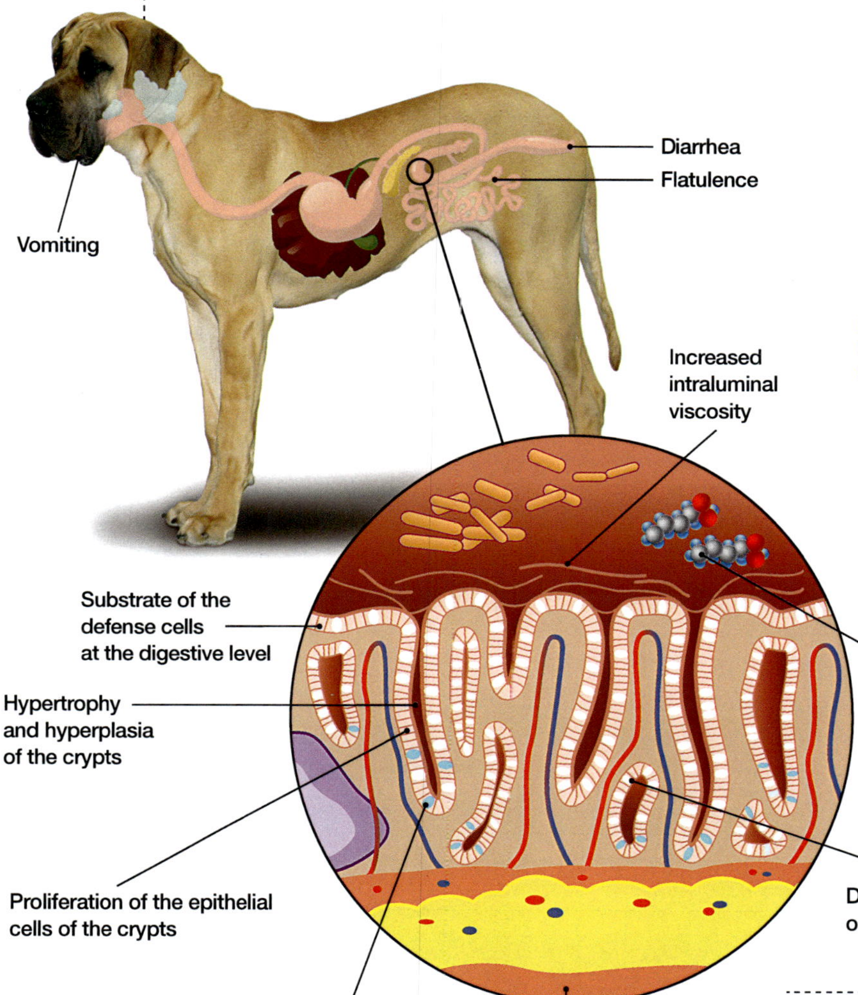

3 Effects on the digestive microflora

It has been observed that the quality of the protein, the type and amount of fiber and the class of carbohydrates (resistant starch, oligosaccharides and non-starch polysaccharides) present in the food rations are related with the modifications in the digestive microflora (see image).

How should I do it?

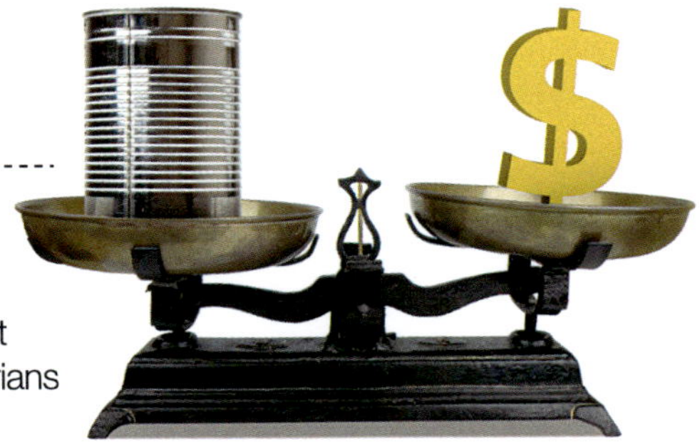

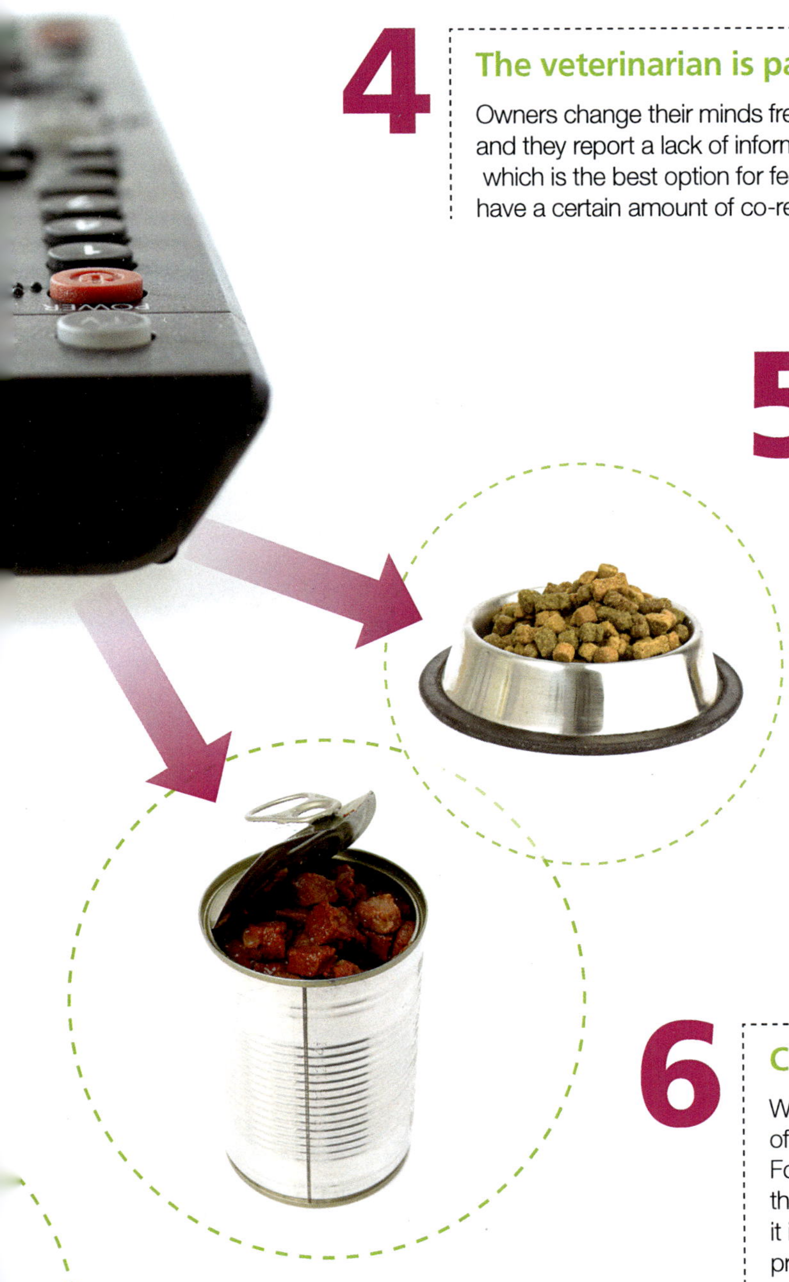

4 The veterinarian is partially responsible

Owners change their minds frequently regarding their pet's diet, and they report a lack of information received by their veterinarian about which is the best option for feeding their pet and the cost: we veterinarians have a certain amount of co-responsibility in this decision.

5 Any change must be gradual

It is recommended to change the type of food for at least 3 days, removing gradually larger amounts of the normal diet and simultaneously increasing the new diet in the same amount, giving the intestinal flora a chance to adapt adequately. If the composition of the new diet causes us to doubt its possible digestive impact or because it is a food that is poorly accepted by our patient, this period should be prolonged up to 7 or 10 days.

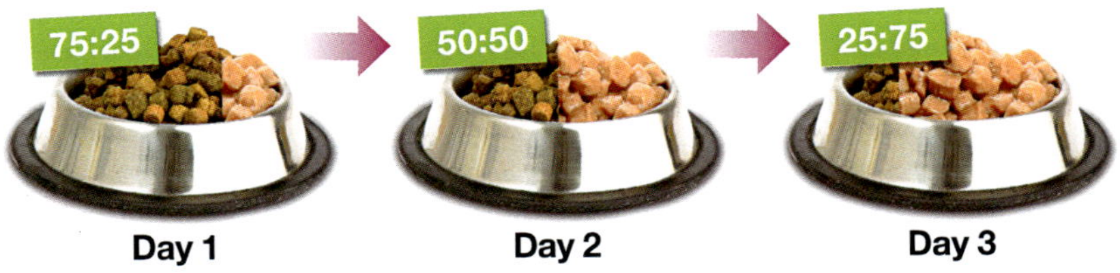

6 Cats require more time to adapt

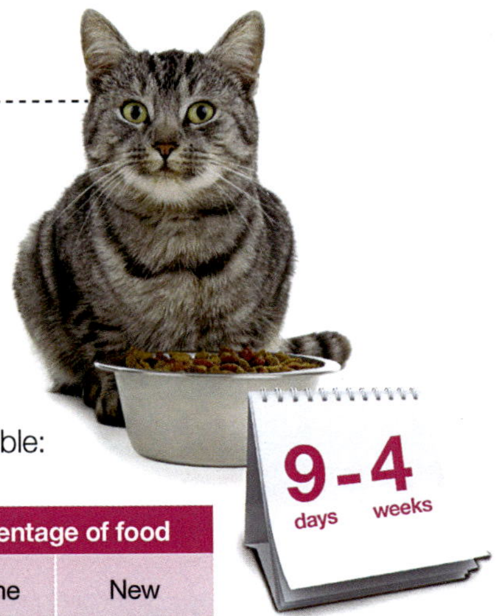

We must keep in mind that the ingestive behavior of cats is more complicated than that of dogs.
For this reason, in this species, and when faced with the possibility of an absolute rejection of the new diet, it is recommended that the food transition process be prolonged.

We can see how this should be done in the following table:

Short transition	Long transition		Percentage of food	
Dogs and cats (days)	Dogs (days)	Cats (weeks)	Routine	New
1.2	1-3	1	75	25
3.4	4-6	2	50	50
5.6	7-9	3	25	75
7	10	4	0	100

7 Continued rejection on behalf of the animal

The animal may continue to reject the food ration in any of the previously mentioned situations. In these cases, we will have to diagnosis the cause, correct it or find alternatives that increase the animal's appetite.

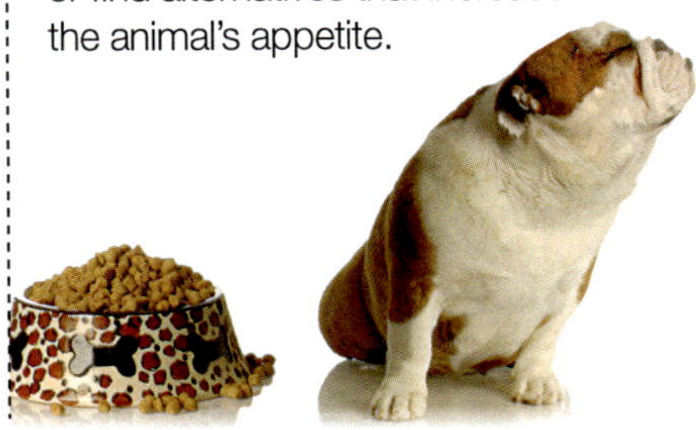

To be taken into account

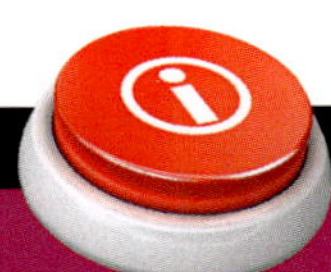

In daily clinical practice, it is very simple, and comfortable for the owner, to use a mixture of 50 % of the two foods for 5 days and from the 6th day on, administer 100 % of the new food.

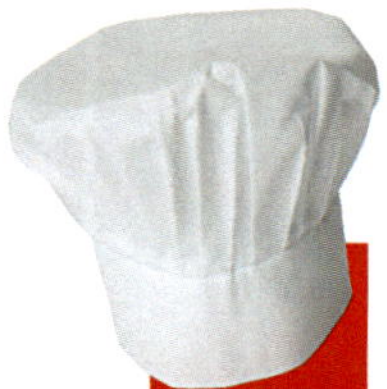

Homemade food

10-25 %

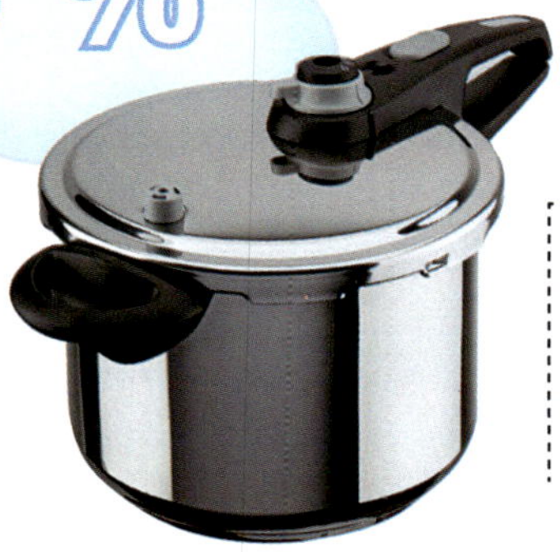

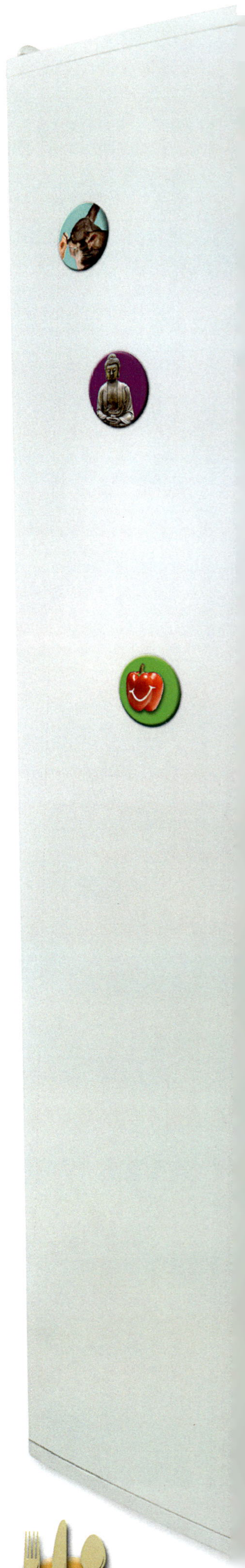

Between 10 and 25 % of pet owners prefer to "cook" for their pet

This figure does not include food leftovers, which are commonly offered to pets.

Why may a pet owner choose a homemade diet?

1 Country's food culture

In countries with a long culinary tradition –Spain, France and Italy–, the use of homemade food is more common.

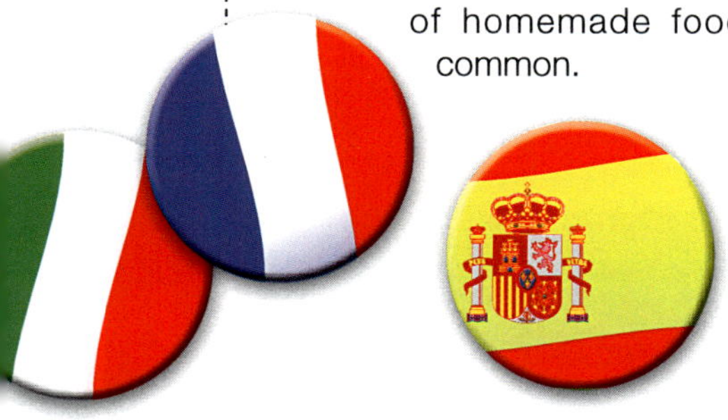

2 Perceived as healthy and ecological

Homemade food is perceived as non-artificial, healthier, whole, fresh and natural food. Owners can decide how and when they purchase the raw materials for this "healthier" and ecological diet, free from chemical substances.

3 Greater owner-pet interaction

Food is used as a result of overprotection or of trying to compensate for a lack of attention: the concepts of love and food are synonyms. A particular case is that of animals with end-stage diseases: this is the last gesture of love and compassion towards a beloved animal.

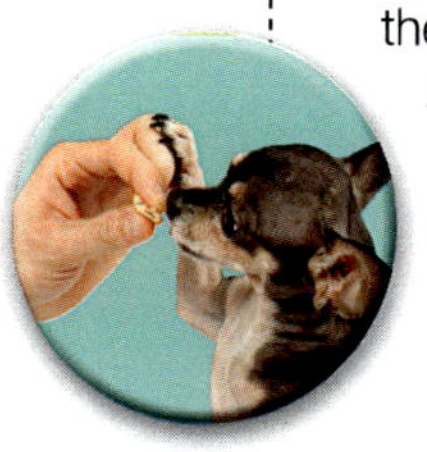

4 Beliefs

Personal, religious or ethical beliefs or philosophical reasons. For example, this would be the case of vegetarians, vegans and people with a holistic approach to health.

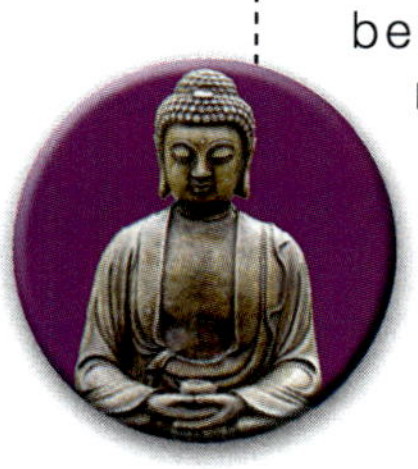

5 Lower cost

Particularly when they are compared with high-end products and with veterinary prescription diets.

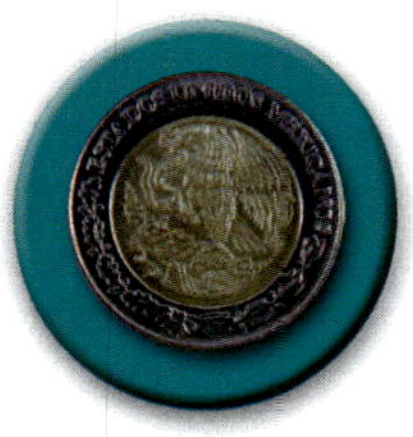

6 Labelling

Poor interpretation of the labels on commercial food.

7 Poor acceptance of commercial food by patients

This situation occurs with prescription diets: the variety of flavours is not as wide as with usual pet food.

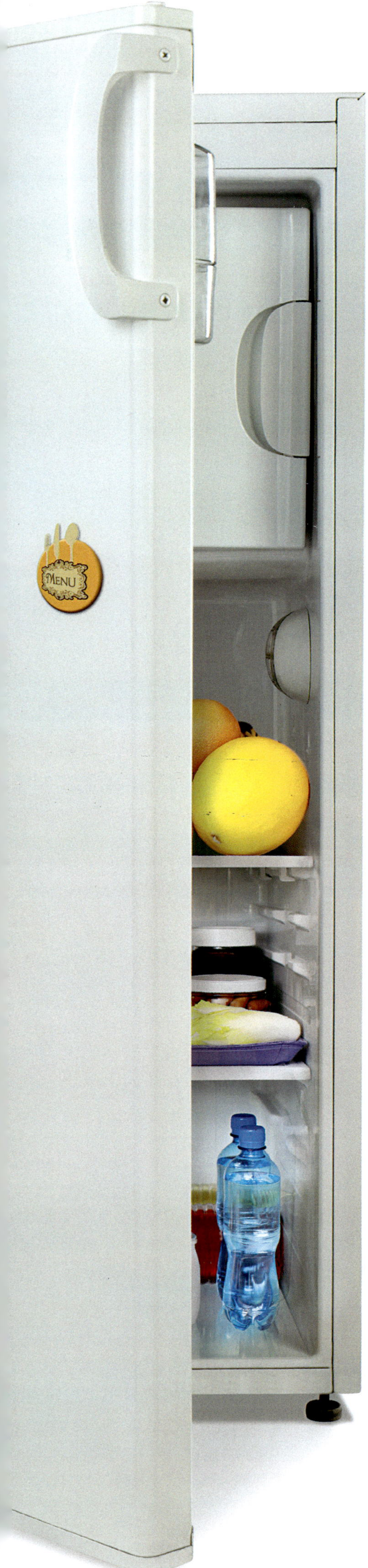

Use of homemade food

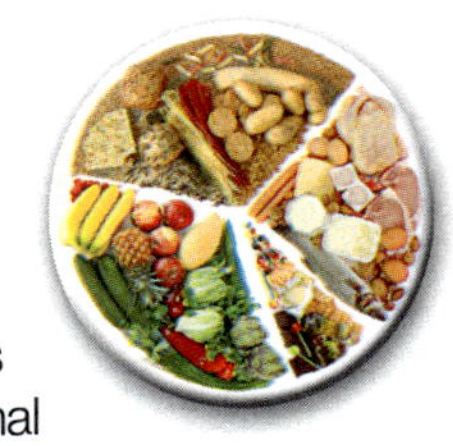

Feeding homemade food is correct provided nutritional requirements are covered and food composition tables for the species are used. In this regard, the diet should be based on the different studies available on animal nutrition and the veterinary surgeon should be responsible for its design.

Risks

Some owners prepare diets incorrectly based on:

- ✔ False ideas about correct human nutrition.
- ✔ Erroneous perception about the pet's nutritional needs.
- ✔ Choice and substitution of raw materials.
- ✔ Previous experience with other pets.
- ✔ Information obtained through non-specialised channels: Internet forums, other owners, breeders, non-specialised publications...

This practice entails risks for the dog and the cat associated with:

EXCESS OF NUTRIENTS
Excess of proteins or abnormal calcium:phosphorus proportions

DEFICIENCY
Energy, vitamins or fats

ANTI-NUTRITITIONAL
Thiaminase in raw fish

TOXIC
Sulfur derivatives in garlic and onions

This fact has been demonstrated using formulation programmes:

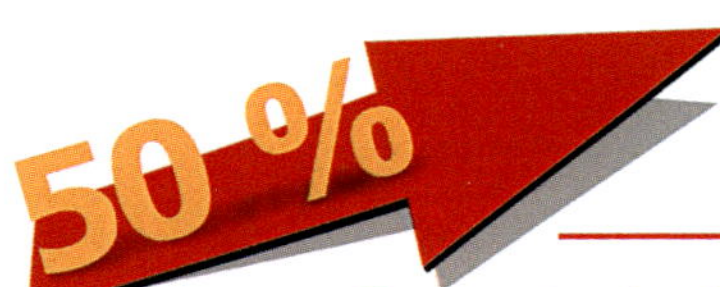

More than 50 % of homemade recipes do not cover the nutritional needs of pets.

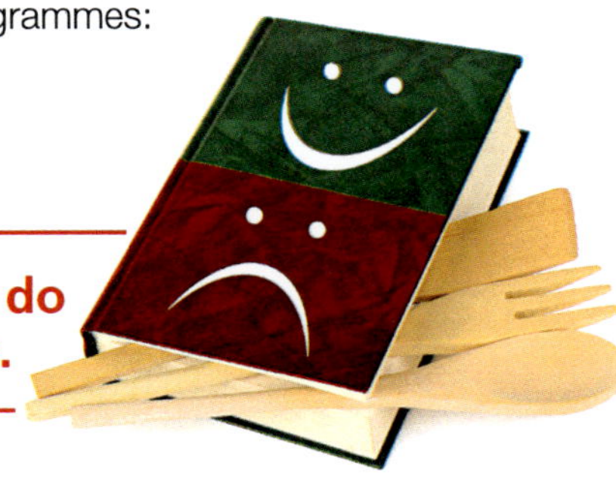

The explanation is simple: owners design diets based on the main nutrients (approximately six) but computer programmes include minor nutrients (macro and microminerals, vitamins, taurine, essential amino acids...).

We can create complete and balanced homemade diets for the two species and their different life stages, with a quality comparable to that of commercial food. This depends on:

- ✔ The veterinarian's qualifications in the field of nutrition.
- ✔ The method chosen to design the diet ("by hand" or, preferably, using a specific computer programme). Computer programmes for diet formulation are usually found in research centres, animal nutrition companies or at universities due to their high cost.
- ✔ Compliance with the rules for the selection, preparation and processing of the ingredients.

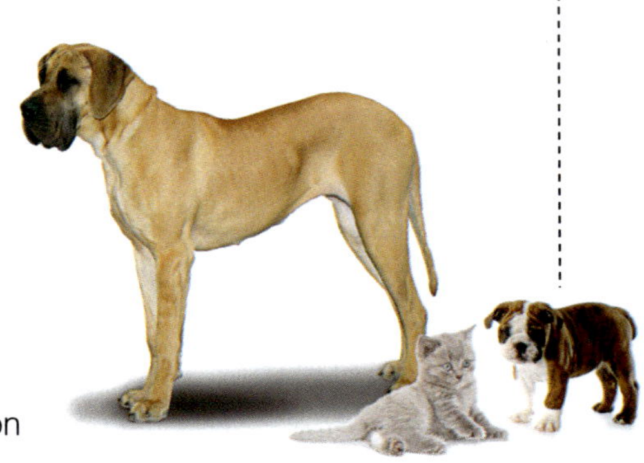

Aspects to take into account

From the veterinary point of view, the use of homemade food is justified as a diagnostic method (in elimination diets in case a food allergy or intolerance is suspected), for the treatment of some diseases or when wanting to increase food intake in animals with chronic or end-stage diseases.

Recipes for a home cooked diet
made "by hand"

1 Selection of the ingredients and the amounts

- The food pyramid should serve as a foundation for the base of the food you make.
- It is a good guide for omnivore diets (dogs) but inadequate for carnivores (cats).

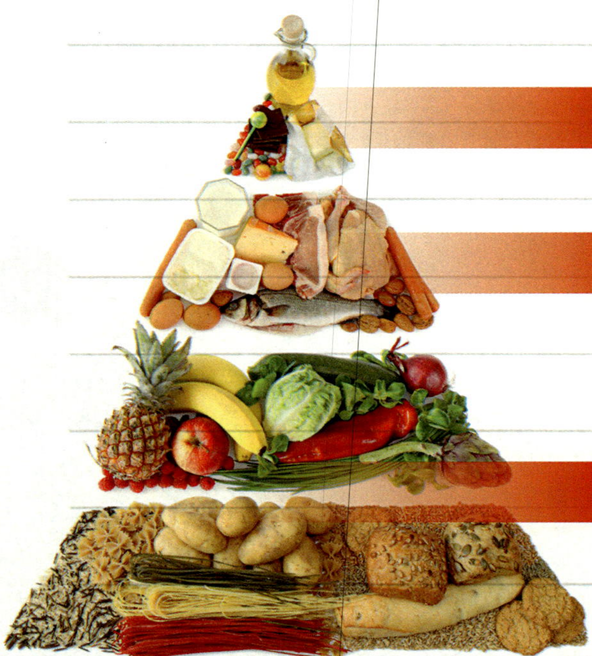

FATS and OILS → **Fats and oils incorporate fatty acids and are a source of energy.**

ANIMAL-BASED
Meat, fish, milk and eggs
→ **They provide protein with a high biological value.**

PLANT-BASED
Grains, legumes, fruit and vegetables
→ **They provide sources of fiber and carbohydrates.**

MACROMINERALS (especially calcium) | **MICROMINERALS and VITAMINS**

Traditionally

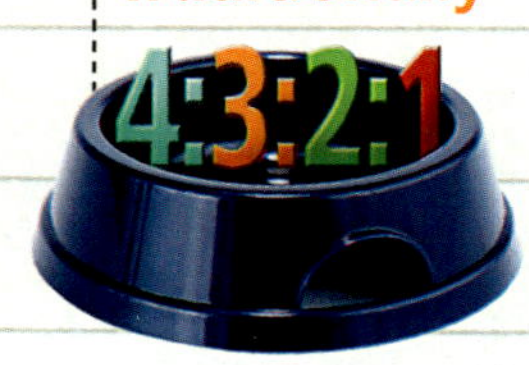

- The proportion of a food ration is made of **CARBOHYDRATES: PROTEIN: FIBER: FAT**.
- The minerals and the vitamins represent an independent group that must be provided, without exceptions, every single day.

Currently, the following is considered to be more adequate: **5:3:1:1** (dog) **3:3:1:3** (cat)

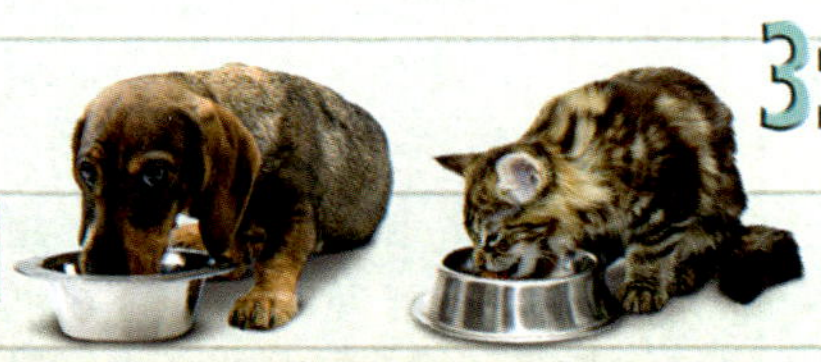

Ingredients	Principal nutrient	Dog (%)	Cat (%)
Grains	Carbohydrates	55	33
Meat	Protein	25	28
Fats and oils	Fats and EFA	10	27
Vegetables	Fiber	10	12

This type of simplified rationing decreases the possible deficiencies based on the overlapping of the nutrients provided by the different ingredients. It is valid for adult and healthy geriatric animals, however it must be kept in mind that it does not offer the ideal profile of nutrients.

Recommendations for the owner

- ✓ *Weigh the recommended amounts of each ingredient with precision. Measurement systems that include a cup, spoon, glass, or piece of food X should be avoided. It is recommended that the owners be encouraged to purchase a scale with a precision of 0.1 g. They can therefore tare a simple unit of measurement (cup) and use it daily to make it easier to prepare the food rations.*
- ✓ *Respect the ingredients proposed by the veterinarian, avoiding any substitutions of one ingredient for another in accordance with the ease of purchasing or availability in the home. The owner must purchase foods thinking about what their pet must eat.*

2 Specifications according to the different ingredients

Carbohydrates:protein (grains:meat). The grains used should always be cooked.

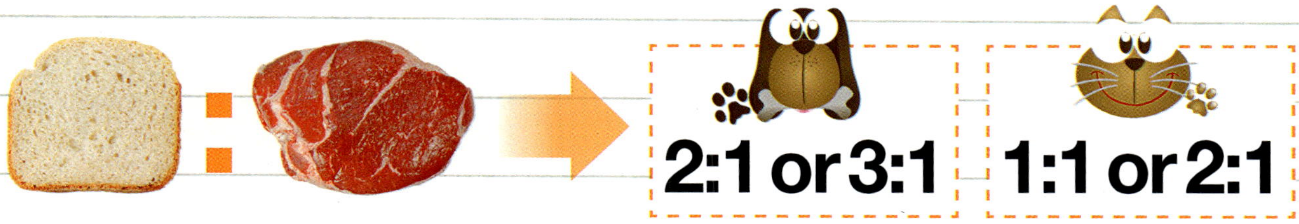

Protein

Protein can come from certain plants and, primarily, from animal-based foods. The amino acid profile of muscle is very similar between different animal species (mammals and birds), and for this reason, except for certain exceptions related with some pathologies, there are no preferences.

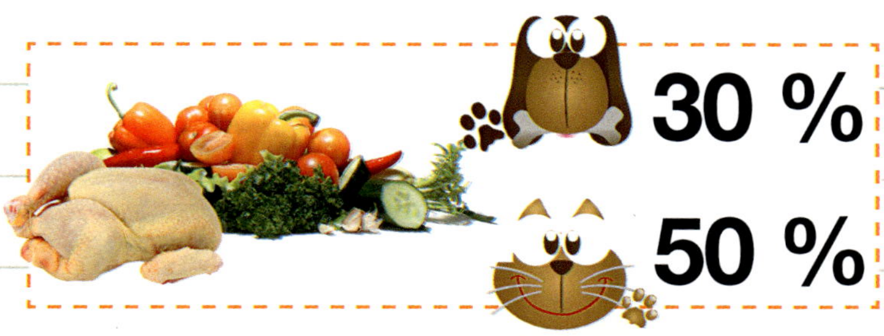

Source of protein	Lean:fatty
White fish, lean meats (beef, pork, rabbit, chicken, turkey, dear, duck), cheese	High
Meat (lamb, pork, duck and goose for foie), blue fish (tuna, salmon, sardines)	Medium
Beef, lamb and pork (ribs, breast, skirt), fatty cheeses (tetilla, gouda, cheddar, brie)	Low

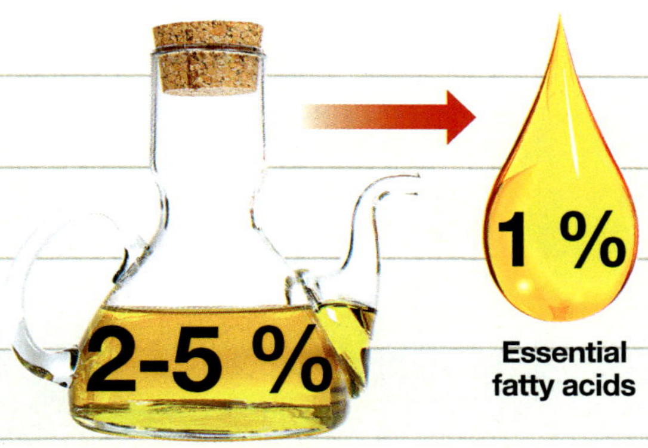

Fat

The levels of fat should oscillate between **2 and 5 %** of the total weight of the food ration, ensuring a minimum of **1 % essential fatty acids** (arachidonic and linoleic).
It can be obtained from plant-based sources, rich in unsaturated fatty acids (FA), or animal-based sources, rich in saturated FA. Also, the lean:fatty proportion provided by animal-based foods must be kept in mind when adding the fat/oil to food.

Vegetables and fruits

Vegetables, fruits, roots, and tubers provide dietary fiber in different proportions and types (soluble/fermentable or insoluble/non-fermentable).

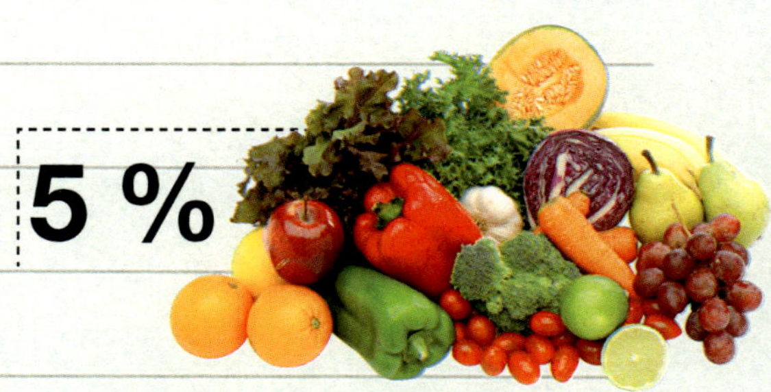

Vitamins and minerals

Home cooked recipes are usually unbalanced regarding minerals when the amount of meat is equal to or greater than that of carbohydrates, especially for calcium: the proportion Ca:P is inverted. For this reason, the daily incorporation of calcium carbonate is recommended with an approximate dose of 0.11 to 0.13 g/kg of the body weight of the dog or cat.

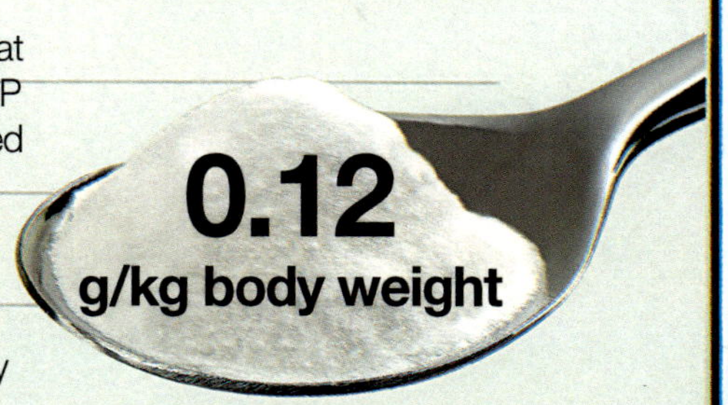

Lastly, the daily administration of a multivitamin and mineral supplement for veterinary or human use is indispensable. The products of this type for human medicine ensure that we cover, without problems of overdosing, the nutritional recommendations for our pets. The range of coverage of the veterinary products is somewhat controversial.
These multi-vitamin compounds are administered directly to the animal and they should not undergo thermal treatment of any kind.

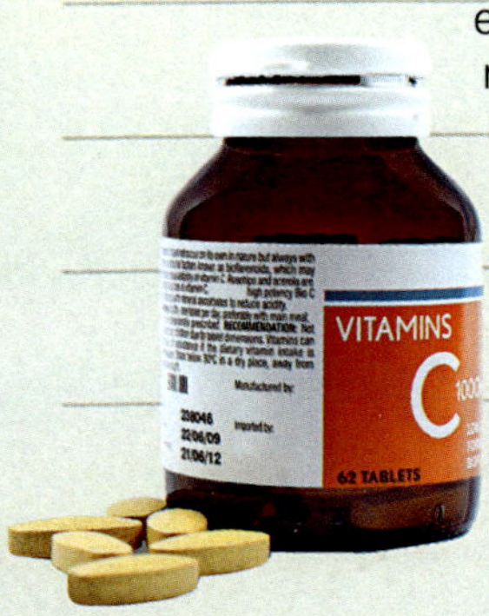

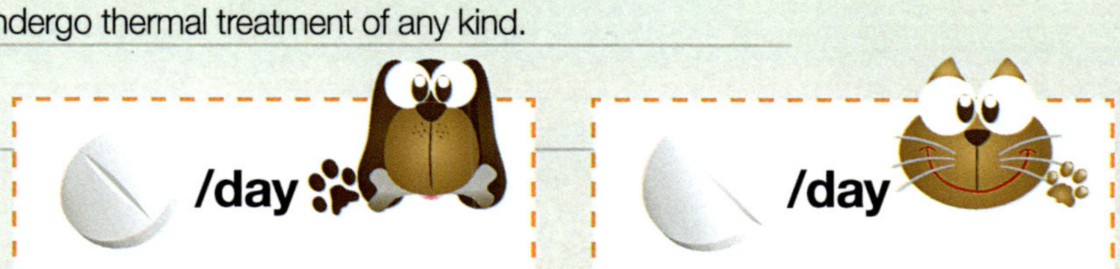

Elaboration of the food

1 All of the ingredients must be cooked

Cooking has various important effects:

- Improves the digestibility of carbohydrates.
- Inhibits anti-nutritive substances.
- Eliminates pathogenic organisms: *Salmonella* spp., *Staphylococcus aureus, E. coli, Clostridium* spp., *Yersinia* spp., *Campylobacter* spp., *Toxoplasma gondii, Cryptosporidium* spp.

2 Cooking should be done separately

The temperature and the cooking time will depend on each ingredient. Vegetables need more time than meat for the correct pre-digestion of starch, although the digestibility of the fiber is not affected. That said, these longer cooking times cause denaturation of the proteins resulting in vitamin loss.

3 Posterior addition of the source of fat

Once the ingredients are cooked, the source of fat should be added (it is done at this time to not interfere with the digestion of the starch during cooking and to increase the palatability of the food) and everything is then mixed together with a blender. This makes it hard for the animal to choose which ingredient it eats, which could lead to a food imbalance. In cats, this type of "blended" food is not well accepted.

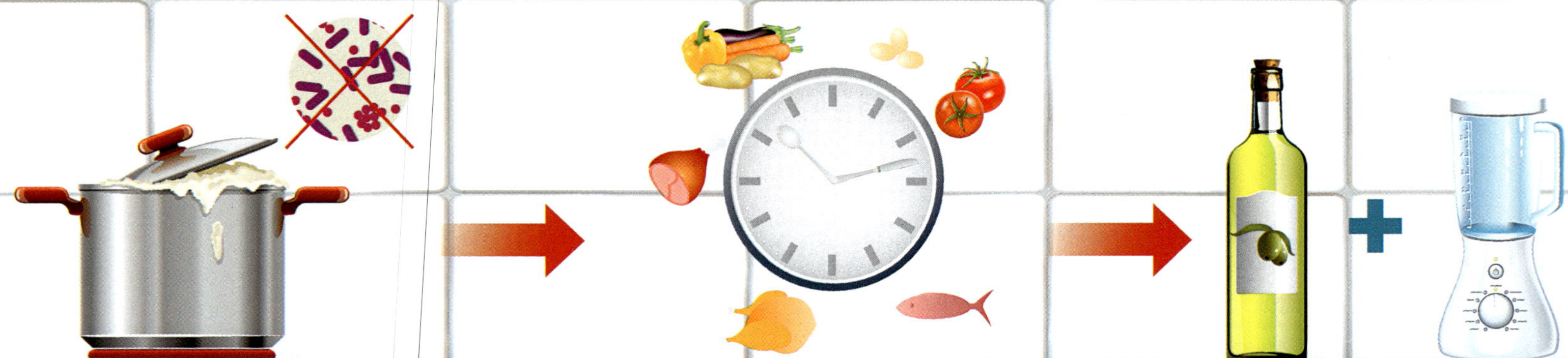

What is needed for this type of feeding to be correct and balanced?

As we have already seen, homemade cooking for pets can be a perfectly correct and balanced option as long as certain premises are kept in mind such as the following:

Aspects to be taken into account

- ✓ *The pet's requirements.*
- ✓ *Composition and nutritional value of the foods for this species, specifically.*
- ✓ *Incorporation of other ingredients: vitamins, minerals...*
- ✓ *Correct formulation of the ingredients.*
- ✓ *Exactness and precision when preparing the food ration.*
- ✓ *Processing of the raw material (cooking).*
- ✓ *Presentation of the food ration (blending).*
- ✓ *Palatability and acceptance.*
- ✓ *Digestibility.*
- ✓ *Storage conditions.*
- ✓ *The half life of the product.*
- ✓ *Temperature of the food at meal time.*

These criteria must be evaluated by the veterinarian, who will determine the proportions and total daily food ration.

Will the pets be well fed with a homemade diet?

Cooking for a pet is not as easy as many owners think it would be. Each and every point to be followed must be emphasized and understood before choosing this type of feeding. Knowledge about these bases provides us with arguments to explain the benefits and inconveniences of this type of diet compared to commercial diets. In spite of this, we have patients fed this way for long periods of time, and we wonder: are they well fed?
In these cases, we can evaluate the nutritional state of the pet as follows:

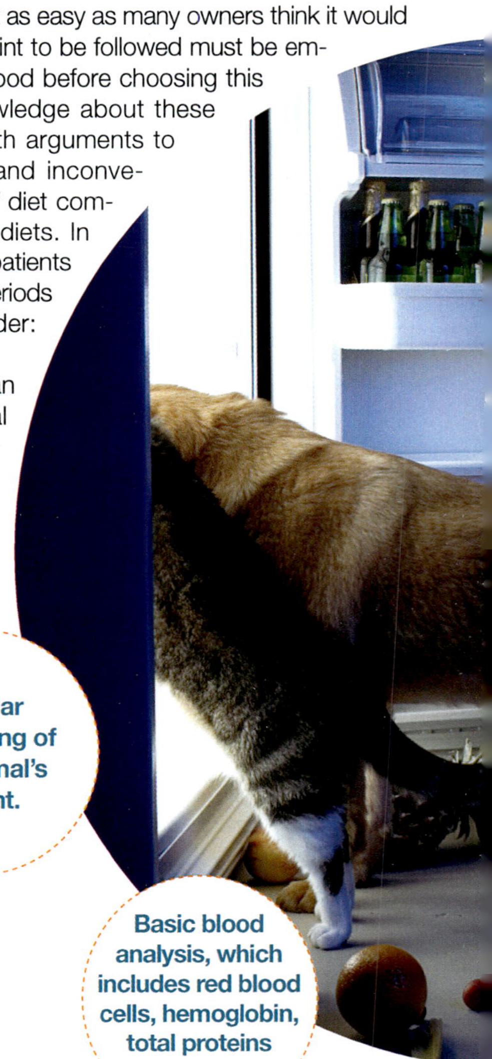

Regular monitoring of the animal's weight.

Basic blood analysis, which includes red blood cells, hemoglobin, total proteins and albumin.

ration and results

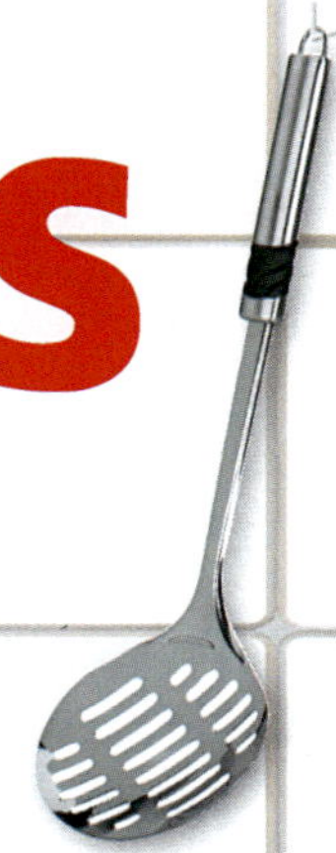

4 Storage at 4 °C for a maximum of one week

Due to the elevated moisture and the absence of additives to these cooked foods, preparing food for no more than 7 days at a time is recommended and it should be stored at 4 °C.

5 Administration of the food ration at 30-37 °C

Before administering the food ration to the pet, it should be heated in a microwave or using a double boiler, to an approximate temperature of 30-37 °C, as this improves voluntary ingestion.

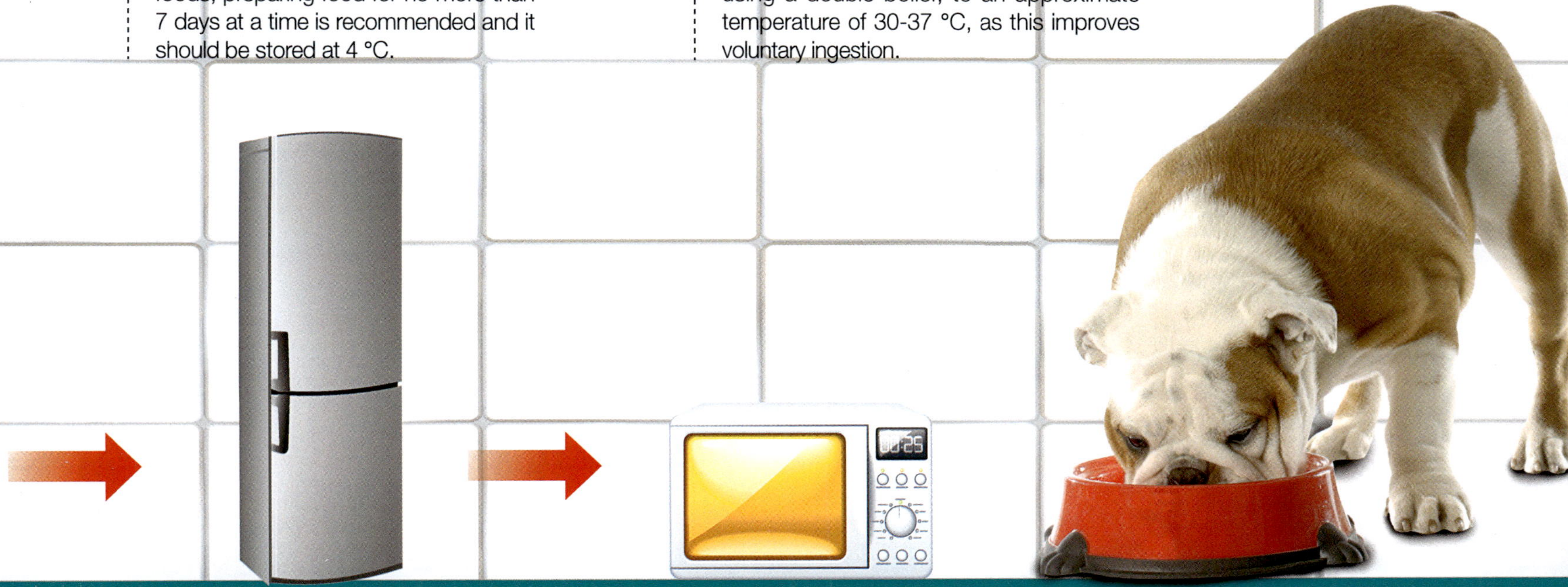

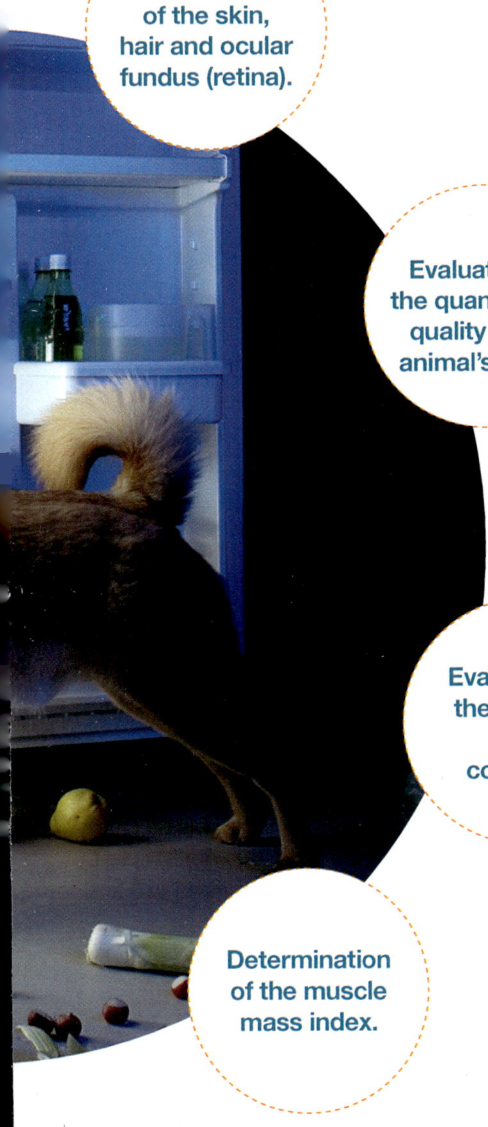

Examination of the skin, hair and ocular fundus (retina).

Evaluation of the quantity and quality of the animal's feces.

Evaluation of the animal's body condition.

Determination of the muscle mass index.

Why do these types of diets not work in practice?

Reality shows us that these factors are not met. We think, without external advice, that we are well fed, but this is not true. Many owners think that their beliefs (e.g. low fat, no cholesterol, veganism...) are the same as their requirements and they extrapolate this concept to their pets. This is where the first error is produced. The requirements or needs of an adult cat or dog are not the same as those of an adult human. That is, we are not the same in any of the previously described sections. Lastly, the owners try to cook according to ease and comfort. For example: they substitute foods, they do not weigh ingredients precisely, they do not blend homogeneously, they do not use the correct ingredients appropriately, they underestimate/overestimate certain sources of minerals, they get bored with the strict processing of the food rations... All while thinking that they are following correct hygiene measures when processing and storing the foods: washing the eggs, soaking vegetables in bleach that is suitable for consumption...

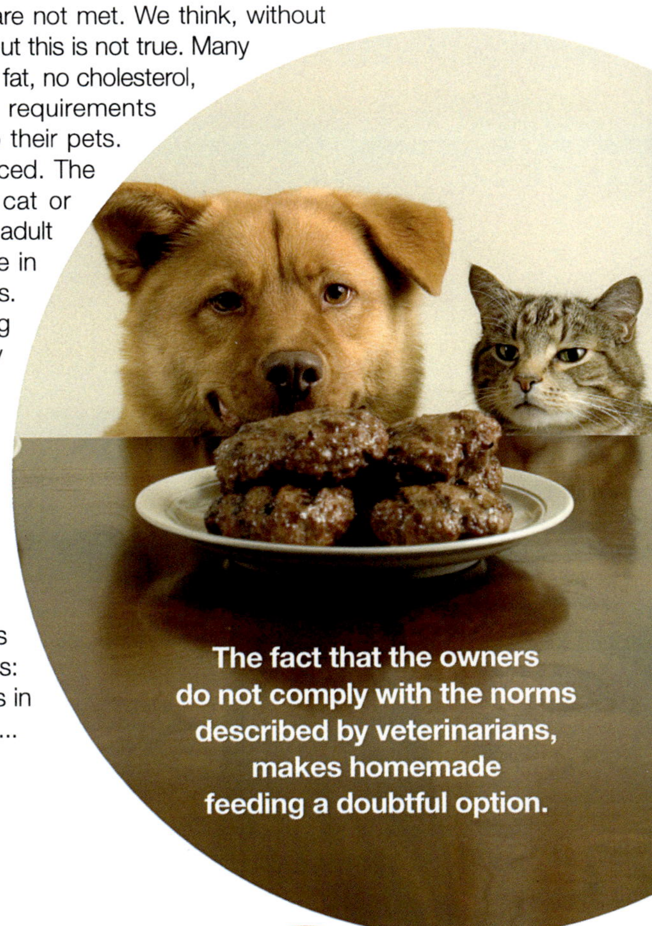

The fact that the owners do not comply with the norms described by veterinarians, makes homemade feeding a doubtful option.

To be taken into account

These animals should be seen by a veterinarian 3 or 4 times per year, coinciding with, for example, the vaccine or deworming programs.